STUDENT WORKBOOK

FOR

D1305926

Pearson's Comprehensive Dental Assisting

Lori Tyler, MS, Editor
Martha L. McCaslin, CDA, BSBM
Roxanne Medinger, CDA, RDA, BSHS
Eleanor D. Vanable, CDA, RDH, BS, MA, EdD

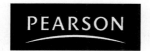

PEARSON

Upper Saddle River, New Jersey 07458

Notice: The authors and the publisher of this volume have taken care that the information and technical recommendations contained herein are based on research and expert consultation, and are accurate and compatible with the standards generally accepted at the time of publication. Nevertheless, as new information becomes available, changes in clinical and technical practices become necessary. The reader is advised to carefully consult manufacturers' instructions and information material for all supplies and equipment before use, and to consult with a healthcare professional as necessary. This advice is especially important when using new supplies or equipment for clinical purposes. The authors and publisher disclaim all responsibility for any liability, loss, injury, or damage incurred as a consequence, directly or indirectly, of the use and application of any of the contents of this volume.

Pearson® is a registered trademark of Pearson plc.

Pearson Education Ltd., London
Pearson Education Singapore, Pte. Ltd.
Pearson Education Canada, Inc.
Pearson Education—Japan

Pearson Education Australia Pty, Limited
Pearson Education North Asia Ltd., Hong Kong
Pearson Educatión de Mexico, S.A. de C.V.
Pearson Education Malaysia Pte. Ltd.
Pearson Education, Inc., Upper Saddle River, New Jersey

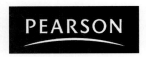

10 9 8 7 6 5 4 3 2 1
ISBN-13: 978-0-13-229413-3
ISBN-10:   0-13-229413-3

Contents

INTRODUCTION

This student workbook is designed to accompany *Pearson's Comprehensive Dental Assisting* as a study guide and practice tool. Complete each exercise in the chapters of this workbook as they correspond with chapters of the textbook to help reinforce and supplement what you have learned. Each chapter includes the following:

Chapter Outline: A quick refresher of the topics that were covered in this chapter. If you can't clearly remember one of the topics, it may be a good idea to go back to the textbook and look over that section.

Chapter Review: A short summary of the chapter. Again, if anything seems unclear, go back to that section in the textbook.

Learning and Study Aids: These questions and small tasks assess whether or not you learned and retained the information in the chapter.

Medical Terminology Review: Terms from the chapter that can be practiced by using a dictionary and/or in-text definitions.

Critical Thinking: These questions allow you to think through the material that you have been learning.

Chapter Review Test: Short multiple choice quizzes that present practice for the certification exams. True/False and Fill in the Blank questions are also provided for versatile practice and assessment.

Skill Building Competency Sheets: These procedures give you a chance to demonstrate the skills needed to become a dental assistant. They include a space for your instructor to document that you have completed the skill. They are provided in an appendix and can be torn out from the student workbook to save in a portfolio.

CHAPTER 1
History of Dentistry

CHAPTER OUTLINE

Review the Chapter Outline. If any content area is unclear, review that area before beginning the workbook exercises.

    A.   Early Times

    B.   The Renaissance

    C.   Early America

    D.   Educational and Professional Development in the United States

    E.   Community Dental Health Program

CHAPTER REVIEW

The following is a summary of the chapter. If any of this material is unclear, review it in the textbook again.

Evidence from historical records indicates that tooth ailments have plagued mankind since prehistory. In response, preventive, curative, and magic-based treatments arose. As dental knowledge increased, treatments became more scientifically sound, ethical, and less offensive to the persons being treated. Historically, dentists were trained through preceptorship. Dental education was formalized in the United States in 1840 when the first dental school was established. Because of the contributions of many dedicated men and women, dentistry is now firmly based on scientific knowledge and has blossomed into education, training, credentialing, and community service systems that seek the best for dental patients and the dental profession.

LEARNING ACTIVITIES AND STUDY AIDS

Review the following study aids and/or complete the activities to ensure that you have achieved the learning objectives for this chapter.

1. What did Hippocrates contribute to the field of dentistry?

2. Explain the dental contributions of Pierre Fauchard and G. V. Black.

3. Who was the first woman to receive a formal dental education in the United States?

4. In your own words, describe the role the American Dental Association serves in the dental profession of the United States.

5. What does the Commission on Dental Accreditation do, and why is this important to the public?

6. What does the seal of acceptance on a dental product indicate?

7. List three community dental health programs that benefit the public, and state why they are beneficial.

8. Describe the formation of the American Dental Assistants Association.

CHAPTER 1   *History of Dentistry*   **3**

9. On one side of a flash card, list the names of the following women: Juliette Southard, Lucy B. Hobbs, Ida Gray, and Irene Newman. On the other side, list why each is historically important. Turn your flash cards in to your instructor as part of your grade for completing the activities in this lesson.

10. On one side of a flash card, list the names of the following men: Horace Wells, William C. Roentgen, Josiah Foster Flagg, and C. Edmund Kells. On the other side, list the contribution each made to the advancement of dentistry. Find a classmate to study with and have a review session where the flash cards created in activity #9 and #10 are used to quiz each other. Turn your flash cards in to your instructor as part of your grade for completing the activities in this lesson.

MEDICAL TERMINOLOGY REVIEW

Use a dictionary and/or your textbook to define the following terms.

accreditation _____

acupuncture _____

amalgam _____

Centers for Disease Control _____

certification _____

confidentiality _____

deciduous teeth _____

dental implant _____

exfoliated _____

fluoridation _____

Hippocratic oath _____

impacted _____

periodontal disease _____

preceptorship _____

pulpitis _____

restorative dentistry _____

stem cell _____

The Surgeon Dentist _____

veneer _____

ABBREVIATIONS

ADA _____

ADAA _____

BCE _____

CDC _____

CE _____

DANB _____

DDS _____

DMD _____

NCDHM _____

CRITICAL THINKING

1. Considering all the differing historical factors surrounding dentistry, why is it important to have an entire month dedicated to National Children's Dental Health?

2. Why is it important for a dental assistant to learn the history of dentistry?

3. Compare and contrast the difficulties the first woman dentist may have faced with the difficulties women dentists may face today. Explain how this may or may not affect the field of dental assisting.

4. What impact do professional organizations have on the field of dental assisting?

CHAPTER REVIEW TEST

MULTIPLE CHOICE

Circle the letter of the correct answer.

1. Which historical group pioneered the use of chewing sticks to clean teeth?
   a. Romans
   b. Chinese
   c. Greeks
   d. Babylonians

2. Which group used acupuncture to treat tooth pain almost 5,000 years ago?
   a. Etruscans
   b. Chinese
   c. Renaissance monks
   d. Egyptians

3. Early bridges to replace missing teeth were constructed of:
   a. stone and carved stone teeth
   b. wood and carved wooden teeth
   c. silver and extracted human teeth
   d. gold and extracted animal teeth

4. Which TWO groups of tradesmen also practiced dentistry?
   a. barbers
   b. blacksmiths
   c. coopers
   d. weavers

5. During the Middle Ages dentistry was most commonly practiced by:
   a. magicians
   b. itinerant harpers
   c. monks
   d. acupuncturists

6. _____ prescribed oil of cloves, a sedative filling material that is still used today.

   a. Fauchard   c. Revere

   b. Aristotle   d. Flagg

7. The National Museum of Dentistry is appropriately located at the dental school associated with this university.

   a. Harvard University   c. University of Maryland

   b. Clemson University   d. University of Virginia

8. What was a "lady in attendance," and why was she so helpful in a dental office?

   a. dental hygienist; her preventive work decreased the need for fillings and extractions

   b. dental assistant; it became respectable for a woman to go to a dental office alone

   c. woman dentist; early women dentists were more ethical than their male counterparts

   d. dental receptionist; a woman was available if financial questions arose

9. Why did Dr. C. Edmund Kells commit suicide?

   a. his shame over the failure of his anesthetic injections to relieve his patients' pain

   b. his realization that the mercury used in silver paste fillings caused harm to his child patients

   c. his ineffective cleaning methods that resulted in his passing infections to his patients and himself

   d. his suffering from the pain caused by radiation-induced cancer of his hand

10. Who is the patron saint of dentistry?

   a. Saint Apollonia   c. Saint Theresa

   b. Saint Francis   d. Saint Thomas

TRUE/FALSE

Indicate whether the statement is true (T) or false (F).

_____ 1. Stem cells have been found in exfoliated deciduous teeth.

_____ 2. The ADA works primarily to educate dental professionals, such as dentists and dental assistants.

_____ 3. The Centers for Disease Control and Prevention is an arm of the government that promotes fluoridation as one of its activities.

_____ 4. Men have more teeth than women.

_____ 5. Porcelain veneers are used to hide unsightly teeth.

_____ 6. G. V. Black's great contribution to dentistry was publishing a book, *The Surgeon Dentist*, that standardized dental practice.

_____ 7. Tooth-drawers were thought of as an educated elite who performed the most complicated dental surgeries.

_____ 8. The silver paste used to fill dental cavities in ancient times is still used today in the form of amalgam filling material.

_____ 9. Celsus first categorized the teeth into central incisors, cuspids, and molars.

_____ 10. Pierre Fauchard believed that sugar was bad for the teeth and should be limited in the diet.

FILL IN THE BLANK

Using words from the list below, fill in the blanks to complete the following statements.

Black	Greenwood	NCDHM
Chinese	Hesi-Re	Wells
Etruscans	Hippocrates	
Flagg	laser	

1. _____ is considered to be the first recorded dentist.

2. A month-long celebration of children's oral health held every February is called _____.

3. Removal of dental decay without necessarily using a local anesthetic may be accomplished with _____ treatment.

4. The Greek physician _____ rejected the notion that spirits or demons caused illness and began to teach a more scientific approach to medicine.

5. Dentures were first made by the _____.

6. The son of an early dentist in the Boston area, who became one of George Washington's dentists and constructed Washington's famous denture, was _____.

7. This group invented the modern toothbrush: _____.

8. _____ allowed dental patients to become more comfortable during treatment by inventing the dental chair.

9. _____ discovered a way to use nitrous oxide gas to provide pain relief for his patients who were undergoing extractions.

10. This American dentist advocated for an independent dental profession and standardized cavity preparations, creating preparation classes that are still used today: _____.

CHAPTER 2
The Dental Team

CHAPTER OUTLINE

Review the Chapter Outline. If any content area is unclear, review that area before beginning the workbook exercises.

 A. Dental Assistant
  1. Responsibilities
  2. Characteristics
  3. Credentialing, Professional Growth, and Development
 B. Dentist
  1. Dental Specialist
 C. Registered Dental Hygienist
 D. Dental Laboratory Technician
 E. Support Staff

CHAPTER REVIEW

The following is a summary of the chapter. If any of this material is unclear, review it in the textbook again.

Dental treatment is provided through the actions of a team whose members work together to ensure patients receive excellent care. Dental assistants provide chairside and administrative assistance to the dentist, dental hygienist, and other auxiliary members. Assistants also aid, comfort, and communicate with patients. Dentists are the head of the team. They diagnose oral health and disease, plan and complete treatment, and oversee all office activities. Dental specialists receive extra education and training in a particular part of dentistry and limit their practices to that area. Dental hygienists provide preventive, therapeutic, and educational services to patients. On the dentist's direction, dental laboratory technicians replace missing teeth and soft tissue. Support staff, such as office managers, and dental aides, complete a variety of tasks that assist patients and all other members of the team as needed.

LEARNING ACTIVITIES AND STUDY AIDS

Review the following study aids and/or complete the activities to ensure that you have achieved the learning objectives for this chapter.

1. In your own words, define a dental assistant and state what functions a dental assistant typically performs.

2. Describe the difference between a dental assistant and a dental hygienist.

3. What type of training is required to become a dentist?

4. Make a list of 10 characteristics that a professional dental assistant exhibits.

5. What is a CDA, and how can a dental assistant earn this credential?

6. Differentiate a dental assistant, a certified dental assistant, a registered dental assistant, and a dental aide.

7. What is the difference between an oral and maxillofacial surgeon and an oral pathologist?

8. Your patient has a toothache the dentist has determined is caused by a disease of the pulp. To what type of dental specialist would this patient be referred?

9. What does a dental laboratory technician do, and how can someone become one?

10. On one side of a flash card list all of the dental team members discussed in this chapter. On the other side, list the major tasks each member completes to make the team run smoothly. Create these cards and turn them into your instructor for a grade. Use these flash cards as a study tool to prepare for exams.

11. Because dental assisting differs from state to state, each dental assistant needs to learn about the functions and requirements of dental assistants in his/her state. Go online to the DANB Web site (http://www.danb.org), and click on State-Specific Information. On the state-specific page, click on your state abbreviation. This takes you to a page that contains a list of the types of dental assistants recognized in your state. Then click on your state's Dental Assisting Functions and Requirements Chart. This brings up a chart you can print out and use for reference regarding what types of assistants your state recognizes, what functions can legally be performed by whom, and, equally as important, which functions are prohibited to dental assistants. This reference will be invaluable as you read each chapter in your textbook and learn about the many functions dental assistants perform. Write a short summary of what you learned about your job responsibilities in the state in which you plan to work and summit this summary for a grade.

MEDICAL TERMINOLOGY REVIEW

Use a dictionary and/or your textbook to define the following terms.

alginate _____

base _____

calculus _____

dental dam _____

endodontist _____

fabricate _____

general practitioner _____

gingival retraction cord _____

liner _____

malocclusion _____

mastication _____

matrix band _____

maxillofacial _____

occlusion _____

operatory _____

orthodontic appliance _____

orthodontics _____

palatal expander _____

pediatric dentist _____

periodontal probing _____

periodontist _____

prosthodontist _____

provisional crown _____

pulpectomy _____

pulpotomy _____

scrubs _____

space maintainer _____

sutures _____

temporomandibular joint dysfunction _____

Tofflemire _____

varnish _____

ABBREVIATIONS

AMT _____

CDA _____

CDPMA _____

CDT _____

EDDA _____

EFDA _____

HIPAA _____

PPE _____

RDA _____

RDH _____

CRITICAL THINKING

1. Why is it important for a dental assistant to know exactly what is accomplished in each dental specialty?

2. Why is it important for a dental assistant to practice good oral heath care? What examples can you provide of ways in which a dental assistant may set the standards for oral health care for his/her patients? (Explain your answer.)

3. Although each state has differing regulations regarding the registration or certification of dental assistants, why is it important for a dental assistant to become nationally or state certified? What benefits are there to either or both?

4. Who would you contact regarding information about professional organizations for dental assistants? How would you locate these organizations or groups?

CHAPTER REVIEW TEST

MULTIPLE CHOICE

Circle the letter of the correct answer.

1. What is the major role of the Dental Assisting National Board in the dental assisting profession?
   a. education
   b. training
   c. credentialing
   d. practice oversight

2. Which TWO groups of dental professionals must successfully complete education, training, and written and clinical examinations to earn a license to practice?
   a. dentists
   b. dental laboratory technologists
   c. registered dental hygienists
   d. dental assistants

3. Which characteristics below would be considered inappropriate for a professional dental assistant to exhibit?

   a. tattoo art
   b. artificial fingernails
   c. long, unbound hair
   d. all of the above

4. Which dental team member would you ask to help with an equipment maintenance problem?

   a. dental supply salesman
   b. dental service technician
   c. dental aide
   d. office bookkeeper

5. A specialist in providing dental care to children is a/an:

   a. periodontist
   b. pediatric dentist
   c. prosthodontist
   d. orthodontist

6. What great advantage does employment of a dental assistant provide to a dentist?

   a. prevents dentist fatigue
   b. enables dentist oversight of team members
   c. saves dentist time for patient care
   d. blocks dentist treatment error

7. A circulating assistant provides help to these dental team members.

   a. dentist
   b. dental assistant
   c. front desk personnel
   d. both a and c
   e. all of the above

8. A Certified Dental Assistant must complete _____ hours of continuing education annually to maintain the credential.

   a. 5
   b. 6
   c. 12
   d. 18

9. Who determines the qualifications an Expanded Function Dental Assistant must have and the duties this assistant may perform?

   a. each state's Board of Dental Examiners
   b. American Dental Association
   c. American Medical Technologists Association
   d. Dental Assisting National Board
   e. American Dental Assistants Association

10. Which of the following is considered an expanded function for dental assistants in many states?

    a. sterilizing instruments
    b. setting up and disassembling the operatory
    c. making and confirming appointments
    d. placing and removing dental dam

TRUE/FALSE

Indicate whether the statement is true (T) or false (F).

_____ 1. The dental hygienist is licensed to place restorations, crowns, and bridges, and to make dentures.

_____ 2. An alternate term for a pediatric dentist is a pedodontist.

_____ 3. General dental practitioners are licensed to perform any of the tasks dental specialists perform.

_____ 4. Dental and dental auxiliary licensure and registration are state functions, although national agencies may administer the required tests.

_____ 5. A laboratory prescription is an optional order from the dentist to the laboratory technician asking that an appliance be made a certain way.

_____ 6. An examination to become certified in radiography is not available through DANB and must be taken as a separate examination from another agency.

_____ 7. Most states allow dental assistants to scale teeth.

_____ 8. Patient confidentiality is of the utmost importance in dental assisting practice.

_____ 9. Dental assistants wear PPE to prevent transfer of disease among patients and personnel.

_____ 10. An EFDA has very different duties than an EDDA.

FILL IN THE BLANK

Using words from the list below, fill in the blanks to complete the following statements.

endodontist	oral pathologist	periodontist
general practitioner	orthodontist	prosthodontist
office administrator	pediatric dentist	public health dentist
oral and maxillofacial surgeon		

1. The _____ diagnoses and treats diseases of the dental pulp.

2. A statewide dental health program would likely be under the direction of the _____.

3. Operative dentistry such as crowns, bridges, restorations, and veneers is usually done by the _____.

4. This dentist diagnoses and treats malpositions of the teeth and problems in jaw development: _____.

5. Diagnosis of oral diseases, treatment of disease or injury, and removal or reshaping of oral structures when indicated are completed by the _____.

6. The _____ is normally responsible for completing all front desk procedures.

7. Staff members in the office of a/an _____ may wear child-friendly clothing to make their patients feel at ease.

8. Replacement teeth are often made by the dental laboratory technician based on a prescription from the _____, who specializes in making oral replacements.

9. The _____ diagnoses oral diseases and conditions by observing a sample of tissue termed a biopsy.

10. The _____ treats the supporting structures of the teeth rather than the teeth themselves.

CHAPTER 3
Dental Ethics and Law

CHAPTER OUTLINE

Review the Chapter Outline. If any content area is unclear, review that area before beginning the workbook exercises.

    A.   Applying Ethical Principles in Dentistry

    B.   Professional Code of Ethics

    C.   State Dental Practice Act

    D.   Dental Jurisprudence

    E.   Risk Management

    F.   Confidentiality

    G.   Dentist–Patient Relationship

    H.   The Patient Record

CHAPTER REVIEW

The following is a summary of the chapter. If any of this material is unclear, review it in the textbook again.

Dental personnel, patients, and society expect dental assistants to provide patients with care that meets high ethical and legal standards. Ethical standards are voluntary obligations dental assistants accept personally. Legal expectations are imposed by society through the laws of the state in which the dental assistant practices. When a dental assistant's conduct is in question, the law recognizes that a patient can be harmed if an improper action is committed, or if the professional fails to act when action was rightly expected. Either an individual or society as a whole may be harmed from improper actions or failure to act. If harmed, the individual or society must be compensated. It is the dental assistant's responsibility to minimize risk for the dental practice by adhering to the dental assisting code of ethics and state dental practice laws.

LEARNING ACTIVITIES AND STUDY AIDS

Review the following study aids and/or complete the activities to ensure that you have achieved the learning objectives for this chapter.

1. Define and explain nonmaleficence and beneficence.

2. Why is the dental assistant's practice of veracity an important underpinning to the implementation of patient autonomy?

3. Differentiate legal and ethical standards.

4. What is the purpose of a state dental practice act?

5. How does implied consent differ from written or oral consent?

6. Explain the difference between civil and criminal law.

7. The dentist is not due to arrive at the office until 8:30 a.m., but the dental assistant is removing sutures from the 8:00 a.m. patient who had surgery five days ago. At 8:15 a.m., the assistant is scheduled to take a full series of radiographs for another patient. Under what type of supervision is the assistant working?

8. Is the type of supervision under which the assistant is working in question #7 legal?

9. Yesterday the dental assistant wrote on a chart that an adult patient had tooth #27 removed. The tooth actually removed was #28. What should the assistant do to correct the chart?

10. Describe the differences between negligence and malpractice.

11. In July 2005, The District Court of Appeal of the State of Florida, Fourth District, found a dentist guilty of negligence because his dental assistant had injured a patient. The decision of the court is posted at http://www.4dca.org/Nov%202005/11-02-05/4D05-149.op.c.pdf. After reading the court's decision, write a short summary of the case, as it pertains to both the original hearing and the appellate hearing. Be sure to answer the following questions:

    Who committed the negligent act?

    What was the negligent act?

    Why was the dentist at fault?

    Who won the case originally?

    Who won the case on appeal?

Why was this simple negligence rather than medical malpractice?

Why was there no standard of care for the negligent action?

What could the dental assistant have done differently to have avoided the problem altogether?

What would you guess would be the next step in the proceedings when the case returns to the lower (circuit) court?

What do you think would be the effect of this decision on the dentist's reputation?

MEDICAL TERMINOLOGY REVIEW

Use a dictionary/or your textbook to define the following terms.

abandonment _____

autonomy _____

beneficence _____

civil _____

criminal _____

due care _____

duty _____

ethics _____

fraud _____

informed refusal _____

jurisprudence _____

justice _____

malpractice _____

negligence _____

nonmaleficence _____

reciprocity _____

res gestae _____

res ipsa loquitor _____

respondeat superior _____

slander _____

standard of care _____

statute _____

tort _____

veracity _____

ABBREVIATIONS

HHS _____

HIPAA _____

PHI _____

CRITICAL THINKING

1. Why do dental assistants need to be aware of ethics and jurisprudence? Is it legally possible that the dental assistant could be held personally liable for damages to a patient?

2. Is it possible to have committed "legal negligence"? Explain your answer.

3. What types of treatment may be covered under an implied contract? What types of treatment must be covered through the use of an expressed or written contract?

4. Each state has a governing body that is responsible for the actions of that state's dental professionals. Describe in detail the duties or expanded functions the state practice act for your state allows dental assistants to perform.

CHAPTER REVIEW TEST

MULTIPLE CHOICE

Circle the letter of the correct answer.

1. For which of these situations should the dental assistant obtain written consent from the patient?
   a. examining the patient's mouth intraorally
   b. use of the patient's photograph in a public presentation
   c. use of standard materials, drugs, and equipment
   d. copying of the patient's radiographs

2. Failure to do which of the following would be considered abandonment?
   a. provide treatment within a reasonable time period
   b. disclose use of new drugs in patient treatment
   c. provide accurate and clear post-treatment instructions
   d. provide treatment without adequate notice and referral

3. A dental assistant accidentally drops a surgical knife on the patient's chin and says "Oops, I'm sorry!" The patient heals, but has a scar and sues the dentist and assistant for compensation for the scarring. Under what legal doctrine would the assistant's words be admissible as court evidence against the dentist?

   a. res ipsa loquitor
   b. respondeat superior
   c. res geste
   d. reciprocity

4. Select the legal doctrine that specifically enables the assistant's words to be admissible as evidence against the assistant.

   a. res ipsa loquitor
   b. respondeat superior
   c. res geste
   d. reciprocity

5. Select all of the elements below that must be present if the legal system is to determine that malpractice occurred.

   a. duty was owed
   b. practitioner was derelict in performing the duty
   c. damage occurred
   d. the dereliction was the direct cause of the damage

6. Informed consent is agreement the patient gives after understanding the following:

   a. proposed treatment
   b. risks and benefits of the treatment
   c. treatment cost and healing time
   d. reasonable alternative treatments
   e. all of the above

7. A patient should be referred to another practitioner for treatment when the treatment needed:

   a. is beyond the knowledge and skill of the referring dentist
   b. is of an experimental nature
   c. requires the use of drugs as well as materials and devices
   d. does not receive the informed consent of the patient

8. Which of the following patient data is protected health information?

   a. any information that can be used to identify the patient
   b. any information assigned by an official agency
   c. information the patient requests be kept confidential
   d. information the dental practice assigns

9. Who owns the original of a patient's dental record?

   a. patient
   b. billing company
   c. insurance company
   d. dentist

10. Which federal agency handles complaints about HIPPA violations?

    a. Department of Elderly Affairs
    b. Indian Health Service
    c. Office of Civil Rights
    d. Health Education Department

TRUE/FALSE

Indicate whether the statement is true (T) or false (F).

_____ 1. The dentist is responsible for the acts of his/her employees.

_____ 2. A dentist's license may lapse as long as the period of lapse does not exceed one year.

_____ 3. The patient is expected to provide the dental practice with an accurate health history.

_____ 4. Patients have the right to review their charts and request copies of their records and radiographs.

_____ 5. Paper records should be signed by the person entering the data; this is not necessary for electronic records.

_____ 6. Fraud is the intentional misrepresentation of facts.

_____ 7. The state board of dental examiners writes the state dental practice act.

_____ 8. A dental professional must have not taken an expected action to be found guilty of negligence.

_____ 9. Civil law deals with wrongs to individuals; criminal law deals with wrongs against society.

_____ 10. A dental assistant may perform any duty that has been delegated to the assistant by the supervising dentist.

FILL IN THE BLANK

Using words from the list below, fill in the blanks to complete the following statements.

autonomy	jurisprudence	reciprocity
due care	justice	risk management
express consent	legal document	veracity
implied consent	nonmaleficence	

1. A patient record is a _____.

2. The obligation to keep one's knowledge and skills current arises out of the principle of _____.

3. The principle of _____ obligates the dental assistant to avoid discriminating against any patient because of prejudice.

4. _____ in dental advertising is an ethical obligation because it enables patients to make informed judgments.

5. A dental assistant is obligated to practice _____ to protect the dental practice.

6. Society expects the dental patient to have the privilege of _____ in decision making.

7. _____ consent is inferred from actions, whereas _____ consent is spoken or written agreement.

8. Dental _____ is a system of law that codifies what society expects of dental practitioners.

9. When an individual licensed in one state is granted a license in another on the basis of a good practice record rather than retesting, the second license was gained by _____.

10. The standard of care, also termed _____, is what any reasonable or prudent person of similar knowledge and skill would do in similar circumstances.

CHAPTER 4
General Anatomy and Physiology

CHAPTER OUTLINE

Review the Chapter Outline. If any content area is unclear, review that area before beginning the workbook exercises.

    A. Planes and Body Directions

    B. Structural Units
        1. Cells
        2. Tissues
        3. Organs
        4. Systems

    C. Body Cavities

    D. Body Regions

    E. Introduction to Major Body Systems
        1. Skeletal System
        2. Muscular System
        3. Cardiovascular System
        4. Lymphatic System
        5. Nervous System
        6. Respiratory System
        7. Digestive System
        8. Endocrine System
        9. Urinary System
        10. Integumentary System
        11. Reproductive System

    F. Interaction of the Eleven Body Systems

CHAPTER REVIEW

The following is a summary of the chapter. If any of this material is unclear, review it in the textbook again.

The mouth is an integral component of the body. As such, it is affected by what happens to the body overall. Ordinarily, body systems work together to create a smooth functioning, balanced whole. When a particular tissue, organ, or system does not function as expected, a disease or disorder may develop. A dental assistant needs to be aware of normal body structure and function, as well as common diseases and disorders, in order to understand patient dental histories and to adapt treatment when indicated to accommodate specific patient conditions.

LEARNING ACTIVITIES AND STUDY AIDS

Review the following study aids and/or complete the activities to ensure that you have achieved the learning objectives for this chapter.

1. Differentiate anatomy and physiology.

2. Make flash cards that list each of the four types of tissue on the back of the card to indicate the tissue's function. Turn your flash cards into your instructor for a grade. Flash cards are a great study tool that can be used to study either independently or with others.

3. List the eleven body systems. Then use only one or two words to describe each function the system performs. Example: integumentary system—covering, lining, gland secretion, skin coloring, protection, heat regulation.

4. Explain why it is important that a standard position be used to describe body planes, directions, and cavities.

5. What is the difference between a tissue and an organ?

6. Dental assistants are responsible for reviewing the medical history of each patient and alerting the dentist to any disease, condition, or treatment of concern to dental care. Go online to http://www.webmd.com, and research the following conditions that may appear on a patient's health history: ADHD, autism, bipolar disorder, transient ischemic attacks, Lyme disease, rosacea, lupus erythematosus, and chronic fatigue syndrome. For each condition, note the definition; cause, if known; and treatments, if available. Then complete the following table to help you remember what you learned about each condition.

Table 4-2

Condition	Summary
ADHD	Definition: Cause: Treatments:
Autism	Definition: Cause: Treatments:
Bipolar disorder	Definition: Cause: Treatments:

(continued)

(continued)

Transient ischemic attack	Definition: Cause: Treatments:
Lyme disease	Definition: Cause: Treatments:
Rosacea	Definition: Cause: Treatments:
Lupus erythematosus	Definition: Cause: Treatments:
Chronic fatigue syndrome	Definition: Cause: Treatments:

7. Make a series of electronic flash cards to review the diseases and conditions studied in this chapter. To make an electronic flash card, open an Excel program. Type the name of the disease or condition in a cell and enter it. Then return to the same cell and select Insert Comment. A box will appear. Type the definition, cause, and treatment for the disease and then click in any other cell. In the cell in which you were working, you will see one side of the "card," which will have the name of the disease or condition. If you go to that cell and place your cursor over the red triangle in the upper-right hand corner, you will see the "other side" of the card, which will have the definition, cause, and treatment. If you do not have access to Excel, make a series of regular flash cards. On one side list the name of the disease or condition, on the other list its definition; cause, if known; and treatments, if available. You should include the following in either type of flash card series you make: arthritis, gout, osteoporosis, fracture, osteomyelitis, strain, sprain, muscular dystrophy, myasthenia gravis, fibromyalgia, coronary artery disease, atherosclerosis, angina pectoris, hypertension, heart failure, pericardial disease, endocarditis, hemophilia, Alzheimer's disease, Bell's palsy, brain tumor, CVA, epilepsy, migraine headache, MS, Parkinson's disease, trigeminal neuralgia, emphysema, bronchitis, sarcoidosis, asthma, tuberculosis, bulimia, anorexia nervosa, xerostomia, hemorrhoids, GERD, hepatitis, Crohn's disease, hyperthyroidism, hypothyroidism, Cushing's syndrome, diabetes, incontinence, cystitis, PID, HIV/AIDS, HPV, syphilis, chlamydia, gonorrhea, genital herpes, toxic shock syndrome, dysmenorrhea, basal cell carcinoma, squamous cell carcinoma, acne, blister, callus, burn, melanoma, lymphoma, leukemia, infectious mononucleosis, allergy, anaphylaxis, and inflammation. Either series of flash cards will serve you well as you review for your externship and/or exams. Turn your flash cards into the instructor in order to receive a grade for your efforts.

8. Which two components of the human body make up most of its weight?

9. If bone structure were likened to a sandwich, which type of bone would be the bread (outer portion), and which type would be the filling?

10. Describe the five basic warning signs of basal cell carcinoma.

MEDICAL TERMINOLOGY REVIEW

Use a dictionary and/or your textbook to define the following terms.

adenoids _____

allergy _____

angina pectoris _____

anorexia nervosa _____

antagonist _____

antigen _____

bulimia _____

capillary _____

cytoplasm _____

erythrocyte _____

esophagus _____

estrogen _____

glucose _____

homeostasis _____

hormone _____

hypertension _____

infection _____

inflammation _____

insulin _____

leukocyte _____

marrow _____

mitosis _____

nucleus _____

organ _____

peristalsis _____

phagocytosis _____

plasma _____

ptyalin _____

puberty _____

Purkinje fibers _____

sinus _____

synovial fluid _____

testosterone _____

thrombocyte _____

thrombosis _____

trachea _____

xerostomia _____

ABBREVIATIONS

ACTH _____

ADH _____

AIDS _____

CVA _____

DNA _____

FSH _____

GERD _____

GH _____

HIV _____

HPV _____

LH _____

MS _____

PID _____

PR _____

RICE _____

RNA _____

STD _____

TSH _____

CRITICAL THINKING

1. Why is it important for a dental assistant to have a thorough understanding of general anatomy and physiology?

2. Why does a dental assistant need to know the four different types of tissue found within the body? List the four types and some of the functions they perform within the oral cavity.

3. What are the tissue layers found within the osseous tissue of the oral cavity? What is the importance of these different layers (remember their consistency and function)? Why is it important for a dental assistant to be able to recognize these layers and identify them?

4. Considering the bony structures found within the oral cavity, what is the only movable bone of the skull, and why is it necessary for this bone to move? If it didn't move, what would be the result?

CHAPTER REVIEW TEST

MULTIPLE CHOICE

Circle the letter of the correct answer.

1. Why does a child have more bones than an adult?

   a. small bones break apart more easily

   b. some bones have not yet fused

   c. adult bones change size and shape

   d. children's bones are not remodeled

2. This tissue produces erythrocytes.

   a. red marrow

   b. nerve tissue

   c. muscle tissue

   d. thyroid gland

3. The master gland of the body, so called because it controls other glands, is the:

   a. adrenal gland

   b. pineal gland

   c. pituitary gland

   d. thyroid gland

4. The major function of insulin is participation in:

   a. oxygen transport

   b. phagocytosis

   c. carbon dioxide removal

   d. glucose metabolism

5. Separation of the epidermis and dermis of the skin may cause:

   a. tissue burn

   b. blister formation

   c. deeper skin color

   d. wrinkles.

6. These systems remove body waste.

   a. integumentary

   b. digestive

   c. urinary

   d. both a and c

   e. all of the above

7. A permeable cell membrane acts as a cell:

   a. gateway

   b. barrier

   c. marker

   d. growth center

8. When a dental assistant moves from a center front tooth of the upper jaw to a center front tooth of the lower jaw, the movement is in this direction.

   a. lateral

   b. anterior

   c. medial

   d. inferior

9. Which cranial nerve provides sensory information from the upper and lower jaws to the brain?

   a. olfactory

   b. optic

   c. trigeminal

   d. trochlear

10. Which disease causes progressive degeneration of the parts of the brain that control memory, thought, and language?

    a. Alzheimer's disease

    b. bulimia

    c. Cushing's disease

    d. diabetes

TRUE/FALSE

Indicate whether the statement is true (T) or false (F).

_____ 1. The acoustic nerve provides sensation for hearing and balance.

_____ 2. A stroke is a common seizure disorder caused by dysfunction of the nervous system.

_____ 3. Patients who eat a lot, then force themselves to vomit so the food is not retained in their bodies, suffer from anorexia nervosa.

_____ 4. The pancreas exercises control of calcium levels in body functioning.

_____ 5. Basal cell carcinoma is a common skin cancer that should be removed but is not considered to be particularly dangerous.

_____ 6. A transverse plane divides the body into upper and lower sections.

_____ 7. Homeostasis is the preferred state in which the body's cells, tissues, organs, and systems operate together to create a smoothly functioning whole.

_____ 8. DNA and RNA contain the genetic information of the cell.

_____ 9. Smooth muscle is under the patient's voluntary control.

_____ 10. Cardiac muscle contracts like other types of muscle but also conducts electricity.

FILL IN THE BLANK

Using words from the list below, fill in the blanks to complete the following statements.

cardiovascular	lymphatic	respiratory
digestive	muscular	skeletal
endocrine	nervous	urinary (excretory)
integumentary	reproductive	

1. This body system controls breathing: _____.

2. This system was developed to ensure continuation of the species: _____.

3. Secretion of melanin is one of the functions of this system: _____.

4. Use and storage of food, including elimination of excess, are functions of this system: _____.

5. This system generates and conducts messages to and from the brain and spinal cord: _____.

6. This system controls growth, stimulates sexual development, causes insulation production, and regulates water balance and organ function by sending chemical messages through the blood: _____.

7. This system filters wastes, toxins, and excess nutrients from the bloodstream and excretes excess water: _____.

8. Components of these two systems work together to enable movement: _____ and _____.

9. If the major muscle of this system fails, the brain will be deprived of oxygen and shortly thereafter all body systems will fail: _____.

10. This system develops the white blood cells that confront and destroy foreign substances that enter the body: _____.

CHAPTER 5
Head and Neck Anatomy

CHAPTER OUTLINE

Review the Chapter Outline. If any content area is unclear, review that area before beginning the workbook exercises.

A. Regions of the Head

B. Bones of the Skull

C. Temporomandibular Joints

D. Muscles of the Face and Oral Cavity

E. Structure and Function of the Salivary Glands and Ducts

F. Sinuses

G. Structures of the Tongue

H. Lymph Nodes in the Face and Neck

I. Nerves of the Face and Neck

J. Circulatory System of the Face and Neck

CHAPTER REVIEW

The following is a summary of the chapter. If any of this material is unclear, review it in the textbook again.

A dental assistant provides clinical assistance to the dentist when working in the oral cavity and on nearby oral and maxillofacial structures. These areas function with support and assistance from all of the structures of the head and neck: bones, joints, muscles, nerves, arteries, veins, lymph nodes, and the tongue and salivary glands. Bones provide support and work with the muscles and joints to provide movement. Nerves transmit electrical signals to receive incoming sensory information and send outgoing directions. Arteries and veins provide transportation, oxygen, and nutrients to structures throughout the body and take waste products to areas where they can be permanently eliminated. Lymph nodes filter out unwanted fluid components, thereby returning fresh, clean fluid to the circulatory system. Knowledge of how this occurs is critical to providing safe, effective intraoral services and educating patients with both normal and abnormal function in the head and neck area.

LEARNING ACTIVITIES AND STUDY AIDS

Review the following study aids and/or complete the activities to ensure that you have achieved the learning objectives for this chapter.

1. Using the line art as provided of the cranium and face, locate each bone and write the name of the bone at the line where the bone is indicated.

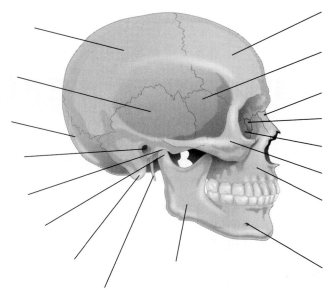

Figure 5-1

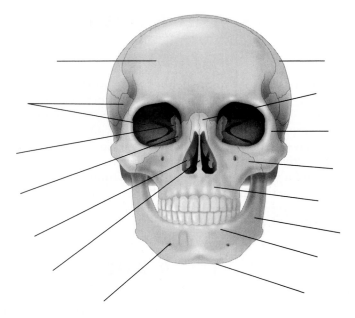

Figure 5-2

2. Describe how the tongue moves from one area to another.

3. Using the line art provided of the external muscles of the tongue, place the name of the muscle by the line shown on the drawing where the muscle is located. Aslo indicate the location of the hyoid bone.

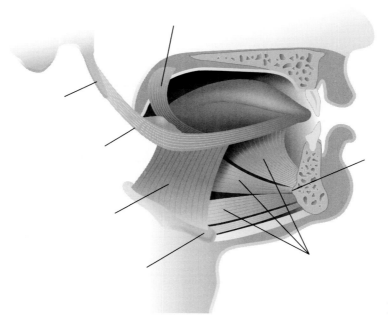

Figure 5-3

4. Complete the following table by indicating the branches of the trigeminal nerve and the areas each supplies.

Table 5-1

Branch of the Trigeminal Nerve	Further Branches	Areas Supplied

5. For each salivary gland listed in the following table, indicate its location, the name of the duct that empties it, and whether the saliva it produces is serous, mucous, or mixed serous and mucous.

Table 5-2

Gland	Location of Gland	Duct that Empties That Gland	Type of Secretion
Parotid			
Submandibular			
Sublingual			

6. Differentiate the external and internal carotid arteries, and list two areas each supplies.

7. Describe how the mandible and temporal bone articulate.

8. Locate the internal and external jugular veins, and name three structures each drains.

9. Define xerostomia, and describe how it can develop.

10. List the paranasal sinuses, and describe their function.

11. Using the drawings of the skull and palate provided, locate and lable the following landmarks: zygomatic, frontal, palatine and alveolar processes, median palatine suture, maxillary tuberosity, and infraorbital foramen. You should place the name of each of these landmarks by the line that best indicates the location.

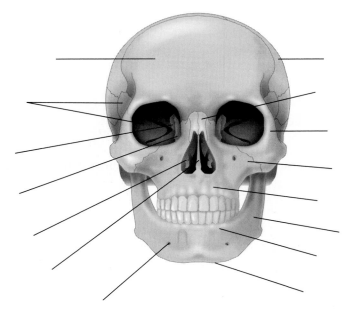

Figure 5-5

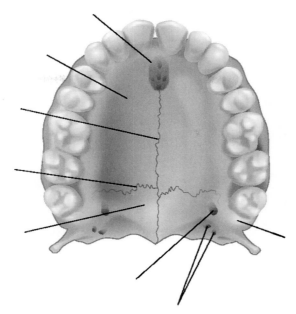

Figure 5-4

12. Using the drawings of the mandible, locate and label by the lines provided the following landmarks: border of the mandible, ramus, mental protuberance, mental foramen, external and internal oblique ridge, retromolar area, mandibular angle, coronoid process, condyle, mandibular notch, genial tubercles, internal oblique ridge, mandibular foramen, mylohyoid groove, submandibular and sublingual fossae, and lingual foramen.

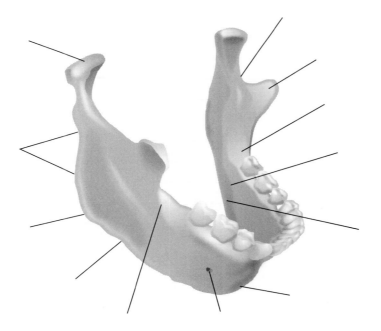

Figure 5-6

CHAPTER 5 *Head and Neck Anatomy* **43**

Figure 5-6 (*continued*)

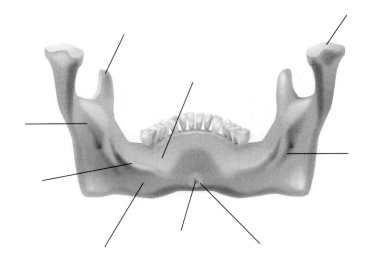

MEDICAL TERMINOLOGY REVIEW

Use a dictionary and/or your textbook to define the following terms.

analgesic _____

articular eminence _____

buccinator _____

cranium _____

deglutition _____

depression _____

elevation _____

hematoma _____

inferior turbinate _____

innervate _____

lateral excursion _____

lymphocyte _____

macrophage _____

malar bone _____

mastoid process _____

median _____

meniscus _____

mucin _____

neuron _____

neurotransmitter _____

palpation _____

parotid gland _____

periosteum _____

protrusion _____

pterygoid plexus _____

pterygopalatine fossa _____

remineralize _____

retrusion _____

styloid process _____

sublingual gland _____

submandibular gland _____

synapse _____

thoracic duct _____

transverse _____

vomer _____

zygomatic arch _____

ABBREVIATIONS

SCM _____

TMD _____

TMJ _____

CRITICAL THINKING

1. How does understanding head and neck anatomy help a dental assistant perform his/her job successfully?

2. What is the muscle that circles the mouth and is required to pucker the lips? What other functions does this muscle have? Why is this muscle of importance to a dental assistant?

3. If you had a patient who complained he/she were having drooping of the lower lip, what muscle(s) or nerve(s) may be involved, and what may be the cause of this condition?

CHAPTER REVIEW TEST

MULTIPLE CHOICE

Circle the letter of the correct answer.

1. If a patient has had a stroke and can no longer pull the maxillary lip up to smile on one side of the face, what cranial nerve was affected?

   a. trigeminal
   b. facial

   c. glossopharyngeal
   d. hypoglossal

2. This bone forms the middle cranial fossa of the skull.

   a. ethmoid
   b. maxilla

   c. sphenoid
   d. zygomatic

3. Which salivary gland is located in a small depression on the medial surface of the mandible below the canine?
   a. sublingual
   b. submandibular
   c. parotid
   d. mucosal

4. In which area does a hematoma sometimes develop as a result of a misdirected local anesthetic injection needle?
   a. pterygopalatine fossa
   b. infratemporal fossa
   c. orbit
   d. external auditory meatus

5. This artery provides blood to the deep structures of the face.
   a. lingual
   b. temporal
   c. internal carotid
   d. maxillary

6. This nerve innervates the skin and mucosa of the cheeks and gingiva.
   a. inferior alveolar
   b. mylohyoid
   c. buccal
   d. auriculotemporal

7. Maxillary premolar teeth are innervated by this branch of the trigeminal nerve.
   a. zygomatic
   b. ophthalmic
   c. pterygopalatine
   d. middle superior alveolar

8. Neurons send signals using this type of transmission:
   a. thermal
   b. electrochemical
   c. magnetic
   d. digital

9. All of the following EXCEPT _____ are signs of infected lymph nodes.
   a. softness
   b. tenderness
   c. enlargement
   d. warmth

10. The most likely site for a sialolith to develop is in this gland.
   a. palatine
   b. sublingual
   c. submandibular
   d. parotid

TRUE/FALSE

Indicate whether the statement is true (T) or false (F).

_____ 1. Arteries and nerves tend to travel together.

_____ 2. Radiation-induced xerostomia is usually temporary but chemotherapy-induced xerostomia is usually permanent.

_____ 3. During swallowing, the palatoglossus muscle raises the tongue so it touches the soft palate.

_____ 4. The muscle that tilts the head to the side is the sternocleidomastoid.

_____ 5. Nonverbal communication is a major function of the muscles of facial expression.

_____ 6. The zygomatic muscle compresses the cheeks against the side of the teeth to keep food in contact with the teeth.

_____ 7. The lateral pterygoid muscle inserts in the coronoid process and functions to pull the mandible up and forward.

_____ 8. To effect mandibular movement, the mandibular condyle rotates and slides on a cartilage disk in the TMJ.

_____ 9. The vomer bone forms the lower part of the bony nasal septum.

_____ 10. The parietal region forms the base of the skull.

FILL IN THE BLANK

Using words from the list below, fill in the blanks to complete the following statements.

alveolar process	greater wing	occipital
encase the brain	lacrimal	retromolar area
ethmoid	maxilla	synovial
glenoid fossa	maxillary tuberosity	

1. Paranasal sinuses are found in the frontal, ethmoid, and sphenoid bones, and in the _____.

2. The _____ holds the teeth in the jaw bones.

3. The TMJ is a _____ joint.

4. The major function of the frontal, ethmoid, parietal, sphenoid, temporal, and occipital bones is to _____.

5. The depression on the undersurface of the temporal bone that articulates with the condyle of the mandible in the TMJ is the _____.

6. The _____ of the sphenoid bone forms part of the side of the skull.

7. The _____ bone forms the upper part of the bony nasal septum.

8. The foramen magnum is a large opening in the _____ bone that allows the spinal cord to pass through the bone and into the brain.

9. The _____ is behind the last molar on the maxilla and the _____ occupies the same position on the mandible.

10. The _____ bone contains the tear ducts.

CHAPTER 6

The Face and Oral Cavity

CHAPTER OUTLINE

Review the Chapter Outline. If any content area is unclear, review that area before beginning the workbook exercises.

- A. Landmarks of the Face
- B. The Oral Cavity
  1. Lips
  2. Oral Vestibules
  3. Buccal Mucosa
  4. Alveolar Mucosa and Gingiva
- C. The Oral Cavity Proper
  1. Palate
  2. Structures of the Tongue
  3. Floor of the Mouth
  4. Oral Cancer and Other Conditions

CHAPTER REVIEW

The following is a summary of the chapter. If any of this material is unclear, review it in the textbook again.

A dental assistant spends many hours working with the tissues of the face and oral cavity. Nearly all clinical assisting tasks, and the majority of education concepts presented, stem from the need to teach patients how to keep these areas healthy. Each portion of the face and oral cavity has a structure that enables efficient completion of the functions it performs. The old adage that "two pairs of eyes are better than one" holds true in dentistry. The operator and assistant both need to observe abnormalities, protect sensitive tissues while worked on, and educate patients regarding their personal conditions. Anatomy knowledge enables the assistant to help the operator provide the best, most comprehensive service to patients.

LEARNING ACTIVITIES AND STUDY AIDS

Review the following study aids and/or complete the activities to ensure that you have achieved the learning objectives for this chapter.

1. Define intraoral and extraoral.

2. Explain the location of the oral cavity and what is considered to be the oral cavity proper.

3. Next to the lines provided on the figure, locate and label the following structures: inner canthus, outer canthus, philtrum, ala of the nose, and tragus of the ear.

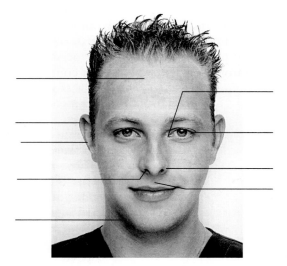

Figure 6-1

4. The oral cavity performs various functions. Create a flash card for each function. On one side of the flash card, list a function. On the other side, list the structure that performs that function. Turn the flash cards in to your instructor in order to receive a grade for completion of this activity. Use these flash cards to study the functions and structure of the oral cavity.

5. Differentiate the locations of the buccal frenum, oral vestibule, and vestibular fornix.

6. Explain the location of the buccal mucosa, alveolar mucosa, and gingiva.

7. Differentiate the free gingiva, attached gingiva, gingival papilla, and free gingival groove.

8. Explain gingiva and alveolar mucosa in terms of appearance.

9. On the following figure, lable the landmarks of the dorsum of the tongue at the lines provided.

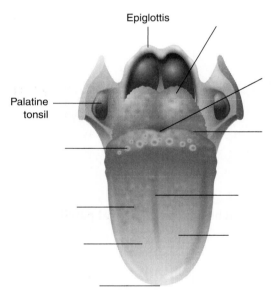

Figure 6-2

10. Using materials from the school's dental lab, mix a batch of white plaster and pour a rubber mold of the maxillary arch. After the plaster has reached final set (about 24 hours), label each part of the palate using watercolors and a paintbrush, or paint each of the parts a different color. Parts to include are the hard palate, soft palate, area where the uvula begins, vault, incisive papilla, palatine rugae, and median palatine raphe. Turn your labeled mold into your instructor to receive a grade for this activity.

MEDICAL TERMINOLOGY REVIEW

Use a dictionary and/or your textbook to define the following terms.

alveolar mucosa _____

alveolar ridge _____

ankyloglossia _____

benign _____

buccal mucosa _____

candidiasis _____

cleft lip _____

cleft palate _____

ducts of Rivinus _____

Fordyce's granules _____

frenum _____

gingiva _____

incisive papilla _____

keratinized _____

labial commissure _____

leukoplakia _____

linea alba _____

median sulcus _____

mucogingival junction _____

mucous membrane _____

orifice _____

palatine raphe _____

papilla _____

plica fimbriata _____

sublingual caruncle _____

terminal sulcus _____

tonsillar pillars _____

ulcerative colitis _____

uvula _____

vermilion border _____

vermilion zone _____

vestibular fornix _____

vestibule _____

ABBREVIATIONS

There are no abbreviations for this chapter.

CRITICAL THINKING

1. Why does a dental assistant need to know what "normal" facial structures/features look like?

2. What techniques may be used by dental healthcare providers to examine patients for normal function and structure of facial features, muscles, and nerves? What are the differences and similarities between these various techniques?

3. Name all the functions of the oral cavity and the different structures that play a part in these functions. (Hint: there are five.) Why is it important for a dental assistant to know all these functions and structures?

4. If a patient is "tongue tied" and the dentist recommends a frenectomy for correction, how might a dental assistant help address a patient's fear of the upcoming procedure?

CHAPTER REVIEW TEST

MULTIPLE CHOICE

Circle the letter of the correct answer.

1. This structure forms the entrance to the oral cavity.
   a. vestibule
   b. vermilion zone
   c. frenum
   d. sublingual caruncle

2. Gingiva is the type of oral mucosa that surrounds the:
   a. cheek
   b. alveolar ridge
   c. lip
   d. teeth

3. The tongue can best be described as a:
   a. bony structure that is attached to the neck and pharynx
   b. nerve system that provides outgoing messages
   c. muscular organ covered with mucous membrane
   d. tendon that enables speech and swallowing

4. All of the following types of papillae contain taste receptors EXCEPT:
   a. filiform
   b. foliate
   c. fungiform
   d. circumvallate

5. Fordyce's granules are:
   a. folds of tissue that connect the labial mucosa with the lip or cheek
   b. oil glands located in the buccal mucosa
   c. projections of tissue into the spaces between the teeth
   d. a type of trench surrounding the circumvallate papilla

6. Normal gingival tissue has a/an _____ texture.
   a. ribbed
   b. grooved
   c. smooth
   d. orange peel

7. The area where the lighter-colored gingiva meets the darker-colored alveolar mucosa is termed the:

a. free gingival groove   c. gingival papilla

b. mucogingival junction   d. median raphe

8. Describe the mucosa of the hard palate. Select all that apply.

a. thick   c. firmly attached to underlying bone

b. keratinized   d. movable

9. The soft palate and tongue are raised during swallowing to:

a. prevent choking on large pieces of food

b. keep food from entering the nasopharynx

c. allow the food to be formed into a ball

d. move the food toward the front of the mouth

10. Which of the following may occur if intraoral jewelry is worn? Select all that apply.

a. tooth fracture   d. infection

b. swelling   e. pain

c. allergic reactions to metal

TRUE/FALSE

Indicate whether the statement is true (T) or false (F).

_____ 1. Although alveolar mucosa is thin, it is fixed firmly to the underlying bone.

_____ 2. The only known danger from wearing oral jewelry is swelling.

_____ 3. The anterior borders of the oral cavity proper are the lips and cheeks.

_____ 4. The palate provides a floor to the nasal cavity and a roof to the oral cavity proper.

_____ 5. Mucosal tissues are smooth, shiny, wet, and thin.

_____ 6. Buccal frenula are found on both jaws between the cheeks and the first or second molars.

_____ 7. Linea alba is most frequently seen on the alveolar mucosa.

_____ 8. The ducts of Rivinus empty saliva from the sublingual glands into the sublingual caruncle in the floor of the mouth.

_____ 9. The incisive papilla covers the incisive foramen on the anterior palate.

_____ 10. The uvula marks the boundary between the nasal and oral cavities and the oropharynx.

FILL IN THE BLANK

Using words from the list below, fill in the blanks to complete the following statements.

alcohol	gag reflex	pharynx
attached gingiva	leukoplakia	record anatomic structures
circumvallate	lingual vein	tobacco
free gingiva	nonkeratinized	

1. A thick, white patch on the oral mucosa termed _____ may be precancerous.

2. The _____ may be seen as a bluish structure on the ventral surface of the tongue.

3. The lighter gingiva that is firmly bound to the underlying alveolar bone is _____.

4. The darker gingiva that is not attached to the underlying alveolar bone is _____.

5. The _____ is a passageway for both food and air.

6. _____ mucosal tissue covers the soft palate.

7. Placing the high-volume evacuator too near the back of the mouth may activate the patient's _____.

8. _____ papillae are found on the base of the tongue and provide taste sensation.

9. Consumption of _____ and _____ is frequently considered to be a factor in the development of leukoplakia.

10. Failure to remove the patient's oral jewelry prior to exposing a radiograph may result in failure to _____.

CHAPTER 7
Oral Embryology and Histology

CHAPTER OUTLINE

Review the Chapter Outline. If any content area is unclear, review that area before beginning the workbook exercises.

    A. Oral Embryology
        1. Primary Embryonic Layers
        2. Development of Facial Structures
    B. Formation and Growth of the Teeth
    C. Oral Histology
        1. Tissues of the Tooth
    D. Supporting Structures
        1. Attachment Apparatus
        2. Gingival Unit

CHAPTER REVIEW

The following is a summary of the chapter. If any of this material is unclear, review it in the textbook again.

Embryology is the study of how and when structures form. Histology is the study of cell structure and function. General body development begins with conception, extends over a 38- to 40-week period, and progresses through three major stages. Tooth development begins during the sixth week and extends through birth and beyond. All teeth and their supporting structures are derived from three embryonic germ layers. Tissues of the tooth include enamel, dentin, pulp, and cementum. Cementum, alveolar bone, and the periodontal ligament comprise the supporting structures. Primary teeth are expected to erupt and be lost at reasonably predictable ages. They are shed because of root resorption. Permanent molars erupt posterior to the primary teeth, an important fact because parents do not always realize a tooth erupting in the back of the mouth is a permanent tooth.

LEARNING ACTIVITIES AND STUDY AIDS

Review the following study aids and/or complete the activities to ensure that you have achieved the learning objectives for this chapter.

1. Create an illustration or find one online that outlines the three embryologic stages.

2. Using the following table, list the three embryologic stages with the major events that occur during each stage.

Table 7-1

Embryologic Stage	Major Events

3. Describe the three primary germ layers and why the timing of their appearance and development is so important.

4. Describe the development of the face.

5. Differentiate the bud, cap, and bell stages of tooth development.

6. On one side of a flash card, list the tissues of the teeth and supporting structures. On the other side, list the function of each tissue, the germ layer from which it is derived, and the structure(s) that form it. Turn the flash cards in for a grade and use the flash cards to study either individually or with another classmate.

7. Using Internet resources, conduct research to further understand the process of tooth eruption. Write a short paragraph to present what was discovered and learned through your research. Suggested Internet sites include:

    http://www.uic.edu/classes/osci/osci590/9_1Mechanisms.htm
    http://www.research.lsu.edu/newsletter/archives/2007autumn/teeth.html

8. Differentiate ameloblasts, odontoblasts, cementoblasts, and osteoclasts.

9. Looking at the following figure of the tooth, on the lines provided label each: enamel, dentin, pulp, alveolar bone, and cementum.

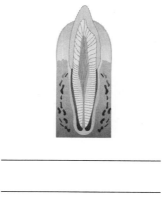

_____

_____

_____   Figure 7-2

10. Explain the difference between a primary, permanent, and mixed dentition.

11. Describe how the tooth repairs itself in a limited manner when it has been worn away or injured.

MEDICAL TERMINOLOGY REVIEW

Use a dictionary and/or your textbook to define the following terms.

alveolar crest _____

ameloblast _____

anatomic crown _____

anatomic root _____

apical foramen _____

attached gingiva _____

bifurcation _____

cementoblast _____

cementoenamel junction _____

cementum _____

clinical crown _____

clinical root _____

conception _____

cribriform plate _____

dental lamina _____

dental papilla _____

dental sac _____

dentin _____

dentinal tubule _____

dentoenamel junction _____

ectoderm _____

embryo _____

enamel _____

enamel organ _____

endoderm _____

eruption _____

exfoliation _____

fallopian tube _____

fetal stage _____

free gingiva _____

gestation _____

lamina dura _____

mandibular arch _____

maxillary process _____

meiosis _____

mesenchyme _____

mesoderm _____

mixed dentition _____

nasal pits _____

odontoblast _____

osteoblast _____

periodontal ligament _____

pharyngeal arch _____

premaxilla _____

primary palate _____

pulp _____

pulp canal _____

pulp chamber _____

secondary dentin _____

Sharpey's fibers _____

stomodeum _____

succedaneous _____

tertiary dentin _____

tooth bud _____

trifurcation _____

uterus _____

ABBREVIATIONS

CEJ _____

DEJ _____

PDL _____

CRITICAL THINKING

1. Why is it important for a dental assistant to know and understand the different stages of development of the oral structures?

2. Why is it important for a dental assistant to be able to differentiate between succedaneous and permanent teeth?

3. Name the four types of tooth structures that are common to all teeth. Also include whether these are considered to be hard structures or soft. As a dental assistant, why is it important to know the difference?

CHAPTER REVIEW TEST

MULTIPLE CHOICE

Circle the letter of the correct answer.

1. Which of the following tissues are derived from the dental papilla?

   a. enamel and dentin
   b. dentin and pulp
   c. pulp and cementum
   d. cementum and periodontal ligament
   e. periodontal ligament and enamel

2. What is the first permanent tooth to erupt into the oral cavity?

   a. maxillary central incisor
   b. mandibular canine
   c. maxillary second premolar
   d. mandibular first molar

3. The major tasks of the fetal period during gestation are:
   a. travel to and implantation in the uterus
   b. establishing the major organs and organ systems
   c. development of the face and palate
   d. growth and maturation

4. All of these structures will be derived from the mandibular (first pharyngeal) arch EXCEPT the:
   a. mandible
   b. maxilla
   c. temporal bone
   d. muscles of mastication
   e. zygomatic bone

5. Covering, lining, and communication tissues such as the skin, nervous system, enamel, and oral epithelium develop from:
   a. endoderm
   b. mesoderm
   c. mesenchyme
   d. ectoderm

6. These structures are embedded in the alveolar bone and cementum to ensure the tooth is held in the correct position in the jaw.
   a. Sharpey's fibers
   b. cementoblasts
   c. dental lamina and oral epithelium
   d. dental and successional laminae

7. Tooth movement to attain a working position in the oral cavity is known as:
   a. exfoliation
   b. eruption
   c. layering
   d. succession

8. Primary teeth are shed because the:
   a. tooth root has been resorbed
   b. tooth moves too far past a working position
   c. alveolar bone that holds them in place is not replaced
   d. dental sac did not make adequate supporting tissue

9. Children with a mixed dentition have:
   a. primary teeth only
   b. permanent teeth only
   c. both primary and permanent teeth
   d. succedaneous teeth only

10. The clinical crown of a tooth is the part of a tooth that is:
    a. covered with enamel
    b. visible in the mouth
    c. covered with cementum
    d. not visible in the mouth

TRUE/FALSE

Indicate whether the statement is true (T) or false (F).

_____ 1. Succedaneous teeth include incisors, canines, and premolars.

_____ 2. Osteoclasts destroy bone, whereas odontoblasts destroy dentin and cementum.

_____ 3. Cementum, periodontal ligament, and alveolar bone form a functional unit termed the attachment apparatus.

_____ 4. Dentin is translucent but enamel is not.

_____ 5. Enamel and cementum can be distinguished clinically by their colors: white for enamel and yellow for cementum.

_____ 6. The two tissues that are of approximately the same hardness are cementum and bone.

_____ 7. Like enamel, dentin cannot transmit sensations.

_____ 8. Tissues of the periodontium support, nourish, and protect the teeth.

_____ 9. As a tooth ages, it forms secondary dentin that decreases the size of the pulp chamber.

_____ 10. Gingival tissues are specialized connective tissues derived from endoderm that cover and protect the teeth.

FILL IN THE BLANK

Using words from the list below, fill in the blanks to complete the following statements.

ameloblast	clast	epithelial
anatomical	clinical	oral epithelium
bell	connective	pulp
blast	dentin	zygote

1. The initial one-celled organism from which the entire child ultimately develops is a _____.

2. Enamel is developed by this type of specialized cell: _____.

3. Tissue builder cells have names that end in _____, whereas those that break down tissue have names that end in _____.

4. Tooth development begins with thickening and downgrowth of the _____.

5. When teeth develop, assumption of the future shape of the tooth and histodifferentiation take place during the _____ stage.

6. Enamel is a/an _____ tissue, whereas all of the other tissues of the tooth and periodontium are _____ tissue.

7. The _____ crown is covered with enamel.

8. The _____ root is covered so is not visible in the mouth.

9. _____ provides nutrition and sensation to the tooth.

10. This tissue forms the bulk of the tooth crown and root: _____.

CHAPTER 8
Tooth Morphology

CHAPTER OUTLINE

Review the Chapter Outline. If any content area is unclear, review that area before beginning the workbook exercises.

    A. Histology of Tooth Development
        1. Stages
        2. Abnormalities

    B. Hard Tissues of the Teeth
        1. Enamel
        2. Dentin
        3. Pulp
        4. Cementum

    C. Formation of the Periodontium
        1. Periodontal Membrane
        2. Alveolar Bone
        3. Gingiva

    D. Dentition Periods
        1. Primary Dentition
        2. Mixed Dentition
        3. Permanent Dentition

CHAPTER REVIEW

The following is a summary of the chapter. If any of this material is unclear, review it in the textbook again.

Prenatal growth is an important time in the oral cavity's development. This is when the stages of teeth development begin as well as the formation of other organs in the body. It is very important that the entire dental team is aware of the structures and functions that occur throughout a lifetime. Dental assistants must be conscious of the different stages of tooth development. Having knowledge of prenatal growth patterns, development of oral embryology, eruptions patterns, and tooth function enables the dental assistant to communicate effectively with his/her dental patients, parents, and their families about changes occurring in the oral cavity. This knowledge also enables the dental assistant to more accurately record patient dental histories for charting and diagnosis of abnormalities.

LEARNING ACTIVITIES AND STUDY AIDS

Review the following study aids and/or complete the activities to ensure that you have achieved the learning objectives for this chapter.

1. Identify the order for eruption of the deciduous teeth.

2. Using a separate piece of paper, write two or three paragraphs describing tooth morphology, and how this knowledge, helps the dental assistant perform his/her job.

3. Explain the differences between the primary and permanent teeth, and between posterior and anterior teeth.

4. Using a practice set of dental radiographs or panograph provided by your instructor (comparing primary and permanent teeth), make a list of the differences you can identify between the maxillary arch teeth and the mandibular arch teeth. If there are any missing teeth on either set of x-rays, annotate these teeth. Also note if there are any unerupted teeth, and which teeth they will replace when fully erupted. If more space is required for your information than is provided here, use an additional piece of paper.

5. Using the figure provided of the permanent dentition, label each of the following for the mandibular and maxillary teeth:

 Central incisor

 Lateral incisor

 Cuspid

 1st Premolar

 2nd Premolar

 1st Molar

 2nd Molar

 3rd Molar or wisdom tooth

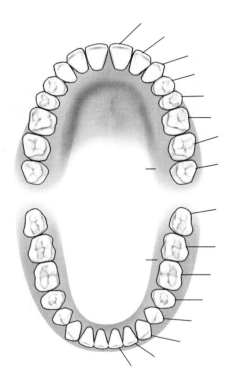

Figure 8-1

6. Describe the formation of the periodontuim and the three separate tissues that aid in its purpose to anchor, support, and protect the teeth.

7. A number of tooth abnormalities can occur during the development stages. To further understand these abnormalities, select two abnormalities and conduct research using the Internet and/or materials from the school or local library. Utilizing a separate piece of paper, write a paragraph on each abnormality, and explain what was learned from your research. Be sure to describe the abnormality, the signs and symptoms, causes, and treatment(s).

8. Describe the fifth stage in the process of odontogenesis.

9. Using a separate piece of paper, create a table listing all the teeth from primary dentition. List the characteristics for the primary teeth. Example: How many of each primary teeth are there? Is the tooth itself larger or smaller?

10. On the lines provided under each image, list the stage of tooth development.

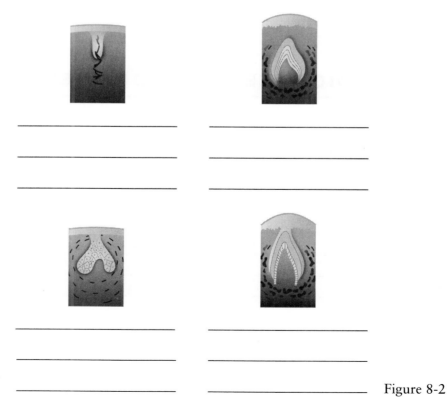

_____   _____

_____   _____

_____   _____

_____   _____

_____   _____

_____   _____ Figure 8-2

Figure 8-2 *(Continued)*

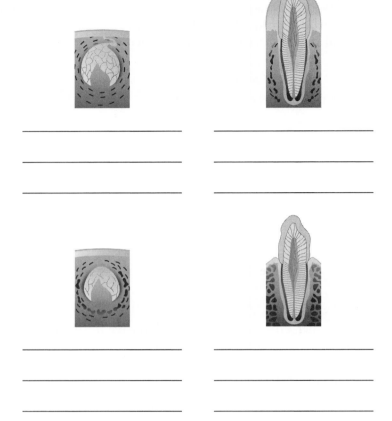

_____   _____

_____   _____

_____   _____

_____   _____

_____   _____

_____   _____

MEDICAL TERMINOLOGY REVIEW

Use a dictionary and/or your textbook to define the following terms.

amelogenesis imperfecta _____

apposition _____

attrition _____

calcification _____

dens in dente _____

dentin dysplasia _____

dentinogenesis imperfecta _____

dentition _____

differentiation _____

eruption _____

exfoliate _____

fluorosis _____

fusion _____

germination _____

hyperdontia _____

hypodontia _____

initation _____

macrodontia _____

microdontia _____

mixed dentition _____

odontogenesis _____

permanent dentition _____

primary dentition _____

proliferation _____

succedaneous _____

supernumerary _____

ABBREVIATIONS

(There are no abbreviations for this chapter.)

CRITICAL THINKING

1. As a dental assistant who may be working in a pedodontic office, you have a $6^1/_2$-year-old-patient who presents for dental care. What primary and permanent teeth would you normally expect to see erupted at this age? Why is it important for the dental assistant to know the normal eruption patterns of primary and permanent teeth?

2. Which teeth found in the maxillary arch may be bifurcated? Why does a dental assistant need to realize the difference between bifurcated and trifurcated teeth?

3. How does having the knowledge of prenatal growth and the course of development of oral embryology help the dental assistant do his/her job effectively?

CHAPTER REVIEW TEST

MULTIPLE CHOICE

Circle the letter of the correct answer.

1. The main function of these teeth is to pulverize food into small pieces that can be swallowed comfortably.
   a. wisdom teeth
   b. molars
   c. central incisors
   d. canines

2. The first tooth/teeth that normally erupt(s) when a baby is approximately six months of age is:
   a. maxillary central incisor
   b. maxillary six-month molar
   c. mandibular central incisor
   d. mandibular six-month molar

3. A child's first permanent tooth generally appears about this age:
   a. three years old
   b. four years old
   c. six years old
   d. twelve years old

4. Another term that can be used for premolars is:
   a. dragon tooth
   b. eye tooth
   c. canines
   d. bicuspids

5. How many teeth are found in permanent dentition?
   a. twenty
   b. twenty-two
   c. thirty
   d. thirty-two

6. How many teeth are found in primary dentition?
   a. twenty
   b. twenty-two
   c. thirty
   d. thirty-two

7. The CEJ (cemento enamel junction) is also know as the:
   a. head of the tooth
   b. neck of the tooth
   c. waist of the tooth
   d. tongue of the tooth

8. Attrition occurs when:
   a. the tooth is in the second stage of eruption
   b. the occusal surfaces of the teeth begin to wear down from normal functions such as chewing and speaking
   c. the facial surfaces of the teeth begin to wear down from normal functions such as chewing and speaking
   d. the first primary molar is lost

9. Deciduous teeth are the first set of teeth. They are also called:
   a. succedaneous teeth
   b. permanent teeth
   c. primary teeth
   d. cat teeth

.0. Periodontium consists of which components?
   a. periodontal membrane and alveolar bone
   b. periodontal membrane and gingiva
   c. periodontal membrane, gingival, and alveolar bone
   d. periodontal membrane, teeth, and alveolar bone

TRUE/FALSE

Indicate whether the statement is true (T) or false (F).

_____ 1. Mammelons are not present on primary teeth.

_____ 2. The developmental groove that forms when the lobes form is called the fissure.

_____ 3. A convex surface means the surface is projected.

_____ 4. There are 16 primary teeth and 32 permanent teeth.

_____ 5. Fluorosis occurs from lack of fluoride during tooth development.

_____ 6. Macrodontia means teeth are smaller than a normal-size tooth of the same type.

_____ 7. In human dentition there are five types of teeth.

_____ 8. The enamel matrix is produced by enameloblasts.

_____ 9. Dentin is a hard outer covering of every tooth.

_____ 10. Alveolar bone is found only in the alveoli linings of tissues.

FILL IN THE BLANK

Using words from the list below, fill in the blanks to complete the following statements.

supernumerary teeth	microdontia	fluorosis
exfoliation	anodontia tooth	eruption
periodontium	dentinogenesis	cementogenesis
odontogenesis	hyperdontia	macrodontia

1. _____ is the presence of extra teeth, more than the normal amount of teeth.

2. _____ are uncommonly small teeth.

3. _____ occurs when excessive fluoride is consumed during tooth development, causing yellowing of teeth, white spots, and pitting or mottling of enamel.

4. A rare genetic disorder that appears at birth resulting in a complete lack of tooth development is termed _____.

5. _____ is the process of a tooth breaking through the gum tissue to grow into place in the mouth and become visible.

6. The supporting structure of the tooth is known as the _____.

7. _____ is known as the development of dentin.

8. _____ is the formation of cementum.

9. Tooth production or development, termed _____, is the process or creation of each tooth

10. The process of taking the place of the primary teeth through the natural pushing or falling out of primary teeth is termed _____.

CHAPTER 9
Dental Charting

CHAPTER OUTLINE

Review the Chapter Outline. If any content area is unclear, review that area before beginning the workbook exercises.

A. The Dental Arches
B. Dentition Periods
C. Types and Functions of Teeth
D. Tooth Surfaces
E. The Morphology of Teeth
F. Stabilization of the Arches
G. Tooth Numbering Systems
H. Cavity Classification
I. Charting Procedures

CHAPTER REVIEW

The following is a summary of the chapter. If any of this material is unclear, review it in the textbook again.

Dental personnel record patient conditions and treatment needed. This visual format saves time and provides information rapidly to anyone who can read the symbols. Because dental assistants do the recording while dentists dictate the information, assistants must be thoroughly familiar with the symbols dentists use and be able to record conditions rapidly. There are three major systems, two of which are used extensively in the United States: Universal Charting and Palmer Notation. Both systems use numbers to designate the permanent teeth, letters to designate the primary teeth, and blue and red pencil to designate specific conditions. Palmer Notation adds quadrant symbols to designate specific areas of the mouth.

LEARNING ACTIVITIES AND STUDY AIDS

Review the following study aids and/or complete the activities to ensure that you have achieved the learning objectives for this chapter.

1. Using the line drawing below of the primary dentition, label one complete quadrant of the teeth.

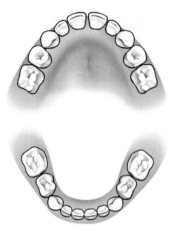

Primary Dentition   Figure 9-1

2. Using the line drawing below of the permanent dentition, label one complete quadrant of the teeth.

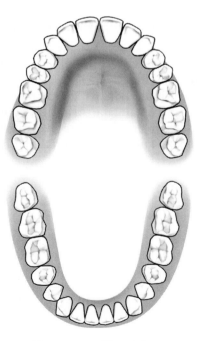

Permanent Dentition   Figure 9-2

3. State which teeth are classified as anteriors, and which are classified as posteriors.

4. Using the drawing for Activity #2 of the permanent dentition, draw two lines to separate the four quadrants, and then label each quadrant.

5. List and describe the location of each surface found on the anterior and posterior teeth.

6. Label each of the following on the line drawings provided below: cusp, distal marginal ridges, triangular ridge, transverse ridge, oblique ridge, supplemental grooves, pits, fossa, cingulum, mamelon, line angle, and point angle.

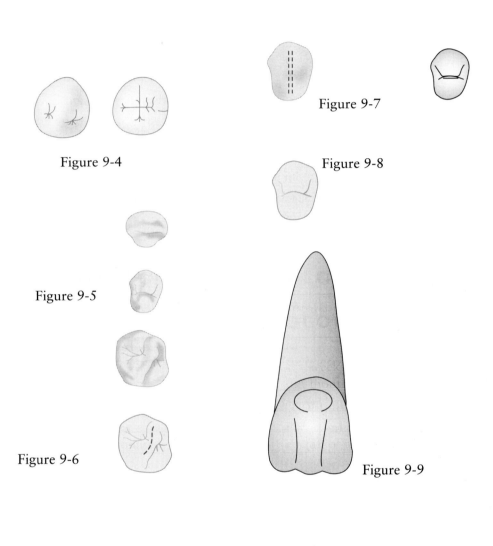

Figure 9-4

Figure 9-7

Figure 9-8

Figure 9-5

Figure 9-6

Figure 9-9

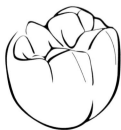

Figure 9-10

7. Explain what the curve of Spee is, and why it is important.

8. Differentiate occlusion and malocclusion.

9. Using the following drawing, divide and label the tooth into thirds vertically and horizontally.

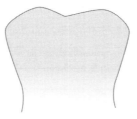

Figure 9-11

0. State the sequence of primary tooth eruption.

11. Describe the characteristics of Dr. Edward H. Angle's three classes of malocclusion.

MEDICAL TERMINOLOGY REVIEW

Use a dictionary and/or your textbook to define the following terms.

anterior _____

buccal _____

canine _____

caries _____

complex cavity _____

compound cavity _____

crossbite _____

curve of Spee _____

cusp _____

deciduous teeth _____

distal _____

distoclusion _____

embrasure _____

facial _____

fissure _____

incisal _____

incisor _____

labial _____

line angle _____

lingual _____

malocclusion _____

mandibular arch _____

maxillary arch _____

mesial _____

mesioclusion _____

mesognathic _____

molar _____

neutroclusion _____

occlusal _____

occlusion _____

overbite _____

overjet _____

pit _____

point angle _____

posterior _____

premolar _____

prognathic _____

proximal _____

quadrant _____

retrognathic _____

simple cavity _____

underbite _____

ABBREVIATIONS

For tooth surfaces:

B _____

D _____

F _____

L _____

M _____

O _____

For Angle's classes of malocclusion:

Class I _____

Class II _____

Class III _____

For types of cavity preparations:

Class I _____

Class II _____

Class III _____

Class IV _____

Class V _____

Class VI _____

CRITICAL THINKING

1. How might a dental assistant explain the difference between primary teeth and permanent teeth to a child?

2. Which surfaces of the teeth are most prone to collecting plaque, bacteria, and becoming decayed (carious)? Why are these surfaces more prone than any other?

3. Why are primary teeth important?

4. How can you tell if a patient has an overbite or an overjet? How might these two malpositions be corrected?

CHAPTER REVIEW TEST

MULTIPLE CHOICE

Circle the letter of the correct answer.

1. In the Universal Charting system, which of the following is a posterior tooth?
   a. 4
   b. 7
   c. 22
   d. 25

2. In the FDI System, which tooth is 42?
   a. maxillary right second molar
   b. mandibular left second premolar
   c. maxillary right canine
   d. mandibular right lateral incisor

3. What color is used to chart restorations?
   a. red
   b. blue
   c. green
   d. black

4. What color is used to chart dental caries?
   a. red
   b. blue
   c. green
   d. black

5. If your patient's mandibular canine is facial to his maxillary canine, what occlusion condition does he have?
   a. overbite
   b. overjet
   c. crossbite
   d. supraeruption

6. If your patient's mandible is retruded when considered in relation to the maxilla, what type of profile does she have?
   a. prognathic
   b. mesognathic
   c. retrognathic
   d. none of the above

7. If your patient has a Class III cavity on #9, what surface and tooth are affected?

a. incisal of primary canine
b. distal of permanent central incisor
c. occlusal of maxillary premolar
d. lingual of mandibular molar

8. This tooth has a strong, heavy root and forms the corner of the dental arch.

a. incisor
b. premolar
c. canine
d. molar

9. Which of the following denotes a quadrant?

a. mandibular left
b. anterior
c. maxillary
d. arch

10. Which of the following denotes a compound cavity?

a. D
b. BOL
c. MODBL
d. MO

TRUE/FALSE

Indicate whether the statement is true (T) or false (F).

_____ 1. The permanent dentition has twenty teeth.

_____ 2. Chewing surfaces of posterior teeth are occlusal surfaces.

_____ 3. Interproximal areas are located between adjacent teeth in the same arch.

_____ 4. A human being normally receives three sets of teeth during his or her lifetime—primary, mixed, and permanent.

_____ 5. On posterior teeth, embrasures curve away from the contact areas in cervical, facial, lingual, and occlusal directions.

_____ 6. There are eight molars in each arch of the permanent dentition.

_____ 7. The first permanent molar normally erupts when a child is about eight years old.

_____ 8. Canines hold and tear food.

_____ 9. Premolars crush food to prepare it for grinding by the molars.

_____ 10. According to Angle's classes, if the mesiobuccal groove of the mandibular first molar is distal to the mesiobuccal cusp of the maxillary first molar, the patient has Class III occlusion.

FILL IN THE BLANK

Using words from the list below, fill in the blanks to complete the following statements.

canine	groove	premolar	drifting	mamelon
pit	fissure	overjet	two	four

1. There are no _____ teeth in the primary dentition.

2. In each quadrant, the _____ is immediately posterior to the lateral incisor.

3. A defective groove is termed an _____.

4. An _____ is found at the junction of grooves.

5. Mandibular molars have _____ roots.

6. Molars have _____ major cusps for grinding food.

7. Premature tooth loss may cause _____ of teeth posterior to the lost tooth.

8. A curved prominence located on the incisal surface of an anterior tooth is termed a _____.

9. An _____ is a linear depression on the tooth surface.

10. An _____ is present when the maxillary anterior teeth extend too far over the mandibular teeth in a horizontal direction.

CHAPTER 10
Oral Pathology

CHAPTER OUTLINE

Review the Chapter Outline. If any content area is unclear, review that area before beginning the workbook exercises.

A. Diseases and Conditions Affecting the Oral Cavity
B. Oral Lesions
C. Conditions of the Tongue
D. Oral Cancer
E. Oral Conditions Due to HIV and AIDS
F. Developmental Disorders
G. Miscellaneous Disorders
H. CDC Rankings of Evidence
I. Environmental Infection Control

CHAPTER REVIEW

The following is a summary of the chapter. If any of this material is unclear, review it in the textbook again.

Oral pathology is the study of diseases and conditions of the mouth and nearby tissues. As an integral part of the body, the mouth exhibits manifestations of many systemic diseases. Additionally, some diseases and conditions occur only in the mouth. Dentists categorize pathologic lesions on the basis of size, appearance, texture, mobility, location, and color. Dental assistants who conscientiously learn and apply knowledge of oral pathology to recognize tissue abnormalities assist the dentist in establishing a timely diagnosis and providing needed care. The dental assistant also provides patient education to ensure the patient understands any pathologic condition the patient may have and any home care measures that should be completed.

LEARNING ACTIVITES AND STUDY AIDS

Review the following study aids and/or complete the activities to ensure that you have achieved the learning objectives for this chapter.

1. To further understand the roles of both the oral pathologist and the oral and maxillofacial surgeon, conduct research online and/or at your school's library or local library to learn more about each of these fields. On a separate piece of paper, write a short report comparing and contrasting these two specialties. At the end of your report cite your sources.

2. During the inspection of the patient's mouth prior to taking a full mouth series of radiographs, a dental assistant notices a thick patch of white tissue on the posterior palatal mucosa adjacent to the right second molar. Closer inspection reveals that three other palatal areas exhibit similar but smaller white patches. Upon questioning the patient, the dental assistant learns the patient is a smoker and is aware that the patches have been present for several months. The patient explains that ordinarily they do not bother her, but sometimes if she hits them with her toothbrush or brushes hard, they bleed. What action should the dental assistant take?

3. Discuss the role of inflammation in the body and list its signs and symptoms.

4. List six methods dentists may use as aids to diagnosis.

5. Describe how information from a patient's medical dental history can contribute to establishing a diagnosis.

6. Describe the process a dentist uses to establish a final diagnosis.

7. Using the following table, explain the signs and symptoms of each condition.

Table 10-1

Condition	Signs and Symptoms
Torus	
Mucocele	
Varix	
Herpes labialis	
Aphthous ulcers	
Abscess	
Pustule	
Attrition	
Abrasion	
Leukoplaki	

8. In years past, dental professionals were more concerned about the presence of leukoplakia in the mouth than erythroplakia. In recent years, new research has reversed that opinion. Go online and research why both conditions are still of concern but erythroplakia is often of greater concern. Good sites to begin your research are: the American Cancer Society Web site, *http://www.cancer.org/ docroot/CRI/content/CRI_2_4_1X_What_is_oral_cavity_and_oropharyngeal_cancer_60.asp*; the Diseases Database references Web site, *http://www.diseasesdatabase.com/ddb30783.htm*; and the cancer research site for the United Kingdom, *http://www.cancerhelp.org.uk/help/default.asp? page=13033*. On a separate piece of paper, write a half-page report detailing your conclusions.

9. Differentiate carcinoma and sarcoma.

10. List the signs and symptoms of Bell's palsy. What are the special considerations when providing dental care to a patient with Bell's palsy?

MEDICAL TERMINOLOGY REVIEW

Use a dictionary and/or your textbook to define the following terms.

abrasion _____

abscess _____

actinomycosis _____

adenocarcinoma _____

amalgam tattoo _____

ameloblastoma _____

amelogenesis imperfecta _____

anaerobic _____

angular cheilitis _____

ankyloglossia _____

anodontia _____

anorexia nervosa _____

aphthous ulcers _____

attrition _____

Bell's palsy _____

benign _____

biopsy _____

bruxism _____

bulimia _____

bulla _____

carcinoma _____

concrescence _____

cyst _____

dens en dente _____

dentinogenesis imperfecta _____

ecchymosis _____

enamel pearl _____

epulis fissuratum _____

erythematous _____

erythroplakia _____

exudate _____

fibroma _____

fistula _____

fusion _____

gemination _____

geographic tongue _____

glossitis _____

granuloma _____

hairy tongue _____

hematoma _____

herpes labialis _____

herpetic gingivostomatitis _____

herpetic whitlow _____

hyperplasia _____

hypodontia _____

Kaposi's sarcoma _____

Koplik's spots _____

lesion _____

lichen planus _____

macrodontia _____

malignant _____

measles _____

microdontia _____

mucocele _____

multilocular _____

mumps _____

neoplasm _____

nicotine stomatitis _____

nodule _____

obturator _____

osteoradionecrosis _____

papilloma _____

patch _____

periodontitis _____

petechiae _____

purpura _____

pustule _____

pyogenic _____

radiolucent _____

radiopaque _____

sarcoma _____

stye _____

supernumerary _____

teratogen _____

tetanus _____

tolouidine blue _____

torus _____

trauma _____

tuberculosis _____

tumor _____

ulcer _____

varicella _____

varix _____

vesicle _____

ABBREVIATIONS

AIDS _____

ANUG _____

CDC _____

HSV1 _____

NUG _____

PPD _____

TB _____

CRITICAL THINKING

1. Why is it important for a dental assistant to have knowledge of normal and abnormal oral pathology?

2. What is the main function of the Centers for Disease Control and Prevention (CDC)? What is the importance of this organization to a dental assistant?

3. How can a dental assistant work with a patient who has the presence of tori but must have a radiograph taken? What will help with making this procedure more comfortable?

4. What are the main factors of ANUG, and how is this condition treated? Why is this condition of concern to a dental assistant?

CHAPTER REVIEW TEST

MULTIPLE CHOICE

Circle the letter of the correct answer.

1. Herpes zoster is a reemergence of this virus in later years.

   a. actinomycosis
   b. tuberculosis
   c. varicella
   d. herpes

2. An abnormally small tooth, frequently a maxillary third molar, is a:

   a. fibroma
   b. microdont
   c. taurodont
   d. papilloma

3. When the cementum of two teeth is fused together, the resulting condition is known as:

   a. concrescence
   b. gemination
   c. ankylosis
   d. lichen planus

4. Aphthous ulcers are a common, painful condition in which the mucosa exhibits:

   a. multiple vesicles on the lips and their lining mucosa
   b. white patches that cannot be rubbed off
   c. circular depressions with a yellow center and red border
   d. malignant bluish-purple growths of irregular shape

5. The presence of Koplik's spots on the buccal mucosa indicates the patient is in an early stage of:

   a. chicken pox
   b. shingles
   c. mumps
   d. measles

6. When an entire lesion and a small amount of surrounding tissue are removed for study, the procedure completed is a/an:

   a. excisional biopsy
   b. incisal biopsy
   c. punch biopsy
   d. brush biopsy

7. A dentigerous cyst may develop when:
   a. a mucocele is incompletely removed
   b. chemotherapy is used to treat oral cancer
   c. a tooth experiences chronic periodontitis
   d. tooth development does not proceed correctly

8. When hypodontia is suspected, what diagnostic method would provide the most useful information?
   a. brush biopsy
   b. radiographic examination
   c. use of a VELtrix device
   d. clinical observation

9. A patient has asked you to explain what the dentist meant when he said she has an abscess. How would you answer her?
   a. excessive wear on a tooth
   b. a fungus that is growing in the tooth
   c. bone that has overgrown
   d. pus that has collected in a specific area

10. A patch is an area of the mucosa that:
    a. appears to be different in color or texture
    b. has small red or purplish spots
    c. is painful and movable
    d. exhibits a small lump

TRUE/FALSE

Indicate whether the statement is true (T) or false (F).

_____ 1. A Mantoux test is used to determine if a patient has carcinoma.

_____ 2. Common sites for TB infection in the oral cavity are the tongue and palate.

_____ 3. An amalgam tattoo is usually removed to protect the patient's health.

_____ 4. Radiation treatment in children may result in developmental defects of the teeth.

_____ 5. Gingiva that has suffered an aspirin burn appears white and rough-textured.

_____ 6. Dental complications from oral piercing are minimal and last for only a short time.

_____ 7. Nicotine stomatitis appears as an overgrowth of the filiform papillae.

_____ 8. The timing of exposure to a teratogen during pregnancy is critical to the degree of impact the developing child may experience.

_____ 9. Geographic tongue exhibits patchy lesions that move from place to place in an irregular pattern.

_____ 10. Dens en dente refers to a small, often misshapen tooth commonly seen at the maxillary midline.

FILL IN THE BLANK

Using words from the list below, fill in the blanks to complete the following statements.

ANUG	pedunculated	tori
attrition	periapical	tumor
fluoride	petechiae	varix
mucocele	periodontal	

1. Trench mouth, also termed _____, is a painful condition of the gingiva caused by microbial overgrowth.

2. Trauma to a minor salivary gland may result in the formation of a fluid-filled _____.

3. A condition related to varicose veins, _____, may be seen on the ventral surface of the tongue, particularly in elderly patients.

4. Patients with an eating disorder should be encouraged to seek professional treatment, rinse after vomiting, and use _____ on a daily basis.

5. Bone growths with a thin tissue covering that are often seen at the midline of the palate, or on the lingual surface of the mandible in the canine or premolar area, are _____.

6. A _____ is an abnormal growth that can be either benign or malignant.

7. A _____ lesion is attached to the tissue by a slender stalk.

8. Small lesions termed _____ are the result of localized hemorrhage.

9. A _____ abscess is located at the apical end of a tooth root, whereas a _____ abscess is located in the periodontal ligament.

10. Enamel _____ is considered a normal result of aging.

CHAPTER 11
Microbiology

CHAPTER OUTLINE

Review the Chapter Outline. If any content area is unclear, review that area before beginning the workbook exercises.

A. Pioneers in Microbiology

B. Major Groups of Microorganisms
1. Algae
2. Bacteria
3. Fungi
4. Protozoa
5. Viruses

C. Viral Diseases
1. Herpes
2. HIV and AIDS
3. Hepatitis

D. Bacterial Diseases
1. Anthrax
2. Botulism
3. Tetanus
4. Tuberculosis
5. Pneumonia
6. Dental Plaque

CHAPTER REVIEW

The following is a summary of the chapter. If any of this material is unclear, review it in the textbook again.

Microbiology is the study of organisms that are too small to be seen with the naked eye. Major pioneers in microbiology first invented the microscope and described the world of microorganisms, then developed processes to control and study them. In time, methods were developed to harness some microbial processes to inactivate or kill those that cause disease. Microbes can cause disease but also provide many benefits to human life. They are skilled at adjusting to methods of control and continually present new challenges to healthcare providers. Dental assistants should follow procedures to prevent disease transmission, educate patients about microbial diseases, and advocate for implementation of measures that prevent them.

LEARNING ACTIVITIES AND STUDY AIDS

Review the following study aids and/or complete the activities to ensure that you have achieved the learning objectives for this chapter.

1. Dentist researchers have contributed greatly to our understanding of the microbiology of caries, periodontal disease, and the relationship of oral disease to general body health. To further enhance your understanding of pioneering microbiologists, go online and research the contributions of the following dentists: Drs. Russell Bunting, Anne Haffajee, Theodor Rosebury, Sigmund Socransky, and Walter Loesche. Using a separate piece of paper, write a one-page summary or prepare a three- to five-minute PowerPoint presentation of what you have learned. Be sure to cite your sources and include your assessment of whether the foundation theories these people developed still guide our thinking today. A good place to begin your research is *http://jdr.iadrjournals.org/cgi/content/full/85/11/990*, which is the text of an article published in the journal of the International Association of Dental Research that speaks to Dr. Rosebury's contributions and refers to the other contributors as well.

2. List and define the major groups of microorganisms.

3. Complete the following table. For some of the requested information, further research using the Internet and/or other sources may be necessary.

Table 11-1

Disease	Signs and Symptoms	Location	Cause	Vaccine(s) (if available)
Herpes I				
Herpes II				
HIV				

AIDS				
Hepatitis A				
Hepatitis B				
Hepatitis C				

4. Make a series of flash cards. On one side, list the following bacterial diseases: anthrax, botulism, tetanus, tuberculosis, pneumonia, and dental plaque. On the other side, describe the disease. Use these flash cards to either independently study or be quizzed on the material by others in preparation for exams. Turn your flash cards into the instructor to receive a grade for completing this activity.

5. Utilizing a separate piece of paper, write a short paragraph to answer the following questions:

What is plaque?

How would a person know if he/she has plaque?

What problems does plaque create?

Can plaque be eliminated, and if so how?

How can a person prevent plaque buildup from returning?

6. write a short scenario where the microbiology of plaque or Herpes I must be explained to a patient.

7. The mouth is a part of the whole body. The Mouth Body Connection, as it's been called, is currently a subject of intense research interest, particularly in periodontology. Go to the American Academy of Periodontology's Web site, *http://www.perio.org/consumer/mbc.respiratory.htm*, to learn the findings related to periodontal disease and several serious conditions—osteoporosis, heart disease, stroke, low birth weight and preterm babies, diabetes, and respiratory diseases. Locate at least two references for each condition. Then develop either a five-minute oral report or PowerPoint presentation to share with others that explains the results of your research. Be sure to cite references in your presentation.

8. Explain why the oxygen requirements of bacteria are important in disease causation.

9. Discuss why it is important that some bacteria form spores.

10. Describe the procedure and importance of gram staining.

MEDICAL TERMINOLOGY REVIEW

Use a dictionary and/or your textbook to define the following terms.

aerobic _____

algae _____

anaerobic _____

anthrax _____

bacterium _____

biodegradable _____

botulism _____

facultative _____

fungus _____

gonorrhea _____

hepatitis _____

herpes _____

leukemia _____

oral candidiasis _____

pathogenic _____

pneumonia _____

protozoa _____

rickettsia _____

spore _____

syphilis _____

tetanus _____

tuberculosis _____

vaccine _____

virulent _____

virus _____

ABBREVIATIONS

AIDS _____

HAV _____

HBV _____

HCV _____

HIV _____

HSV1 _____

HSV2 _____

TB _____

CRITICAL THINKING

1. Choose one of the many historical individuals mentioned in the textbook for their contribution to the field of microbiology. How do you think the individual's specific contribution has impacted the field of dentistry today?

2. Which one of the main groups of bacteria is the most difficult to destroy, and what effect does this have on the sterilization of dental instruments? How can the dental team eliminate this bacteria in the dental office?

3. Which type of bacteria is of the most concern to the dental assistant regarding sterilization and infection control? What steps can the dental assistant take to maximize infection control from this type of bacteria in the dental office?

4. Which type of infectious disease is of the most concern for a dental assistant? State your reasons for your answer. How might the dental assistant prevent this disease from being passed from person to person (patient to patient, patient to staff, and staff to patient)?

CHAPTER REVIEW TEST

MULTIPLE CHOICE

Circle the letter of the correct answer.

1. These microorganisms can replicate only when they can penetrate and function inside a living cell.

   a. algae
   b. bacteria
   c. fungi
   d. viruses

2. Bacteria that can adapt to living with or without oxygen are:

   a. anaerobic
   b. facultative
   c. aerobic
   d. spore forming

3. Several forms of an infection affect the liver, all known as a type of:

   a. botulism
   b. pneumonia
   c. hepatitis
   d. herpes

4. The first antibiotic to be discovered was:

   a. acromycin
   b. amoxicillin
   c. zithromycin
   d. penicillin

5. Antibiotic resistance develops when:

   a. evolutionary mutations in bacteria allow them to survive powerful drugs
   b. patients do not finish their prescribed courses of antibiotics
   c. physicians prescribe antibiotics for viral infections
   d. a and c
   e. all of the above.

6. Vaccines are available to prevent these types of hepatitis.

   a. Hepatitis A and B
   b. Hepatitis B and C

   c. Hepatitis C and D
   d. Hepatitis I and II

7. Pneumonia is more likely to become serious and perhaps fatal for _____ patients.

   a. very young
   b. female
   c. elderly

   d. a and c
   e. all of the above

8. Gram stain is used to:

   a. determine whether a vaccine is effective
   b. identify the types of bacteria that cause meningitis
   c. differentiate between types of bacterial cell walls
   d. locate protozoa and rickettsia

9. Oral candidiasis is treated with:

   a. antibiotics
   b. specialized mouthwash
   c. antifungal drugs
   d. application of heat and curettage

10. The only difference between HSV1 and HSV2 is the:

   a. vaccine used for prevention
   b. location of the infection
   c. size of vesicles formed
   d. lack of pain associated with HSV1

TRUE/FALSE

Indicate whether the statement is true (T) or false (F).

_____ 1. Opportunistic infections are caused by failure of the immune system to protect the patient from overgrowth of microorganisms that are normally present.

_____ 2. Some cases of hepatitis are caused by inhalation of chemicals that affect the liver.

_____ 3. Virulent microorganisms are somewhat weak and require the assistance of other members of their microbial community to cause disease.

_____ 4. Two diseases that produce toxins that attack the nervous system are anthrax and tuberculosis.

_____ 5. Symptoms of pneumonia include chills, fever, a persistent cough, and chest pain.

_____ 6. Lactobacilli in dental plaque produce fermentable carbohydrates as a waste by-product that is further fermented by such bacteria as actinomyces and streptococci.

_____ 7. *Streptococcus mutans* bacteria can be transferred from caregivers to infants through saliva.

_____ 8. The primary bacteria that cause dental caries are bacilli.

_____ 9. Toothbrushing and flossing are effective measures to prevent formation and growth of dental plaque.

_____ 10. A positive skin test is used to confirm a diagnosis of tuberculosis.

FILL IN THE BLANK

Using words from the list below, fill in the blanks to complete the following statements.

botulism	herpes	tetanus	candidiasis
HIV	tuberculosis	dental plaque	
pneumonia	spore	fungi	

Identify the disease or object that is described in each question below.

1. Forms small, painful vesicles on the lips and mucous membrane: _____.
2. Attacks the central nervous system and causes muscle spasms: _____.
3. Attacks CD4 T-cells that are required for the immune system to function properly: _____.
4. Is a lethal form of food poisoning: _____.
5. Spreads through the air and is the leading cause of death from a single infectious disease: _____.
6. Alters the mucous membrane lining of the respiratory system to permit more bacterial growth: _____.
7. Harbors a bacterial population that initiates demineralization of the tooth surface: _____.
8. Forms creamy white patches on the mucous membrane lining the mouth: _____.
9. Comprised of protein layers that encapsulate a dormant bacterium that can be reactivated to full function: _____.
10. Group that includes mushrooms, yeasts, and molds: _____.

CHAPTER 12
Dental Disease and Infection Control

CHAPTER OUTLINE

Review the Chapter Outline. If any content area is unclear, review that area before beginning the workbook exercises.

A. The Chain of Infection
B. The Immune System
C. Disease Transmission to the Dental Office.
D. Roles and Responsibilities of the CDC and OSHA in Infection Control
E. Infection Control Practices: Waste Management in the Dental Office
F. Additional Infection Control Practices
G. Special Considerations from the Center for Disease Control

CHAPTER REVIEW

The following is a summary of the chapter. If any of this material is unclear, review it in the textbook again.

Infection control is always changing and improving the safety of the dental team and patients. The OSHA Bloodborne Pathogen standard and the CDC guidelines for infection control are important to every dental office and healthcare facility. Various methods are available to protect both the patient and the dental team. These efforts include the wearing of the proper PPE to disposing of waste properly. It is the responsibility of each dental practice to follow the regulations and standards established by both the CDC and OSHA to maintain a safe environment for both the patient and the dental team.

LEARNING ACTIVITIES AND STUDY AIDS

Review the following study aids and/or complete the activities to ensure that you have achieved the learning objectives for this chapter.

1. Interview a dental assistant working in a dental office who serves as the office compliance manager, asking him/her questions about infection control policies, Exposure Control Plan, OSHA regulations and requirements, hazardous material storage policies, MSDS, engineering/work practice controls, and so forth. Then on a separate piece of paper write a one-page report that compares and contrasts the differences and similarities between the office policy and those discussed in Chapter 12 of your textbook.

2. Using the Internet and other available resources, research the duties of a dental assistant, OSHA compliance officer in a general office, an oral surgery office, and a children's dental office. Explain how the duties vary depending on the practice specialty.

3. Describe why all dental staff members need to be concerned with infection control and OSHA policies. Explain the training requirements for each office member. Include the main responsibilities of each group of individuals along with duties that may overlap within each category, and the categories that each office member would fall into depending upon their job classification.

4. Go to the Web site *http://www.osha.gov* and locate the bloodborne pathogen standard. How would you explain this policy to a new employee?

5. Go to the Web site *http://www.danb.org* and locate one article containing information about biofilm in water lines. Write a short summary on the article and what was learned from the article related to what you can do as a dental assistant to prevent biofilm from contaminating patient water supplies. Use an additional piece of paper if needed to record your information.

6. Describe the pathways for disease transmission in a dental office. Be sure to include how the use of universal and standard precautions can be effective in preventing transmission.

7. Describe hazardous waste that is found in a dental office, and explain how these materials must be disposed.

8. Describe each of the following types of waste: general, contaminated, regulated, and unregulated. Describe correct disposal procedures for each.

9. Demonstrate your knowledge of the steps in the chain of infection by creating a drawing that demonstrates this chain. Use of poster board and colored markers is highly encouraged.

10. For each of the terms in the following table's left-hand column, provide the CDC's definition in the right-hand column.

Table 12-1

Occupational Exposure	
Blood	
Other Potentially Infectious Material (OPIM)	

MEDICAL TERMINOLOGY REVIEW

Use a dictionary and/or your textbook to define the following terms.

active immunity _____

bloodborne pathogens _____

droplet transmission _____

engineering control _____

Exposure Control Plan _____

innate immunity _____

latent infections _____

opportunistic infections _____

other potentially infectious material _____

passive immunity _____

personal protective equipment _____

standard precautions _____

universal precautions _____

ABBREVIATIONS

CDC _____

HBV _____

HCV _____

HIV _____

MMWR _____

OPIM _____

OSHA _____

PPE _____

CRITICAL THINKING

1. What are the three primary modes of disease transmission in dentistry? How does an understanding of these modes make a difference in how one might do his/her job as a dental assistant?

2. When preparing for patient care, in what order should PPE be donned? What vitally important task must be completed just prior to donning PPE and immediately after removing PPE?

3. OSHA makes it mandatory for employers in healthcare settings to provide vaccines to employees. Why might an employee decline a vaccine, and what must the employer do if the employee declines? Why is this step important for the employer to do?

4. What are the six main pathways for cross contamination within the dental office, and why are these of concern to the dental assistant?

CHAPTER REVIEW TEST

MULTIPLE CHOICE

Circle the letter of the correct answer.

1. Which of the following is NOT considered to be OPIM?

   a. saliva
   b. skin
   c. blood
   d. pleural fluid
   e. pericardial fluid

2. Which color on a chemical warning label indicates the material in the container is a health hazard?

   a. red
   b. blue
   c. yellow
   d. white

3. Standard precautions should be followed by whom?

   a. housekeeping staff only
   b. all dental care providers
   c. only dental assistants
   d. lab technicians

4. An example of engineering controls would be:

   a. sterile gloves
   b. splash guards on model trimmers
   c. annual training
   d. MSDS
   e. OPIM

5. The government agency (regulating body) that requires employers to protect their employees from blood and OPIM exposure is:

   a. CDC
   b. OSAP
   c. EPA
   d. FDA
   e. OSHA

6. Passive immunity can be best defined as:

   a. immunity from an outside source that lasts for a short time
   b. immunity that is passed from one person to another
   c. immunity from an outside source that lasts for a long time
   d. immunity that is gained by being constantly exposed to a disease

7. Innate immunity is best defined as:

   a. also known as natural immunity: general protection that humans are born with
   b. immunity that is gained by being constantly exposed to a disease
   c. immunity that never really exists
   d. immunity from an outside source that lasts for a long time

8. Diseases are caused by:

   a. microorganisms or pathogens
   b. immunity
   c. not washing your hands
   d. travel to foreign countries
   e. immunizations

9. In order to reduce the number of bacteria found in the oral cavity before dental treatment, you could ask your patient to:
   a. take a shower before attending their dental appointment
   b. use a preprocedural mouth rinse with antimicrobial properties
   c. sit patiently while you apply a rubber dam
   d. open wide while you use an HVE to suction any excess saliva from his/her mouth
   e. chew a breath mint prior to dental treatment

10. Direct contact transmission of a disease occurs when:
    a. the care provider touches an infected lesion or comes into direct contact with contaminated body fluids such as blood or saliva
    b. the care provider comes in contact with inanimate materials such as contaminated instruments, items, and surfaces
    c. occurs only through contaminated spray and spatter from use of a high-speed handpiece.
    d. a host inhales a pathogen.

TRUE/FALSE

Indicate whether the statement is true (T) or false (F).

_____ 1. A cough or sneeze from someone cannot transmit the flu virus.

_____ 2. Protective eyewear and masks are not required to prevent airborne transmission.

_____ 3. Humans have three types of immunity: innate, adaptive, and passive.

_____ 4. OSHA's airborne pathogen standard protects employees who are at risk to exposure of blood or other potentially infectious material.

_____ 5. The employer must provide infection control and safety training to all personnel who may come in contact with blood, saliva, or other infectious materials.

_____ 6. Training records should be kept for thirty to fifty years.

_____ 7. Engineering controls are the use of a device that minimizes the risk of exposure to infectious material.

_____ 8. OSHA and the CDC advise against two-handed needle recapping.

_____ 9. There are five potential surfaces that may be contaminated during patient treatment: transfer surfaces, splash, spatter, aerosol surfaces, and housekeeping.

_____ 10. Cleaning is the first step of any disinfection process.

FILL IN THE BLANK

Using words from the list below, fill in the blanks to complete the following statements.

ADA	hazardous	OSHA	CDC
infectious	sharps	thirty	noninfectious
unregulated	EPA	OPIM	ten

1. _____ accredits educational programs, insuring dentists and all allied dental personnel meet national standards.

2. _____ provides recommendations for best practices to protect health and prevent disease.

3. The _____ is responsible for issuing regulations that promote worker safety.

4. _____ publishes clinical research results, helping dentists to identify high-quality and safe materials for use in patient care.

5. The mission of _____ is to safeguard the environment in which we live.

6. _____ waste should be packaged in easily identifiable bags that must be closed securely before disposal.

7. In accordance with OSHA, employee training records must be kept for _____ years.

8. Employers must provide new employees hazardous material training and the HBV vaccine within _____ days of employment.

9. _____ materials have been contaminated with blood or OPIM.

10. _____ should be placed in specially labeled containers that should be located as close as possible to their point of use.

CHAPTER 13
Dental Caries

CHAPTER OUTLINE

Review the Chapter Outline. If any content area is unclear, review that area before beginning the workbook exercises.

A. The Caries Process
B. The Importance of Saliva
C. Diagnosis of Caries
D. Methods of Caries Intervention
E. Risk Assessment of Caries

CHAPTER REVIEW

The following is a summary of the chapter. If any of this material is unclear, review it in the textbook again.

Dental caries is an infectious disease that causes localized destruction of dental tissue, affects all ages and classes of people, and has been known since prehistoric times. Caries formation is a complex process that results from interaction of the tooth, salivary composition and function, microbial action, and the patient's diet and preventive behaviors. In recent years preventing caries has become possible; as a consequence, caries rates are slowly declining. Diagnosing and preventing caries, as well as intervening to prevent caries formation, is accomplished using a variety of techniques. The dental assistant educates the patient regarding caries prevention, and assists the dentist with caries diagnosis and treatment procedures.

LEARNING ACTIVITIES AND STUDY AIDS

Review the following study aids and/or complete the activities to ensure that you have achieved the learning objectives for this chapter.

1. The Caries Risk Test is used by some dentists. To further learn about this test, go online and find one article on the topic. On a separate piece of paper, write a one-page report on your findings. Be sure to cite your resources at the end of your report. Be prepared to share your information with your classmates in a classroom discussion.

2. Explain how the anatomy of the tooth contributes to, and protects against, caries formation.

3. Describe how dental caries forms.

4. List two types of bacteria implicated in caries formation and describe their contributions.

5. Discuss how pellicle, plaque, and biofilm contribute to caries formation.

6. To further understand the difference between demineralization and remineralization, read one of the following articles found online at: http://www.mizar5.com/demin.htm, http://www.db.od.mah.se/car/data/carprincip.html, or http://www.healthpartners.com/files/34749.pdf. Write a short summary of what you learned from the article.

7. Explain how saliva contributes to tooth protection.

8. List and define the types and locations of carious lesions.

9. List the six methods used by dentists to diagnose caries.

10. List six means of intervening to prevent caries formation.

MEDICAL TERMINOLOGY REVIEW

Use a dictionary and/or your textbook to define the following terms.

biofilm _____

caries _____

cariogenic _____

cariology _____

cavitation _____

cementum _____

chlorhexadine _____

demineralization _____

dentin _____

doxycycline _____

enamel _____

hydroxyapatite _____

incipient _____

occlusal _____

pandemic _____

pellicle _____

plaque _____

prevalence _____

recurrent caries _____

remineralization _____

prism _____

ABBREVIATIONS

CA _____

CRT _____

LB _____

MS _____

PH _____

CRITICAL THINKING

1. Describe demineralization and remineralization, and include their cause as well as their appearance. Why is understanding the difference between demineralization and remineralization of concern for the dental assistant?

2. Name the four primary sites for decay to form. Which site is particularly prone to decay, and why?

3. What is the main reason patients get decay in the interproximal surfaces of teeth, and what can the dental assistant do to help them decrease their risk?

4. What methods can be used for caries intervention?

CHAPTER REVIEW TEST

MULTIPLE CHOICE

Circle the letter of the correct answer.

1. The prevalence of dental caries refers to:
    a. the number of individuals or teeth infected with caries at any one time
    b. the number of individuals or teeth newly infected with caries
    c. the process by which people become infected with caries
    d. a child's initial infection with caries

2. Place these tooth tissues in order, hardest/least susceptible to decay first, softest/most susceptible to decay last.
    a. dentin, cementum, enamel
    b. enamel, dentin, cementum
    c. cementum, enamel, dentin
    d. dentin, enamel, cementum

3. Characterize dental caries.
    a. chemical process
    b. bacterial infection
    c. destruction of hard tissue
    d. a and c
    e. all of the above

4. Caries formation requires the tooth to harbor a highly organized layering of proteins and microorganisms that function as a unit termed:
    a. salivary pellicle
    b. demineralization
    c. plaque or biofilm
    d. remineralization

5. When the tooth is just beginning to experience demineralization, the decay is classified as:
    a. frank
    b. gross
    c. rampant
    d. incipient

6. Older patients are more likely than younger patients to experience caries at this location.
    a. along the margins of a restoration
    b. on the root surface
    c. in pits and fissures
    d. on the smooth surface

7. *Streptococcus mutans* and lactobacilli contribute this to the caries process.
    a. calcium
    b. proteins
    c. carbohydrates
    d. acid

8. Active destruction of tooth structure is caused by:
    a. *Streptococcus mutans*
    b. plaque
    c. lactobacilli
    d. remineralization

9. The diagnodent diagnosis of caries is detected through the use of:
    a. a laser beam
    b. an explorer
    c. a radiograph
    d. clinical observation

10. Root caries is the most suitable description for:
    a. smooth surface caries
    b. cementum caries
    c. pit and fissure caries
    d. baby bottle tooth decay
    e. enamel caries

TRUE/FALSE

Indicate whether the statement is true (T) or false (F).

_____ 1. Salivary fluid flushes acids and carbohydrates away from the tooth surface.

_____ 2. Chewing gum may help to prevent the initiation of caries.

_____ 3. Carbohydrate on the teeth reduces the potential for acid production.

_____ 4. Prescribed medications and radiation therapy commonly increase saliva flow.

_____ 5. Fluoride applied to tooth structure may increase its hardness, thereby reducing its susceptibility to caries.

_____ 6. Radiographs are important aids to the diagnosis of interproximal caries.

_____ 7. An intraoral camera is a significant aid to the diagnosis of recurrent caries.

_____ 8. When caries indicator dye is used as an aid to diagnosis, the dye washes away from the carious lesion but remains in the noncarious areas.

_____ 9. The presence of caries can often be detected using only a mirror and light because enamel is translucent.

_____ 10. Improved oral hygiene is imperative for all patients if they are to avoid caries development.

FILL IN THE BLANK

Using words from the list below, fill in the blanks to complete the following statements.

calcium	explorer	pellicle
chlorhexadine	family	pits and fissures
chronic	fluoride	saliva
doxycycline	likely	

1. *Streptococcus mutans* is introduced into the child's mouth by the _____.

2. A caries risk assessment is used to determine how _____ the patient is to develop caries.

3. The most common _____ disease of childhood is dental caries.

4. Dentin contains less _____ and more water, and therefore is softer than enamel.

5. _____ added in small amounts to a public drinking water supply helps to prevent caries.

6. The traditional means of detecting dental caries is through the use of a handheld _____.

7. _____ mouth rinses and _____ antibiotic are used to help prevent caries.

8. Dental sealants are most effective when placed on the _____ of a tooth.

9. A caries risk assessment is performed on a sample of the patient's _____.

10. _____ protects tooth enamel by providing a cell-free film of proteins that may aid in remineralization.

CHAPTER 14
Periodontal Disease

CHAPTER OUTLINE

Review the Chapter Outline. If any content area is unclear, review that area before beginning the workbook exercises.

    A. Structures of the Periodontium

    B. Prevalence

    C. Types of Periodontal Disease
       1. Description of Gingivitis
       2. Description of Periodontitis
       3. Oral Conditions Linked to Periodontal Disease
       4. Signs and Symptoms

    D. Systemic Conditions Linked to Periodontal Disease
       1. Cardiovascular Disease
       2. Respiratory Disease
       3. Diabetes Mellitus
       4. HIV/AIDS
       5. Genetic Marker for Periodontal Disease
       6. Other Risk Factors

CHAPTER REVIEW

The following is a summary of the chapter. If any of this material is unclear, review it in the textbook again.

Periodontal disease is an infection that slowly destroys the supporting structures of the teeth. There are two basic forms: gingivitis is inflammation of the gingival tissues only; periodontitis extends into the supporting ligament and bone. There are seven types of periodontal disease. Classification is based on location, extent, and severity. Periodontal disease is linked to poor oral hygiene, the presence of plaque and calculus, several serious systemic diseases, and low birth weight and premature infants. Everyone is at risk for periodontal disease and many people are chronically infected. Most forms can be prevented with good oral hygiene.

LEARNING ACTIVITIES AND STUDY AIDS

Review the following study aids and/or complete the activities to ensure that you have achieved the learning objectives for this chapter.

1. List, locate, and state the attachment function of the normal tissues of the periodontium.

2. Fill in the following table by providing the clinical signs and symptoms of both gingivitis and periodontitis.

Table 14-1

Signs and symptoms of gingivitis	Signs and symptoms of periodontitis

3. Complete the following table by providing the names of the seven basic case types of periodontitis with a description of each.

Table 14-2

Types of periodontitis	Description of each type
1.	
2.	
3.	
4.	
5.	
6.	
7.	

4. State how plaque and calculus contribute to the development of periodontal disease.

5. Describe the relationship between poor oral hygiene and periodontal disease.

6. Using research tools such as the Internet and/or materials found in the school library, research information on the role of smoking in periodontal disease. On a separate piece of paper, write a one-page report on your findings.

7. List and describe systemic diseases that have been linked to periodontal disease.

8. Discuss the prevalence of periodontal disease.

9. The periodontium is composed of the gingiva, epithelial attachment, periodontal ligament, cementum, and alveolar bone. To demonstrate your understanding of where these are located, look at the following figure and label each component of the periodontium.

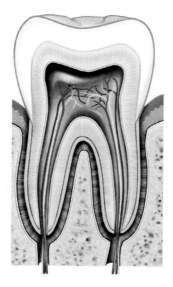

Figure 14-1

10. Provide five descriptive words to describe healthy periodontium, and five other descriptive words to describe diseased periodontium.

MEDICAL TERMINOLOGY REVIEW

Use a dictionary and/or your textbook to define the following terms.

aerobic _____

alveolar bone _____

anaerobic _____

calculus _____

cementum _____

edema _____

epithelial attachment _____

erythema _____

free gingiva _____

furcation _____

gingiva _____

gingivitis _____

periodontal ligament _____

periodontal pocket _____

periodontal probe _____

periodontitis _____

periodontium _____

perioscopy _____

plaque _____

stippling _____

subgingival _____

sulcus _____

suppuration _____

supragingival _____

ABBREVIATIONS

AIDS _____

CVD _____

DNA _____

HIV _____

NUG _____

NUP _____

PST _____

CRITICAL THINKING

1. There is a new test out that helps determine if patients are genetically at high risk for periodontal disease. What is the name of the test, who can administer it, and how well does the test work?

2. What factors contribute to periodontal disease, and what role does the dental assistant play in informing the patient about controllable factors?

3. Periodontal disease includes both gingivitis and periodontitis. What are the differences in these two conditions, and what role does the dental assistant have in the treatment of both?

CHAPTER REVIEW TEST

MULTIPLE CHOICE

Circle the letter of the correct answer.

1. This normal structure of the periodontium is the space between the tooth and the free gingiva.
   - a. epithelial attachment
   - b. sulcus
   - c. periodontal ligament
   - d. attached gingiva

2. This portion of the tooth helps anchor the tooth to the bone by providing an attachment surface for the periodontal ligament.
   - a. enamel
   - b. dentin
   - c. cementum
   - d. none of the above

3. The tooth loss that results from periodontal disease can be avoided with:
   - a. early detection and treatment
   - b. cessation of smoking
   - c. control of blood sugar
   - d. less frequent brushing and flossing

4. Describe common signs and symptoms of gingivitis.
   - a. erythema
   - b. edema
   - c. bleeding on brushing
   - d. a and c
   - e. all of the above

5. The instrument used to measure pocket depth is a(n):
   - a. explorer
   - b. gingival knife
   - c. scaler
   - d. periodontal probe
   - e. curet

6. The term periodontal pocket refers to a(n):
   - a. deepened sulcus
   - b. healed area of gingivitis
   - c. surgical procedure for treating periodontal disease
   - d. area where plaque has accumulated

7. When less than thirty percent of the sites in the mouth are infected with periodontal disease, the condition is described as:
   - a. moderate
   - b. slight
   - c. generalized
   - d. localized

8. The ulcers and periodontal pockets of chronic periodontal disease are created by:
   - a. oozing pus
   - b. abscesses
   - c. tissue necrosis
   - d. plaque

9. Calculus contributes to periodontal disease development by providing:
   - a. calcium bacteria need to survive
   - b. a rough surface for plaque attachment
   - c. suppression of the immune system
   - d. fluid for synthesis of acids

10. The link between periodontal disease and exacerbation of systemic disease appears to be related to:
    a. release of increased numbers of pathogens into the bloodstream
    b. attachment of pathogens to fatty deposits in the bloodstream
    c. increased clot formation in the arteries
    d. a and c
    e. all of the above

TRUE/FALSE

Indicate whether the statement is true (T) or false (F).

_____ 1. Periodontal disease may cause a change in the tissue lining of the respiratory tract, thereby allowing invasion of other pathogens.

_____ 2. When gingivitis bleeds, bacterial pathogens escape into the bloodstream, attach to fatty deposits, and increase the number of clots in the arteries.

_____ 3. Good sugar control unfortunately does not reduce the risk a diabetic will develop periodontal disease.

_____ 4. To date, it is known that periodontal disease is linked to premature birth and low birth weight but the mechanism by which this is thought to occur remains unknown.

_____ 5. A specific gene that is associated with periodontal disease risk has not yet been identified.

_____ 6. Smoking creates an environment in which the bacteria that cause periodontal disease can thrive; it also slows healing.

_____ 7. Calculus usually forms first on the lingual surfaces of premolars and secondly on the labial surfaces of mandibular molars.

_____ 8. All types of periodontal disease are caused by infection with viruses.

_____ 9. Most affected people have no idea they have periodontal disease.

_____ 10. The types of bacteria in plaque that cause periodontal disease differ from those that cause dental caries.

FILL IN THE BLANK

Using words from the list below, fill in the blanks to complete the following statements.

blood disorder
prepubertal
smoking
necrotizing ulcerative gingivitis

generalized
gingivitis
juvenile

necrotizing ulcerative periodontitis
periodontal abscess
stippling

1. This type of generalized disease is often associated with periodontal disease: _____.

2. This aggressive type of periodontitis tends to appear in the late teenage years and manifests as bone loss around the first molars and incisors: _____.

3. This type of periodontal disease manifests as red, swollen, bleeding gingival tissues and is reversible because it does not extend deeper into the supporting ligament and bone: _____.

4. This type of periodontal disease causes suppuration and pustule formation: _____.

5. Patients who have experienced high stress may present with this painful, foul-smelling periodontal disease: _____.

6. This aggressive form of periodontal disease begins before puberty and affects both the primary and permanent teeth: _____.

7. This form of periodontal disease affects more than one-third of the sites in the mouth: _____.

8. This type of periodontal disease causes such extensive destruction that deep pockets are not formed: _____.

9. Healthy gingiva shows _____ on its attached portion.

10. Periodontal disease associated with this risk factor does not appear erythematous because the capillaries are constricted: _____.

CHAPTER 15
Oral Health

CHAPTER OUTLINE

Review the Chapter Outline. If any content area is unclear, review that area before beginning the workbook exercises.

    A. Patient Education
        1. Prevention

    B. Fluoride
        1. History of Fluoridation
        2. Optimum Fluoridation
        3. How Fluoride Works
        4. Encouraging Fluoride Use
        5. The Fluoride Controversy

    C. Nutrition and Dental Caries
        1. Eating for Health

    D. Plaque Control Program
        1. Disclosing Dental Plaque
        2. Toothbrushing
        3. Flossing
        4. Oral Hygiene Aids

CHAPTER REVIEW

The following is a summary of the chapter. If any of this material is unclear, review it in the textbook again.

Proper diet and meticulous plaque control helps preserve teeth for a lifetime, and affects one's general overall health as well as one's dental health. Simple carbohydrates and sugar in any form contributes to the colonization of plaque. The most important plaque control method is toothbrushing, and it should be established as a daily routine from early childhood. Community water fluoridation is cost effective and benefits everyone. It is the most efficient way to prevent one of the most common childhood diseases—tooth decay. Dental diseases are caused by microorganisms found in plaque. These microorganisms cause disease that can destroy healthy tissue and ultimately result in tooth loss. Plaque control is the removal and prevention of all soft deposits on the teeth and gingival tissues. Motivating patients toward the awareness that they are ultimately responsible for improving and maintaining the health of their oral tissues is the primary duty of the dental assistant. Educating patients on the negative effects of poor nutrition, tobacco use, and neglect is part of overall general and oral health.

LEARNING ACTIVITIES AND STUDY AIDS

Review the following study aids and/or complete the activities to ensure that you have achieved the learning objectives for this chapter.

1. Create a chart depicting primary dentition that could be used to explain to a parent the importance of proper oral health care for a child under the age of six. Use colored poster board, pictures, colored markers, or pencils to depict the eruption patterns or describe key terms. Using this poster, create a presentation for the class on the importance of caring for primary teeth.

2. On a separate piece of paper, write an essay describing why oral health care is an important topic to learn about as a dental assistant—be certain to include diet and nutrition, the importance of primary teeth, permanent teeth, edentulous oral care, special care for crown and bridge patients, and any other considerations.

3. Write an explanation for a parent as to why hard candy is more harmful for their child's teeth than candy bar might be.

4. Explain how to use a floss threader under a bridge, floss braces, care for partial or complete dentures, properly brush teeth (what type of toothbrush, angle of toothbrush, what type of toothpaste), and floss properly.

5. Find a friend or family member who will track his/her diet for at least three days to include all meals, including serving sizes on snack foods, beverages, and so forth, then using his/her "food diary," break each meal down into proteins, carbohydrates, sugars, and potential vitamins and minerals consumed. Evaluate his/her daily intake of cariogenic foods. What types of changes might you recommend he/she make in diet to control caries? How would you explain this to a patient? Document all of your information on a separate piece of paper. Turn the information into your instructor for a grade.

6. Contact your local dental association or dental hygiene association and ask them what their involvement is at the local, state, or national level concerning promotion of oral health. Do they provide presentations for parents and children to attend to learn about oral health? Are there arrangements made during National Children's Dental Health Month for screening exams or treatment? Do they participate in Special Olympics—fabricating sport mouth guards or providing oral health care instructions for the athletes? Do they offer any other services on nutritional information, oral health care, or how overall health may affect oral health? On a spearate piece of paper, write a short synopsis of the information you obtained.

7. Using the Internet, go to the Web site http://www.usda.gov and find *MyPyramid*. Calculate your daily nutritional values—what amounts of protein, carbohydrates, and fats should be consumed for an individual of your age and gender? How might you explain to a patient how to use this Web site for nutritional enhancement? Using the plan you developed, track your food intake for a week and then compare your food diary to the actual plan developed. Are there any differences? Similarities? Present the information in a one-page written summary on a separate piece of paper.

8. Take a trip to two of your local drug or department stores—compare the differences between the oral healthcare products for sale. Which store has the largest selection of toothbrushes, toothpastes, and dental adjuncts? Is there a product that may commonly be recommended in a dental office that is easier to find at one store than another? What is their selection of automatic (electric or battery-operated) toothbrushes? What are the prices of their products? Take notes during your visit. On a separate piece of paper, provide a written summary of your visit to your instructor, and be prepared to compare your information with your classmates.

9. If you were working in a dental office and had reason to suspect a patient was bulimic or anorexic, what signs might you have observed to lead you to believe they were having a nutritional problem? What might the patient experience, or even have dental complaints about? What is your role as a dental assistant in treating this patient? What advice might you provide to the patient?

10. Contact your local water company and ask if they add fluoride to the community water supply. If not, why not? How is the community informed of this action? How often is the fluoride level monitored, and to whom is it reported? Is the fluoride level optimum? Too high or too low? What are the effects of too much fluoride in water? Try to determine whether local residents have their water tested for fluoride levels if they have a private well and, if so, who performs the testing? Do these residents request fluoride supplement prescriptions from local dentists? If more space is required for documentation of your information, utilize an additional piece of paper and attach to this one prior to submitting to your instructor.

MEDICAL TERMINOLOGY REVIEW

Use a dictionary and/or your textbook to define the following terms.

baby bottle decay _____

biofilm _____

bridge threader _____

calculus _____

dental plaque _____

fluoridation _____

fluorosis _____

gingivitis _____

halitosis _____

periodontitis _____

sodium hexametaphosphate _____

Streptococcus mutans _____

sulcus _____

systemic fluorides _____

topical fluorides _____

triclosan _____

xylitol _____

ABBREVIATIONS

ADA _____

CDC _____

PPM _____

CRITICAL THINKING

1. What is the dental assistant's role in educating patients concerning oral health?

2. What is the primary bacteria found in dental caries, and how does it work?

3. What age group has the highest rate of dental caries, and what factors do you believe are the cause?

CHAPTER REVIEW TEST

MULTIPLE CHOICE

Circle the letter of the correct answer.

1. Chronic illnesses such as _____ and _____ can affect oral health.
   a. AIDS and cancer
   b. lupus and AIDS
   c. cancer and bronchitis
   d. flu and hepatitis

2. Dental caries and periodontal diseases are caused by _____ found in dental plaque.
   a. fats
   b. microorganisms
   c. staphylococcus
   d. nutrition

3. The primary bacterium in dental plaque (that causes decay) is:
   a. *Flagella mutans*
   b. *bacteria*
   c. *Streptococcus mutans*
   d. *Staphylococcus mutans*

4. The Bass brushing technique requires that the toothbrush be angled at _____ degrees toward the gum line in order to be effective.
   - a. 90
   - b. 40
   - c. 45
   - d. 360

5. When applying toothpaste to a toothbrush, you should use a _____ drop.
   - a. marble-sized
   - b. snowball-sized
   - c. pea-sized
   - d. pinky-finger-sized

6. The ADA recommends toothbrushes be replaced every _____ months.
   - a. one to two
   - b. three to four
   - c. five to six
   - d. ten to twelve

7. To accomplish effective toothbrushing, you should brush for at least _____ minute(s).
   - a. one
   - b. two
   - c. five
   - d. ten

8. The human body is made up of _____ percent water.
   - a. 40 to 50
   - b. 60 to 70
   - c. 70 to 80
   - d. 90 to 100

9. Research has shown that use of products containing _____ actually reduces the incidence of tooth decay.
   - a. sugar
   - b. saccharin
   - c. water
   - d. xylitol

10. The optimal level of fluoride from water fluoridation is:
    - a. 10 ppm
    - b. 1.1 ppm
    - c. 1 ppm
    - d. 0.1 ppm

TRUE/FALSE

Indicate whether the statement is true (T) or false (F).

_____ 1. Periodontal diseases range from mild forms of gingivitis to severe forms of periodontitis that result in tooth loss.

_____ 2. Eighty percent of Americans currently have some form of periodontal disease.

_____ 3. The dental assistant is the only oral health educator in the dental office.

_____ 4. A child with dental caries in her deciduous teeth is at a much higher risk of developing decay in the permanent dentition.

_____ 5. Fluorosis occurs from lack of fluoride during tooth development.

_____ 6. Tooth decay in infants and young children most often occurs in the maxillary anterior teeth but may affect other teeth.

_____ 7. Plaque must be removed from the teeth through the mechanical action of proper toothbrushing.

_____ 8. The surface of the tongue should be scrubbed to prevent bad breath (halitosis).

_____ 9. The ADA recommends that a toothbrush be replaced every three to four months, or sooner if the bristles become frayed.

_____ 10. One of the main reasons people don't brush effectively is because they don't brush long enough.

FILL IN THE BLANK

Bass technique   dental plaque   gingivitis   calculus

oral health   dental plaque   carbohydrates   gingivitis

biofilm   Fones' Technique

1. _____ is a sticky, colorless, almost invisible mass of bacteria and their by-products.

2. _____ is a reversible inflammation of the gingiva.

3. _____ is the most commonly recommended technique for toothbrushing.

4. _____ is essential to the general overall health of the body.

5. If _____ is left untreated it can advance to periodontitis, which affects the bone that supports the teeth.

6. _____ also called tartar, is hardened plaque, a mineralized deposit on teeth formed by saliva, debris, and minerals that can trap stains and cause discoloration.

7. _____ is a sticky, colorless, almost invisible mass of bacteria that contains by-products that constantly form on teeth.

8. The bacteria in plaque use _____ to produce acids that can attack tooth enamel.

9. _____ is a diverse community of microorganisms found on the tooth surfaces.

10. _____ has the teeth closed with the toothbrush placed toward the teeth, and moved in large circles at the tooth and gingiva of both arches, then using circles at the palate and lingual areas.

CHAPTER 16
Oral Nutrition

CHAPTER OUTLINE

Review the Chapter Outline. If any content area is unclear, review that area before beginning the workbook exercises.

    A. Functions of the Six Major Nutrients
        1. Water
        2. Carbohydrates
        3. Fats
        4. Proteins
        5. Vitamins
        6. Minerals

    B. Diet Modification
        1. Diet Modifications for Infants and Toddlers

    C. Diet Analysis

    D. Reading Food Labels

    E. Eating Disorders

    F. Healthy Eating Habits

CHAPTER REVIEW

The following is a summary of the chapter. If any of this material is unclear, review it in the textbook again.

The type of food one consumes as a child and later as an adult can significantly impact one's oral health. Individuals on a daily and weekly basis often consume too much sugar or sodium. To help dental patients monitor their eating, drinking, and exercise habits, a food journal may be suggested. Keeping a daily or weekly journal can assist individuals in monitoring their consumption of water, fruits, vegetables, grains, and dairy products. A food journal also helps people realize where they could decrease their intake of cariogenic foods. This helps to decrease the development of decay in the mouth. The USDA provides a complete and current list of recommendations for children and adults at *http://www.usda.gov.* A dental assistant must have a thorough knowledge of proper nutrition, and its relationship to oral health, in order to keep both themselves and their patients informed. The dental assistant must also realize there are differences in diet for different ethnicities and cultures, and be respectful of these differences when making suggestions or recommendations for diet changes.

LEARNING ACTIVITES AND STUDY AIDS

Review the following study aids and/or complete the activities to ensure that you have achieved the learning objectives for this chapter.

1. Using the Internet, go to the Web site *http://www.usda.gov.* Click on Food and Nutrition, and then MyPyramid, Steps to a Healthier You. Calculate the daily nutritional values for a patient (you choose the age, weight, and gender). If the person you created is overweight, what are the RDAs for him/her to remain at that weight? If he/she wants to lose weight, what are the RDAs (protein, fruits, grains, carbohydrates, and fats) recommended to be consumed? How might you explain this information to your patient? How would you explain this Web site to your patient? Using the plan developed, keep a food diary of your food intake for a week, and then compare this food diary to the actual plan developed for your created patient. Are there any differences? Similarities? How might MyPyramid become a useful tool to recommend to your patients for their personal use? Utilizing a separate piece of paper, write a one-page report about what you learned through this exercise.

2. Fill in the following table by providing the source and purpose of each water-soluble vitamin listed.

Table 16-1

Vitamin	Source	Purpose
Thiamin (B1)		
Riboflavin (B2)		
Pyridoxine (B6)		
Cobalamin (B12)		
Biotin		

Ascorbic acid (Vitamin C)		
Folic acid (folate)		
Niacin		
Antothenic acid		

3. On a separate piece of paper, create a table with the following categories: tired/drowsy, happy, energetic, focused, dizzy, sad, satisfied/full, still hungry, craving something else (salt, sweet, crunchy), or any other combination of categories you can think of that would relate to the way you might feel after eating meals or snacks. The goal is to track the way certain foods make you feel thirty to forty-five minutes after eating them. You will need to create columns in your table to indicate the days of the week, foods eaten, and the feelings associated with those foods. Compare the ways these foods make you feel if consumed in the morning, afternoon, or evening. Do certain foods have a different effect at different times of the day? Do you feel better after eating one type of food than another?

4. Various health issues arise from misuse of carbohydrates. Using the Internet and/or other sources (not including your textbook), conduct research on three health issues that arise due to misuse of carbohydrates. Utilizing a separate piece of paper, write a paragraph for each health issue. Describe the condition, its signs and symptoms, and possible treatment options.

5. Find a friend or family member who will track his/her diet for at least three days to include all meals, paying particular attention to snack foods and beverages that contain sugar or sugary products (even carbohydrates). Based on this food diary, what is his/her daily intake of cariogenic foods? Anticariogenic foods? What types of changes might you recommend they make in their diet to control caries? What types of changes might you recommend for better oral health overall? How would you explain this to a patient? Submit to your instructor your friend/family member's food diary, along with a short paragraph explaining what types of changes you recommended to the individual's diet and oral health, and how you would explain this information to a patient.

6. Gather your local grocery store weekly food sale advertisements. Which types of food products are the best bargains? Healthy foods or "quick fix sugary carbohydrate-type foods"? Now using these sales flyers, create a menu for meals for three days—can you create meals that are considered healthy from these sales flyers? Can you meet the USDA's RDAs using these sales flyers? Is this menu oral-health considerate? What other items might you need to ensure the menu encourages oral health as well as overall health? What type of spending/budget does a patient need to consider eating for good oral health? Submit to your instructor your three-day meal menu, along with your answers to the questions posed in this activity.

7. What are the affects of alcoholism on the oral cavity?

8. Pretend you are already working in a dental office as a dental assistant and have a patient who presents to your office with multiple cervical facial areas of decay. The patient states that he consumes at least one 12-pack of regular highly caffeinated sodas every day, otherwise he doesn't feel well. However, lately he has noticed his teeth are very sensitive to hot, cold, and sweet foods. What do you suspect to be the cause of his complaint? What immediate suggestions might you make for restructuring his diet? How would you explain to the patient why he feels bad on days that he does not consume twelve sodas? Would you recommend a different type of soda? What if you had the same patient scenario, but the patient tells you he/she drinks six to eight glasses of iced tea per day with three tablespoons of sugar in each glass? On a separate piece of paper, write a one-page report answering these questions, and present your thoughts on these issues.

9. What is the difference between Vitamin B1 and Vitamin B2? What are some sources for obtaining vitamin B?

10. Have some fun! Go out for lunch or dinner to your favorite restaurant and ask for a nutrition guide. Before reading the guide, choose your menu item and order. Now read the guide and determine whether or not the meal your ordered was a healthy choice for oral health or not. What was the fat content of your meal? What vitamins and minerals were contained in your choice? What vitamins and minerals were contained in your meal that contribute to good oral health? Is there a lighter menu option that you could have or would have chosen? Why did you choose the meal you selected—did it just sound good, was it your favorite food, or were you just hungry and chose the first item you came across? Now going back to activity #3—how did the food make you feel after eating it? Utilizing a separate piece of paper, write a one-page paper to document your experience. Include the answers to the various questions posed in this activity. Be prepared to discuss your experience in class.

MEDICAL TERMINOLOGY REVIEW

Use a dictionary and/or your textbook to define the following terms.

anorexia _____

bulimia _____

carbohydrates _____

caries _____

cirrhosis _____

diabetes mellitus _____

fats _____

hyperglycemia _____

hypoglycemia _____

macrominerals _____

microminerals _____

minerals _____

nutrients _____

obesity _____

osteomalacia _____

proteins _____

vitamins _____

ABBREVIATIONS

AA _____

DNA _____

DT _____

FPG _____

LPN _____

RD _____

RDA _____

RN _____

USDA _____

CRITICAL THINKING

1. What is the most essential nutrient our bodies need in order to survive? Why is this nutrient so important?

2. Of all the vitamins discussed in the chapter, which one is most important to the formation of healthy teeth and bones? In which types of food products is this vitamin found? Are there other ways to obtain this vitamin?

3. Why is it important for the dental team to have a thorough knowledge of nutrition?

CHAPTER REVIEW TEST

MULTIPLE CHOICE

Circle the letter of the correct answer.

1. Vitamin D and calcium help keep _____ strong.
   a. gingival tissue
   b. periodontal ligaments
   c. alveolar bone
   d. mandibular bone

2. There are _____ essential nutrients that the human body needs every day.
   a. eight
   b. seven
   c. six
   d. five

3. Good eating habits provide the body the ability to:

   a. run a marathon   c. use less energy

   b. prevent sickness and disease   d. brush teeth less often

4. It would not be unusual for a patient who is anorexic to also be bulimic.

   a. true

   b. false

5. _____ is the most essential nutrient in the human body.

   a. Blood   c. Calcium

   b. Vitamin C   d. Water

6. _____ is the primary energy source for the brain.

   a. Protein   c. Glucose

   b. Oxygen   d. Magnesium hydroxide

7. Cariogenic foods may also be referred to as:

   a. quick foods   c. salty foods

   b. healthy foods   d. spicy foods

8. A lack of enzymes to break down milk sugars is termed:

   a. lactose intolerance   c. milk intolerance

   b. sugar intolerance   d. enzyme intolerance

9. _____ is an insufficient amount of insulin secretion.

   a. Diabetes melanoma   c. Diabetes millionitis

   b. Diabetes mellitus   d. Diabanese

10. Another name for fats found in diet is:

   a. cholesterol   c. grease

   b. gumma   d. lipids

TRUE/FALSE

Indicate whether the statement is true (T) or false (F).

_____ 1. Hyperglycemia is associated with diabetes.

_____ 2. Hypoglycemia is associated with diabetes.

_____ 3. Saturated fats become clear when exposed to heat.

_____ 4. There are two types of proteins: complete and partial.

_____ 5. There are two types of vitamins: fat-soluble and water-soluble.

_____ 6. Excess amounts of fat-soluble vitamins can be stored in tissues; excess water-soluble vitamins are excreted from the body.

_____ 7. Plaque forms in the mouth only on teeth.

_____ 8. Vitamins A, C, D, and E are fat-soluble.

_____ 9. Vitamin D is the most essential vitamin for healthy teeth and bone formation.

_____ 10. Osteoporosis is the decalcification of bone, causing the bone to become soft.

FILL IN THE BLANK

Using words from the list below, fill in the blanks to complete the following statements.

osteoporosis	osteomalacia	microminerals
anorexia	Vitamin D	Vitamin E
Vitamin K	macrominerals	Vitamin A
bulimia		

1. _____ is the decalcification of bone, causing the bone to become soft.

2. _____ occurs when the bones lose their inner strength or density.

3. Deficiencies of _____ can cause vision problems, night blindness, and severely dry skin.

4. _____ are essential to healthy teeth and bone formation.

5. _____ helps prevent fatty acids from oxidizing and is great for skin cell regeneration.

6. _____ is essential for natural blood clotting and kidney function.

7. _____ are minerals used by the body in large quantities.

8. _____ are minerals used by the body in small quantities.

9. Signs of _____ include constant exercise, meals found thrown away in the garbage, trouble concentrating, cancellations to appear for group activities, and eating alone.

10. _____ is exhibited by an individual who self-induces vomiting after eating.

CHAPTER 17
Instrument Processing and Sterilization

CHAPTER OUTLINE

Review the Chapter Outline. If any content area is unclear, review that area before beginning the workbook exercises.

A. Introduction to Instrument Processing
   1. Sterilization vs. Disinfection

B. Classification of Patient-Care Items
   1. Patient Protection

C. Transporting and Processing Contaminated Patient-Care Items

D. Instrument Processing Area
   1. Workflow Pattern

E. Precleaning Instruments
   1. Hand Scrubbing
   2. Ultrasonic Cleaner
   3. Washer/Disinfector
   4. Lubrication and Corrosion Control
   5. CDCP Guidelines

F. Prepackaging and Storing Materials
   1. Packaging Materials
   2. Storing of Sterilized Instruments

G. Sterilization Monitoring
   1. Biological Indicators
   2. Sterilization Documentation
   3. CDCP Guidelines for Sterilization Monitoring

H. Methods of Sterilization
   1. Steam Sterilization
   2. Loading and Unloading the Autoclave
   3. Operation and Maintenance of the Autoclave
   4. Flash Sterilization
   5. Dry Heat Sterilization
   6. Chemical Vapor Sterilization
   7. Operation of Chemical Heat Sterilizer
   8. Chemical Solutions for Sterilization
   9. Sterilization Failure

I. Handpiece Sterilization

CHAPTER REVIEW

The following is a summary of the chapter. If any of this material is unclear, review it in the textbook again.

In order to maintain the health and safety of the dental team and patients, it is important for dental assistants to know, understand, and effectively practice the guidelines provided by the Centers for Disease Control and Prevention (CDCP) that address dental infection control. Patient safety and health issues, as well as dental healthcare worker safety, are of the utmost importance when addressing instrument processing, packaging, sterilization, and disinfection. Instrument processing is another extremely important issue when thinking about both operator and patient cross-contamination issues. The future may hold many improvements in the area of instrument processing and sterilization. Dental assistants should not only remain knowledgeable in how to properly handle and process instruments, but also stay abreast of the latest techniques and equipment used to maintain the health and safety of patients and the dental team.

LEARNING ACTIVITIES AND STUDY AIDS

Review the following study aids and/or complete the activities to ensure that you have achieved the learning objectives for this chapter.

1. Recalling the definitions for disinfection and sterilization, think of ways you can compare how dental instruments and surfaces that require either disinfection or sterilization are similar to items or surfaces in your home. What similarities might you make? Can you sterilize items in your home (baby bottle or silverware, for example) and, if so, how might you do this? What methods are available for you to disinfect your countertops or cooking utensils? Are the chemicals used in home disinfection products similar to the ones used in a dental office? What are the differences? Write a short synopsis of your findings and provide the answers to the questions posed in this activity. Use an additional piece of paper if more space for your information is needed.

2. On a separate piece of paper, write an essay (about one page) describing why sterilization is a critical component for quality patient care. What areas within your dental office are considered critical? Noncritical? Semicritical? Why are they different? Do all dental instruments require sterilization? Why or why not?

3. Design an explanation for a patient regarding how and what in your office is sterilized and what is disinfected. Provide this explanation to another classmate—have the classmate ask you questions that a patient without this knowledge might ask. Are your answers sensible, clear, and concise? How might you better answer these questions? Take notes during this activity and turn these in to your instructor. Your notes should reflect what was learned through this activity. Use an additional piece of paper if more space for your information is needed.

4. Outline the CDCP guidelines for receiving, cleaning, and decontaminating patient care items.

5. Describe the advantages and disadvantages of each type of cleaning method in the following table.

Table 17-1

Method	Advantages	Disadvantages
Hand scrubbing		
Ultrasonic cleaning		
Washer/disinfector		

6. Think about dental radiology and the specialized film holders used for taking radiographs. Which film holders must be sterilized between patients? How long does this process take? Can they be heat sterilized, or do they need cold sterilization—what difference in time does this make? Which film holders are disposable? Can these film holders be covered with barriers to prevent the need to sterilize them after each use? What other components of the x-ray machine or developer might you be concerned about contaminating? Would you disinfect these components, or might you use barriers? How often should these barriers be replaced? How would you explain this to a patient? Use an additional piece of paper if more space is needed to record your answers.

7. Obtain a copy of the newest *CDC Guidelines for Infection Control in Dental Health-Care Settings* from the CDC Web site *http://www.cdc.com*. Create a five-minute PowerPoint presentation on one section of this guideline that you feel is important yet may not have been discussed in depth, or in one area you feel you and your classmates may benefit from more information. Turn your presentation in to your instructor, and be prepared to present this information to the class.

8. In your own words, explain the basic steps from the CDCP for sterilization monitoring.

9. Using the Internet, go to the OSAP Web site *http://www.osap.org*. What new guidelines are posted for cleaning contaminated instruments? What types of gloves should you wear when processing instruments in the sterilization room? What other types of personal protection equipment (PPE) should be worn for personal protection when processing instruments? Is there information in this Web site that addresses the bloodborne pathogen standard from OSHA? How does this regulation affect instrument processing?

10. If you were working in a dental office and had reason to suspect a patient was a carrier of a communicable disease, how might you verify this fact? What precautions might you take while treating the patient, or when cleaning the treatment area and processing instruments? Starting from the pretreatment preparations, make a list of how you would ready the treatment area, maintain a clean environment during care, and finally process the instruments through the sterilization area. Would this patient be treated any differently than any other? Why or why not?

MEDICAL TERMINOLOGY REVIEW

Use a dictionary and/or your textbook to define the following terms.

autoclave _____

biological monitor _____

critical items _____

disinfection _____

dry heat sterilizer _____

event-related sterilization _____

flash sterilization _____

holding solution _____

noncritical items _____

semicritical items _____

sterilization _____

time-related sterilization _____

ultrasonic cleaner _____

washer/disinfector _____

ABBREVIATIONS

C _____

CDCP _____

EPA _____

F _____

FDA _____

OSAP _____

PSI _____

CRITICAL THINKING

1. Why is it important for a dental assistant to have knowledge of instrument processing?

2. What is the difference between sterilization and disinfection? As a dental assistant, why is this distinction critical to understand?

3. After dismissing a patient from a routine restorative (amalgam) appointment, what critical, semicritical, and noncritical items must either be disinfected or sterilized? Define each category before you list items that are contained in each.

4. Why is it important to have a "logical flow" when processing instruments?

CHAPTER REVIEW TEST

MULTIPLE CHOICE

Circle the letter of the correct answer.

1. PPE includes all of the following EXCEPT:
   a. face masks
   b. ear plugs
   c. scrubs/gowns
   d. eyewear

2. Another term for a steam sterilizer is:
   a. heater
   b. autoclave
   c. harvey
   d. gluteraldehyde

3. Items such as scalpels, chisels, and surgical forceps are considered:
   a. not critical
   b. semicritical
   c. critical
   d. noncritical

4. _____ items pose the biggest risk of disease transmission and must be sterilized after each use.
   a. Semicritical
   b. Critical
   c. Noncritical
   d. Plastic

5. Mouth mirrors, amalgam condensers, and impression trays are considered to be:
   a. critical
   b. semicritical
   c. noncritical
   d. disposable

6. The sterilization area should be divided into _____ part(s).
   a. four
   b. three
   c. two
   d. one

7. The flooring in the sterilization area should be
   a. carpeted, with softer rugs to stand on for longer periods of time.
   b. carpeted, except for right next to the sink area.
   c. not carpeted; a hard surface.
   d. not carpeted, except for right next to the sink.

8. Another name for the sterilization area might be:
   a. central processing area
   b. dirty instrument area
   c. supply area
   d. clean instrument area

9. The type of gloves worn during instrument processing are:
   a. vinyl
   b. plastic
   c. utility
   d. patient care

10. Which of the following methods is LEAST recommended for cleaning instruments?
    a. hand scrubbing
    b. ultrasonic cleaning
    c. washer/disinfector
    d. finger scrubbing

TRUE/FALSE

Indicate whether the statement is true (T) or false (F).

_____ 1. The sterilization area should be either linear or U-shaped in design to aid the flow of processing instruments.

_____ 2. There is no need to wear PPE after removing instruments from the ultrasonic cleaner.

_____ 3. The ultimate responsibility for sterilization lies with the dentist.

_____ 4. You can use a regular kitchen dishwasher to clean instruments.

_____ 5. Instruments can be placed while still wet into the sterilizer; it will not harm them.

_____ 6. If an interment package is torn or punctured, the instruments are still sterile until the package expiration date.

_____ 7. Packaging material must be FDA approved.

_____ 8. There are two different types of chemical indicators: external and internal.

_____ 9. The CDCP recommends that sterilization monitoring include only mechanical and chemical processes.

_____ 10. One of the main reasons people don't process instruments correctly is they just don't have time.

FILL IN THE BLANK

Using words from the list below, fill in the blanks to complete the following statements.

Time-related	Storage	Ultrasonic cleaner
Instruments	Event-related	Receiving, cleaning, and decontamination
Chemical indicators	Disinfection	Biourden
Sterilization		

1. _____ shelf life means that the sterility of the instrument is maintained indefinitely if packages are handled and stored properly.

2. _____ shelf life means that instruments are identified with an exact expiration date.

3. _____ is a highly contaminated area requiring utility gloves and full PPE.

4. _____ areas are considered to have a low contamination risk and require only clean hands; no gloves are necessary.

5. _____ works with an enzyme solution to clean instruments.

6. _____ should be dried and lubricated to prevent rust and corrosion.

7. _____ should be used in each instrument package.

8. _____ prevent the growth of disease-carrying microorganisms.

9. _____ are blood and saliva left on instruments after patient care.

10. _____ is a process that kills all living microorganisms and destroys all living organisms and endospores.

CHAPTER 18
Occupational Health and Safety

CHAPTER OUTLINE

Review the Chapter Outline. If any content area is unclear, review that area before beginning the workbook exercises.

    A. Types of Safety Standards
        1. Regulatory
        2. Advisory Agencies
    B. Hazardous Chemicals
        1. Chemical Exposure
        2. Hazard Communication Program
    C. Achieving Safety through Personal Action
    D. Waste Handling and Disposal

CHAPTER REVIEW

The following is a summary of the chapter. If any of this material is unclear, review it in the textbook again.

Acceptance and practice of safety procedures is essential to maintaining the health and safety of dental personnel and patients. Specified federal and state agencies issue safety regulations that must be followed. Other government agencies and professional organizations provide recommendations for the best policies and practices for achieving compliance with the regulations. Recommended best practices are influential but voluntary. Materials used and waste generated in dental practice can be harmful, depending on their nature and concentration, the amount and type of exposure an individual receives, and the time period over which the exposure occurs. Dental assistants must ensure that they are in compliance with both state and local regulations and should strive for compliance with the recommendations of the Centers for Disease Control and the American Dental Association.

LEARNING ACTIVITIES AND STUDY AIDS

Review the following study aids and/or complete the activities to ensure that you have achieved the learning objectives for this chapter.

1. Explain the difference between standards, regulations, and recommendations.

2. List the responsibility that each of the following agencies has in safety assurance.

Table 18-1

Agency	Safety Role
OSHA	
EPA	
FDA	
CDC	
NIOSH	
ADA	
OSAP	
CRA	
ADAA	

3. Describe why a chemical may be designated as hazardous, and explain how chemical exposure occurs and can cause harm.

4. List the provisions of the Hazard Communication Standard.

5. Describe hazardous chemical labeling when using the NFPA system.

6. Various resources are available online to obtain free MSDS for various products. Find, print out, and turn in to your instructor three to five completed MSDS sheets. A good site from which to begin your search is the Centrix Dental site, *http://www.centrixdental.com/msds.asp*. Other helpful sites are the Grand Rapids Community College site, *http://igrcc.grcc.cc.mi.us/ShowPage.cfm?PageID=3087* and the Zenith Dental site, *http://www.zenithdental.com/Msdssearch.asp*.

7. Review the waste streams in the following table. Then complete the table by indicating the sterilants and restorative materials for each type. Information to complete this table can be found both on the Internet and in your textbook.

Table 18-2

Dental Practice Waste Streams				
X-ray/ Photography	Office	Medicaments	Sterilants	Restorative Materials
Developer	Paper	Anesthetics		
Fixer	Cardboard	Antibiotics		
Machine cleaners	Toner	Analgesics		
Lead foil	Electronic devices	Administration equipment		
Spent film	Ink cartridges			

8. Describe the procedure for correct disposal of a hazardous material.

9. Differentiate regulated waste and unregulated waste, and describe correct disposal procedures for each.

10. Dental assistants are generally responsible for disposing of amalgam waste generated by a dental practice. The American Dental Association updated its amalgam waste management guidelines in 2007, and it is important that dental assistants be aware of the latest information and recommendations. Go to the ADA Web site (*http://www.ada.org*) and click on A–Z Professional Topics. Then click on Amalgam Waste, Best Practices, which will take you to *http://ada.org/prof/ resources/topics/amalgam_bmp.asp*. Download and watch the four videos describing the best practices. After watching the videos, on a piece of paper write down three important concepts about amalgam waste management that you did not know before you watched the videos and three of the steps a dental assistant must take to manage amalgam waste properly.

MEDICAL TERMINOLOGY REVIEW

Use a dictionary and/or your textbook to define the following terms.

acceptance _____

acute _____

chronic _____

citation _____

compliance _____

contaminated waste _____

Hazard Communication Standard _____

hazardous waste _____

infectious waste _____

material safety data sheet _____

recommendation _____

regulated waste _____

regulation _____

revocation _____

standard _____

ABBREVIATIONS

ADA _____

ADAA _____

ANSI _____

CDC _____

CRA _____

EPA _____

FDA _____

FIFO _____

HAZCOM _____

HBV _____

HIV _____

ISO _____

MSDS _____

NFPA _____

NIOSH _____

OPIM _____

OSAP _____

OSHA _____

PPE _____

CRITICAL THINKING

1. Of the various professional organizations and agencies discussed in Chapter 18 that perform research and testing on occupational health and safety materials for the dental field, which three are the most valuable to a dental assistant? State your reasons why.

2. Why would OSHA require set standards for all organizations rather than allow for a variation of standards that dental practices can choose from? What are some requirements that OSHA mandates employers follow?

3. Are hazardous wastes disposed of differently depending on one's state, or is the method of disposal universal throughout the United States? Why or why not?

CHAPTER REVIEW TEST

MULTIPLE CHOICE

Circle the letter of the correct answer.

1. Official statements of government agencies that must be followed are:
   a. regulations
   b. recommendations
   c. standards
   d. a and c
   e. all of the above

2. This agency issues and enforces standards designed to protect the health and safety of U.S. workers.
   a. EPA
   b. FDA
   c. OSHA
   d. OSAP

3. Most dental office safety compliance inspections occur because:

    a. the office has more than ten employees and was randomly chosen
    b. someone has filed a compliant about the facility
    c. the dentist has requested help with compliance issues
    d. all of the above

4. Which federal agency has the authority to enforce cleanup of hazardous waste sites, require acceptable hazardous material disposal, impose fines, and file criminal complaints?

    a. ADA
    b. CDC
    c. FDA
    d. OSHA
    e. EPA

5. Why should the different waste streams in a dental office be kept separate?

    a. Each hazardous waste disposal company processes only one type of waste.
    b. If mixed, the streams must be separated at additional expense before being processed.
    c. State and federal regulations nationwide require waste stream separation.
    d. The dental office must file additional paperwork if the streams are not separated.

6. Select the TWO statements that describe hazardous and infectious materials.

    a. The material is highly reactive, toxic, carcinogenic, corrosive, contaminated, combustible, or degraded.
    b. The material is restricted to use in certain areas on certain types of patients.
    c. The material may be capable of spreading disease.
    d. The material has not yet been approved by the FDA or ADA as safe and effective.

7. Caustic agents cause:

    a. tissue whitening and severe burns
    b. skin irritation and loss of the sense of smell
    c. kidney and liver damage
    d. coughing and lung damage

8. Chemicals can enter the body in all of the following ways EXCEPT:

    a. inhalation
    b. ingestion
    c. contact with the skin or mucous membrane
    d. crossing heavy nitrile utility gloves

9. The Hazardous Communication Standard is based on the assumption that workers should:

    a. know what they are using and how to use it safely
    b. have employers who value their health
    c. understand Congress wants them to be safe
    d. be prepared to answer any questions their employers have

10. An MSDS provides:

    a. condensed, easily understood information about a chemical
    b. comprehensive information about a single chemical
    c. comparison information about several chemicals that accomplish the same task
    d. general historical information about development of a chemical

TRUE/FALSE

Indicate whether the statement is true (T) or false (F).

_____ 1. FIFO storage requires that new materials be stored behind old materials.

_____ 2. General waste is unregulated.

_____ 3. Infectious waste may be autoclaved and then treated as noninfectious.

_____ 4. Sharps such as needles must be bent before being placed in a sharps container.

_____ 5. Toxic materials are classified as regulated, contaminated waste.

_____ 6. OPIM include pathologic wastes such as extracted teeth.

_____ 7. A 3 in the red diamond of a NFPA label indicates the material does not burn at temperatures less than 200°F.

_____ 8. Hazardous materials should be packaged for disposal in securely closed, fluid-impervious containers with a standard hazardous label on the outside.

_____ 9. Because OSHA is a federally administered agency, a state may not develop and administer its own OSHA program.

_____ 10. ADA acceptance indicates a material has been tested and found to be safe, although it may not necessarily be effective.

FILL IN THE BLANK

Using words from the list below, fill in the blanks to complete the following statements.

ADA	hazardous	OSHA	CDC
infectious	sharps	CRA	noninfectious
unregulated	EPA	OPIM	

1. This agency issues regulations to promote worker safety: _____.

2. This organization provides recommendations for best practices to protect human health and prevent disease: _____.

3. This organization helps to protect the public's oral health by ensuring training programs for dental and allied dental personnel meet quality standards: _____.

4. This organization helps dentists identify high-quality materials by publishing clinical research results: _____.

5. This organization works to safeguard the environment in which we all live: _____.

6. _____ waste should be packaged in fluid-impervious bags that are securely closed.

7. _____ waste can be autoclaved and then treated as _____ waste.

8. The appropriate MSDS should be consulted to learn the proper disposal method for _____ waste.

9. _____ include materials that have been contaminated with blood or other potentially infectious bodily fluids.

10. _____ should be placed in specially designated and labeled containers that are located as close as possible to the point of use.

CHAPTER 19
Dental Unit Waterlines

CHAPTER OUTLINE

Review the Chapter Outline. If any content area is unclear, review that area before beginning the workbook exercises.

A. Introduction to Dental Unit Waterlines
B. History of Waterline Quality
C. Biofilm
D. Methods for Reducing Bacterial Contamination
E. Infection Control and Dental Unit Water

CHAPTER REVIEW

The following is a summary of the chapter. If any of this material is unclear, review it in the textbook again.

Waterlines are used in dentistry to cool and clear debris from the operative site. Water contains bacteria that multiply and form colonies that are resistant to destruction and capable of causing disease. Although no definable public health problem results from bacteria in dental waterlines, the dental profession has voluntarily adopted a waterline quality standard to protect patients from unnecessary exposure to waterborne bacteria. Methods of control include the use of independent water reservoirs, filtration of water entering the lines, chemical treatment regimens, daily line draining and cleaning, and the practice of recommended precautions during patient treatment. Effective control is more likely to be achieved when more than one method is used. Dental assistants are responsible for implementing the control strategies selected by their employers.

LEARNING ACTIVITIES AND STUDY AIDS

Review the following study aids and/or complete the activities to ensure that you have achieved the learning objectives for this chapter.

1. Various agencies set standards for safe drinking water quality. Research at least two of these agencies, and write a short description of what each agency does.

2. In your own words, define biofilm and discuss why some patients may be more at risk from waterborne bacteria than others.

3. List nine reasons why dental unit waterlines in particular encourage bacterial growth.

4. Compare the standards for drinking water and dental unit waterline quality.

5. Discuss why dental assistants should be knowledgeable about maintenance and monitoring of dental unit waterlines.

6. Describe the biofilm formation process.

7. The CDC has written guidelines about water used in oral surgical procedures. Visit the CDC Web site, conduct research on this topic, and write a paragraph to present the guidelines provided by the CDC.

8. Explain the difference between pathogenic and nonpathogenic, and then indicate whether the microorganisms found in dental waterlines are pathogenic or nonpathogenic.

9. List ten procedures the CDC recommends for reducing contamination of the water used during treatment.

10. List four procedures a dental office may use to reduce the number of bacteria in DUWL.

MEDICAL TERMINOLOGY REVIEW

Use a dictionary and/or your textbook to define the following terms.

adhere _____

aerobic _____

aerosol _____

algae _____

anaerobic _____

biofilm _____

compliance _____

immunocompromised _____

laminar flow _____

ozone _____

pathogen _____

protocol _____

protozoa _____

slime layer _____

ABBREVIATIONS

ADA _____

CDC _____

CFU _____

DUWL _____

EPA _____

OSAP _____

CRITICAL THINKING

1. What type of patient is especially sensitive to biofilm contamination that may be found in waterlines on dental units? What potential problem may this present to the patient, and how might this affect decisions related to treatment?

2. Describe what biofilm is, and how it forms. What one example of biofilm can you think of that wasn't listed in your textbook?

3. Discuss the five methods recommended by the CDC for decreasing the production of biofilm in dental unit waterlines. Why are these important to a dental assistant?

4. What methods are most recommended for disinfecting/removing biofilms from dental unit waterlines? What chemical is least recommended for use in performing this, and why?

CHAPTER REVIEW TEST

MULTIPLE CHOICE

Circle the letter of the correct answer.

1. The survival strategies that enable bacteria to form biofilm are:
   - a. adherence to surfaces
   - b. extraction of nutrients from water
   - c. secretion of a slime layer
   - d. both a and c
   - e. all of the above

2. Dental assistants are responsible for waterline:
   - a. maintenance
   - b. selection
   - c. monitoring
   - d. both a and c
   - e. all of the above

3. The cfu standard for dental unit waterline quality is _____ the cfu standard for drinking water quality.
   - a. equal to
   - b. more stringent than
   - c. less stringent than
   - d. double

4. Biofilm is formed where:
   - a. moisture meets a solid surface
   - b. water flow is faster
   - c. water lines have a large diameter
   - d. none of the above

5. Biofilm may develop within:
   - a. minutes to hours
   - b. hours to weeks
   - c. weeks to months
   - d. months to years

6. Select the chemicals listed below that are used for DUWL flushing.
   - a. sodium hypochlorite
   - b. chlorhexadine gluconate
   - c. glutaraldehyde
   - d. a and c
   - e. all of the above

7. The CDC recommends that DUWL be purged of all water at this time.
   - a. at the beginning of each day
   - b. when cleaning the operatory after each patient
   - c. at the end of each day
   - d. at least once per week
   - e. at least once per month

8. Dental unit water quality should be monitored:
   - a. at the beginning of each day
   - b. at the beginning and end of each day
   - c. weekly
   - d. monthly

9. Chemical treatment does this to DUWL:

a. flush
b. disinfect
c. sterilize

d. a and b
e. b and c

10. The primary source of bacteria in dental treatment water is:

a. the dental assistant's hands
b. aerosols generated by handpieces and ultrasonic scalers
c. retraction of saliva into water lines
d. the public water supply

TRUE/FALSE

Indicate whether the statement is true (T) or false (F).

_____ 1. Handpieces used for dental treatment should be flushed for thirty seconds between each patient.

_____ 2. Heating dental unit water assists in reducing the number of bacteria it contains.

_____ 3. Antiretraction valves should be installed to pull oral fluids into the DUWL so they can be properly disinfected.

_____ 4. An independent water reservoir is effective in reducing bacterial contamination, provided it is used in conjunction with chemical treatment.

_____ 5. Waterline antimicrobials must be registered with the CDC.

_____ 6. Dental equipment, such as handpieces and syringe tips, should remain in treatment position while water-monitoring samples are being taken.

_____ 7. If used, water filters should be placed at the point where water enters the DUWL.

_____ 8. It is important to follow an established schedule of DUWL treatment.

_____ 9. Waterline samples taken with an in-office kit should be tested within one week.

_____ 10. Scientific reports have not linked waterborne contaminants directly to an increased incidence of disease in either patients or dental personnel.

FILL IN THE BLANK

Using words from the list below, fill in the blanks to complete the following statements.

30 seconds	manufacturer's directions	water
ethanol	pH strips	wear gloves
high volume evacuator	required	
infection control protocol	voluntary	

1. The ADA standard for acceptable numbers of cfu in DUWL is _____.

2. The EPA standard for acceptable numbers of cfu in drinking water is _____.

3. Use of rubber dam for some dental procedures is recommended to prevent _____ entry into the mouth.

4. The dental assistant should use a _____ to remove oral fluids present during dental treatment.

5. Materials used to make dental equipment should be preserved by following the _____ regarding DUWL disinfection.

6. Ninety-five percent _____ may be used for DUWL.

7. _____ are used to monitor the presence of colorless disinfectant in DUWL.

8. When taking a DUWL sample, the dental assistant should _____ to ensure the samples are not being contaminated.

9. The dental assistant should run each handpiece, air-water syringe, and ultrasonic unit for _____ after each patient.

10. DUWL disinfection is a routine part of the _____ for any dental facility.

CHAPTER 20
The Dental Office

CHAPTER OUTLINE

Review the Chapter Outline. If any content area is unclear, review that area before beginning the workbook exercises.

A. Dental Office Setting
B. Administrative and Reception Area
C. Dentist's Private Office
D. Dental Staff Lounge
E. Daily Routine Care for Dental Assistants
F. Clinical Treatment Rooms
G. Clinical Equipment
   1. Central Vacuum Compressor
   2. Central Air Compressor
   3. Oral Evacuation System
   4. Patient Dental Chair
   5. Operator's Chair
   6. Assistant's Stool
   7. Dental Unit
   8. Operating Light
   9. Dental Cabinets
   10. Dental Radiology Units
   11. Small Equipment
H. Central Sterilization Area
I. Dental Laboratory Area

CHAPTER REVIEW

The following is a summary of the chapter. If any of this material is unclear, review it in the textbook again.

Within a dental practice, consideration must be given to the type of office design and materials needed to operate efficiently. The design, type of equipment chosen, and patient flow depends on the type of dentistry being practiced and the personal preferences of the dentist. The dental assistant must be familiar with all types of equipment that vary between dental offices. Infection control procedures for the cleaning, sterilizing, and maintenance of equipment must be learned and strictly adhered to in order to ensure the safety of the dental patients and the entire dental team. It is always advisable to follow manufacturer instructions on the maintenance and care of dental equipment, including the use of infection control barriers and disinfectants, as well as keeping all patient care areas clean and presentable. Other areas that need to be addressed in a dentist office include the sterilization room, employee break room, and patient waiting area. These areas should be neat and free of debris and clutter not only for the safety of the patients but also to ensure an organized and efficient office. In addition to providing quality dental care, developing an office that is pleasant and inviting for the patient should be the goal of the entire dental team.

LEARNING ACTIVITIES AND STUDY AIDS

Review the following study aids and/or complete the activities to ensure that you have achieved the learning objectives for this chapter.

1. Consider a dental office or other type of medical facility that you have recently visited. How well organized do you think the facility is, and does the office present an inviting environment? What do you base your opinion on? Does it feel organized? Does it feel inviting? Why or why not? Is the waiting room adjacent to the reception area, is there a separate entrance and exit to allow for patient privacy and billing issues, is the sterilization area away from immediate patient view? In considering what you have learned from this chapter on dental office design, write a one-page report on your experience, explain how you believe the office design does or does not meet the needs of the practice, and provide the answers to the questions posed in the activity.

2. Write a brief essay (about a half page) on how the Americans with Disabilities Act of 1990 has impacted the design for dental offices. Use an additional piece of paper if more space is needed for your information.

3. Compare a general practice dental office to an orthodontic office. What differences are there? Now compare a general dental office to a pedodontic practice. What differences are there between these three? Do you find any similarities between the three? (You may have to visit these offices in your local community or use the Internet to search for these three types of offices). Submit your comparisons to your instructor in a written summary. If outside resources were used, note these in your summary.

4. List the eleven design elements required by the Americans with Disabilities Act for a barrier-free office.

5. Go online and look for virtual tours of different office designs. Then write a brief report of your findings, citing your sources. Explain what was learned in your search about various office designs. Describe an office design that you believe best meets the needs of a medium-size dental practice. Utilize an additional piece of paper if more space is needed to record your information.

6. Using the information found in your textbook and other resources (Internet, dental equipment manufacturer catalogs, or representatives), what components are taken into consideration when designing or ordering a dental treatment chair? What features are most important? What types of positions might the patient need to be adjusted to while seated in this chair? What is the average price of a dental treatment chair? How might the chair be maintained? Why is this information important for the dental assistant? Utilize an additional piece of paper if more space is required for recording your information.

7. Why is it so important to follow the manufacturer's care and maintenance instructions on dental equipment?

8. The textbook lists five areas of concern when designing a business office:

   a. Business assistants should face the reception area to be able to make eye contact with patients as they arrive and leave the office.

   b. Items such as appointment cards and patient information should be easily accessible to the dental staff but confined to areas that are secure.

   c. Intercom systems should be placed in appropriate areas to provide effective communication between the administrative and clinical areas.

   d. Master controls for heating and air settings, music volume, and light settings should be within easy reach for quick access.

   e. Storage space for paper, pens and pencils, and telephone message pads should be provided to ensure that these items are available as needed.

   What are the reasons behind these considerations? What is the one thing they all have in common? Are there any other considerations for the business office that you can think of? Consider the office of the dentist you may go to—do you find/see all of these factors? What changes may be possible to recommend for increased efficiency in this one area?

9. Most dental offices have magazines, books, children's toys, perhaps even a television or DVD player. Whose responsibility is it to ensure the toys are safe? The book and magazines are picked up? Who is responsible for the television channels or DVD being played in the waiting room? What types of magazines might you want to subscribe to? Why is the waiting room a concern for the dental assistant?

10. Explain the three different types of delivery systems, and why each type might be selected.

MEDICAL TERMINOLOGY REVIEW

Use a dictionary and/or your textbook to define the following terms.

air abrasion _____

air/water syringe _____

amalgamator _____

central air compressor _____

consultation room _____

curing light _____

dental chair _____

dental operatory _____

dental unit _____

front delivery system _____

handpieces _____

operatories _____

oral evacuation system _____

rear delivery system _____

rheostat _____

side delivery system _____

subsupine position _____

supine position _____

triturate _____

tubehead _____

ultrasonic scalers _____

upright position _____

x-ray _____

ABBREVIATIONS

ADA _____

CDC _____

HIPAA _____

HVE _____

OSHA _____

PPM _____

CRITICAL THINKING

1. What are some considerations for the design of a dental office?

2. Where should the reception area be within a dental office, and why is the location of the reception area important?

3. What are some considerations for planning the reception area?

CHAPTER REVIEW TEST

MULTIPLE CHOICE

Circle the letter of the correct answer.

1. The Americans with Disabilities act ensures that:
   a. strict specifications ensure the dental office designs comply with state and federal guidelines
   b. dental offices are designed for the comfort of the patient and dental office employees
   c. all patients are treated equally, receive the same quality of care, and the same price for that care
   d. none of the above

2. Intraoral cameras can be used for:
   a. taking pictures inside the oral cavity only
   b. documenting oral conditions and patient education only
   c. taking pictures outside the mouth to document skin conditions
   d. patient education, documentation of oral conditions, discussing specific treatment concerns and payment issues, and obtaining informed consent

3. The main characteristics to consider before purchasing a dental curing light are:
   a. intensity or speed of the light, the spectrum generated by the light, and portability
   b. color of the light unit, heat generated, and amount of electricity consumed by the light while in use
   c. spectrum generated by the light, color of light emitted, price of unit
   d. all of the above

4. If a dental radiography unit is not operating properly, the dental assistant should contact a:
   a. RDH   c. CDA
   b. RDT   d. CDT

5. The operating light provides:
   a. a bright light necessary to see into the oral cavity during procedures
   b. enough light to adequately see across the room
   c. a laser-powered light used in operations
   d. a light that works versus one that does not

6. The dental unit typically consists of:
   a. vacuum, compressor, air-water syringes, saliva ejector, and possibly oral evacuator
   b. air-water syringes, saliva ejector, and possibly oral evacuator, handpieces, and other options depending upon the operator
   c. dental chair, control panel, oral evacuator, handpieces, and other options depending upon the operator
   d. all of the above

7. Who should arrive fifteen to thirty minutes earlier to the office than the remainder of the staff?
   a. dentist   c. dental assistant
   b. office manager   d. dental hygienist

8. Why should the above-mentioned person arrive earlier than the remainder of the staff?
   a. to flush dental handpieces and rinse water lines
   b. to set up the dental operatory
   c. to turn on the film developer and all other equipment as required
   d. all of the above
   e. none of the above

9. The pedal that controls the speed and rate of the dental handpieces is called the:
   a. gas pedal
   b. control pedal
   c. handpiece pedal
   d. rheostat

10. The most commonly used position for treating dental patients is:
    a. subsupine
    b. upright
    c. supine
    d. downright

TRUE/FALSE

Indicate whether the statement is true (T) or false (F).

_____ 1. The design and size of a dental office are determined by the type of practice the dentist plans to build.

_____ 2. Patients will judge the quality of the dental care the practice provides by the appearance of the office.

_____ 3. Carpet should never be used in a treatment area because it is difficult to sanitize.

_____ 4. The office manager is the only person who is allowed to enter the front office.

_____ 5. The dental laboratory is an area where blood and other bodily fluids are tested for diseases that affect the mouth.

_____ 6. The operating light is used to cure and set light-curable materials.

_____ 7. An amalgamator is a small machine used to mechanically mix dental amalgam for silver fillings and some dental cements.

_____ 8. The operating light provides bright light necessary to see into the oral cavity during procedures.

_____ 9. The dental unit has three types of dental handpieces: high-speed handpieces, medium-speed handpieces, and slow-speed handpieces.

_____ 10. Air abrasion is the mechanical etching of the surface of a tooth.

FILL IN THE BLANK

Using words from the list below, fill in the blanks to complete the following statements.

Front delivery systems	Rear delivery systems	Sides delivery systems
Ultrasonic scalers	Radiology units	X-rays
View boxes	Saliva ejectors	Air water syringes
HVEs	HIPAA	

1. _____ allow equipment to be used over the patient's chest and in front of the operator and assistant.

2. _____ expose intraoral radiographs and digital radiographs.

3. _____ remove waste and debris from a patient's mouth during dental procedures.

4. _____ allow equipment to be used from behind the patient's head.

5. _____ are used during dental cleanings and produce a vibrating action that removes hard deposits such as calculus and other debris from the teeth.

6. _____ allow equipment to be used from the operator's side. The dental unit is attached to either a fixed or mobile unit that has an extendable arm to aid the operator in gaining access from the dental unit to the patient.

7. _____ remove small amounts of fluid from a patient's mouth, not large amounts of fluid or debris.

8. _____ are used by the dentist to read and diagnose dental radiographs.

9. _____ regulates the privacy of patients.

10. _____ are attached to the dental unit and used to rinse surfaces in the oral cavity.

CHAPTER 21

Examination and Care Planning

CHAPTER OUTLINE

Review the Chapter Outline. If any content area is unclear, review that area before beginning the workbook exercises.

A. Patient Record and Confidentiality
1. Health Insurance Portability and Accountability Act
2. Personal Data
3. Dental and Medical History
4. Clinical Examination and Progress Notes
5. Retention of Records
6. Transfer of Records
7. Faxing Dental Records

B. Creating and Maintaining the Patient Record
1. Electronic Dental Record
2. Recording Information in the Record

C. Patient Record Forms
1. Personal Data
2. Health History and Drug Allergies
3. Visual Dental Chart
4. Care Plan
5. Progress Notes
6. Miscellaneous Reference Data

D. Obtaining the Health History

E. Examination and Diagnostic Techniques
1. Seating the Patient
2. Comprehensive Examination
3. Diagnostic Techniques

F. Clinical Examination of the Patient
1. Extraoral Examination
2. Intraoral Examination

G. Recording the Dental Examination
1. Subjective
2. Objective
3. Assessment
4. Plan

H. Charting

I. The Care Plan
1. Care Plan Presentation

J. Recording Dental Treatment

K. The Digital Patient Record

CHAPTER REVIEW

The following is a summary of the chapter. If any of this material is unclear, review it in the textbook again.

Examination and care planning provides the basis for all dental treatment. Records are the foundation of the examination and treatment process. The dentist, with the aid of the dental assistant, collects pertinent data, then assesses it to determine the patient's needs and formulates a treatment plan. Treatment is based on the likely prognosis if the planned care is provided. The patient is an active participant throughout because informed consent is necessary before any treatment can be rendered.

LEARNING ACTIVITIES AND STUDY AIDS

Review the following study aids and/or complete the activities to ensure that you have achieved the learning objectives for this chapter.

1. Given the progress notes listed in the following table, state what is missing that should be included.

Table 21-1

Date	Progress notes	Initials
12/11/07	Initial examination Restorative charting Paralleled full mouth series: 20, #2 films	RMS
12/11/07	Prophylaxis Periodontal charting: No pockets over 4 mm, gingiva moderately inflamed in maxillary anterior, likely from patient's Class II malocclusion as oral hygiene is fairly good. Demonstrated Bass brushing and spool flossing. Patient practiced both and did well. Patient will return week after next for restorative work and redemonstrate her home care skills for me at that time.	RMS
12/27/07	One carpule lidocaine with 2% epinephrine #15 MOD amalgam with calcium hydroxide liner and zinc phosphate base. Referred to orthodontist for examination and assessment: Dr. James Kirby in Providence.	RMS
1/15/08	One carpule lidocaine with 2% epinephrine #21 full crown preparation. Dual tray impression taken with polyvinylsiloxane.	RMS
1/15/08	#21 acrylic temporary crown	KAW
2/12/08	#21 fit and deliver full PFM crown Recall: 6 months Patient education regarding care of crown	RMS KAW
8/18/08	Recall examination Prophylaxis Restorative and periodontal charting	RMS

2. The dentist completes her clinical examination of the patient, gives him an injection of local anesthetic for a planned composite restoration, and leaves the room to tend to a patient in the next operatory. As soon as the dentist leaves, the patient turns to you and says, "Why did she feel my face in front of my ear and push my lower front teeth back and forth?" In simple language, explain to her why these things were done.

3. Last week another dental assistant in the office charted a full mouth series of radiographs for the school-age patient the dentist saw at that time and you are seeing today. Everything was charted correctly except the size of the film used. Ordinarily the office uses #2 film for older children, but because this patient is petite and has a small mouth, #1 film was used. How can you correct the error appropriately?

4. List and define the components of a SOAP record.

5. Discuss how to obtain a medical history.

6. Define the term chief complaint, and state why it is an important part of the medical history.

7. Describe acceptable means of transferring dental records.

8. List the instruments and materials used for a clinical examination.

9. Describe the order of precedence of the components of a care plan.

10. Explain how to prepare a patient for a dental examination.

MEDICAL TERMINOLOGY REVIEW

Use a dictionary and/or your textbook to define the following terms.

abrasion _____

asymmetry _____

attrition _____

bruxism _____

chief complaint _____

comprehensive oral exam _____

crepitus _____

erosion _____

etiologic _____

HIPAA _____

objective _____

palpation _____

subjective assessment _____

ABBREVIATIONS

ADA _____

EDR _____

HIPAA _____

SOAP _____

CRITICAL THINKING

1. Why is the treatment planning phase of dental care so vitally important, and what role does the dental assistant play in ensuring planning is done correctly?

2. In the dental office, whose responsibility is it to ensure that all patients receive and understand what HIPAA is? What are the four primary administrative safeguards found in a dental office regarding patient records?

3. Can dental records be faxed? If so, what precautions must be taken to ensure patient confidentiality under HIPAA?

CHAPTER REVIEW TEST

MULTIPLE CHOICE

Circle the letter of the correct answer.

1. The primary purpose of care planning is to:
   a. create thorough and precise records
   b. assure the confidentiality of all matters discussed
   c. determine an appropriate sequence of treatment
   d. develop an effective relationship between the patient and dentist

2. If dental records are visible by others, they should be:
   a. placed face down
   b. moved to another area
   c. enclosed in an envelope
   d. any of the above

3. The TWO primary purposes of HIPAA are to:
   a. protect the confidentiality of patient data
   b. ease the recordkeeping burden of healthcare providers
   c. ensure patients know how their information is used
   d. require offices to switch to electronic health records

4. All patients are required to sign an acknowledgement that they have received:
   a. a full accounting of information disclosures
   b. a notice of office privacy practices
   c. secure, reasonable, protected information
   d. all of the above

5. Personal data must include all of the following EXCEPT:
   a. name and date of birth
   b. address and place of employment
   c. name and telephone number of emergency contact
   d. credit rating and history of cooperation with dentist

6. The patient's chief complaint, if present, is the:
   a. concern she found in dealing with her previous dentist
   b. problem that caused her to seek dental care
   c. list of services rendered and actions taken
   d. objective portion of SOAP notes

7. Which of the following is true?
   a. The name, quantity, and strength of all drugs dispensed, administered, or prescribed must be included in the patient's clinical examination and progress notes.
   b. Radiographs, study models, and periodontal chartings must be included in the patient's SOAP notes for a minimum of twelve months.
   c. Patient records must be maintained in the dental office for a minimum of six years following the patient's last examination, prescription, or treatment.
   d. The law recognizes that it is not always possible to protect records from such destructive forces as rodent invasion, water, or theft.

8. The patient's permission to transfer records must indicate whether:
   a. all or a portion of the records should be released
   b. the record to be released is current or archived
   c. the dentist or patient legally owns the records
   d. the patient's account balance is paid in full

9. To maintain the security of faxed information, the dental assistant should:
   a. fax only to secure places such as another doctor's office
   b. use a cover sheet with a warning that the information can be shared only with authorized individuals
   c. call to confirm that the receiver did in fact receive the message
   d. a and c
   e. all of the above

10. A disadvantage of the electronic chart is that:
   a. caries and restorations must be charted at separate times
   b. consistent standard abbreviations cannot be used
   c. norms for information to be included have not been established
   d. it is difficult to retrieve data from computerized charting systems

TRUE/FALSE

Indicate whether the statement is true (T) or false (F).

_____ 1. Manual records should be written in blue or black ink.

_____ 2. Personal data is obtained and maintained in the patient registration form.

_____ 3. The patient's health history must be updated at least annually.

_____ 4. Allergies can range from minor irritations to life-threatening emergencies.

_____ 5. Geometric charts have anatomic representations of the teeth, including depiction of anatomically correct roots, on which the dental assistant can chart the patient's dental conditions.

_____ 6. To avoid unnecessary upset, the patient is not informed of any copay she may owe until after the insurance company has sent an Explanation of Benefits form.

_____ 7. The treatment plan can be presented to the patient by the dentist, administrative assistant, dental hygienist, or chairside dental assistant in accordance with office policy.

_____ 8. All entries placed in the patient's record must be signed or initialed by the healthcare provider.

_____ 9. Patients rarely omit or intentionally distort their answers to questions on the medical/dental history.

_____ 10. The ADA recommends that some new patients, and all established patients who have been away from the office for at least three years, receive a comprehensive examination.

FILL IN THE BLANK

Using words from the list below, fill in the blanks to complete the following statements.

abrasion	diabetes	painful
beneath the patient's chin	erosion	palpation
cocoa butter	eye protection	pocket depths
crepitus	lipstick	tender

1. _____ may be used as a lubricant for the lips during dental procedures.

2. After the patient has been seated and the dental assistant has positioned the chair, the light should be turned on and focused _____, then turned off until the dentist arrives.

3. Patients wearing _____ should be given a tissue to remove it.

4. During all dental procedures, including examination, patients should wear _____, either their own or office-supplied.

5. Medical conditions that may show up in the mouth and be visible during a dental examination are hypertension, sinusitis, oral cancer, and _____.

6. The dentist palpates lymph nodes of the neck, face, and floor of the mouth to see if they are _____ or _____.

7. The periodontal portion of a comprehensive examination includes documentation of tooth mobility, bone loss, hard and soft deposits present, bleeding, swelling, and _____.

8. _____ is a process of examining for disease or abnormality by use of the fingers or hands.

9. _____ refers to cracking or grating sounds made by the TMJ when it moves.

10. Chemical wearing away of tooth structure is _____; mechanical wearing away is _____.

CHAPTER 22
Caring for The Dental Patient

CHAPTER OUTLINE

Review the Chapter Outline. If any content area is unclear, review that area before beginning the workbook exercises.

A. Establishing Patient Rapport
   1. Ways to Build Rapport

B. Reviewing the Patient Record
   1. Quality Assurance
   2. Health Insurance Portability and Accountability Act

C. Preparing the Treatment Area
   1. The Operatory

D. Greeting and Seating the Patient
   1. Escorting the Patient to the Treatment Area
   2. Seating and Preparing the Patient for Treatment

E. Assessing Patient Needs
   1. Considerations for Pregnant Patients
   2. Considerations for Patients who are Sensory Impaired
   3. Considerations for Patients with Language Barriers

F. The Rights of All Patients
   1. Rights as Specified by the ADA

G. The Role of the Dental Assistant
   1. Functioning as a Member of the Dental Team

H. Patients with Special Needs
   1. The Geriatric Patient
   2. Patients in Wheelchairs or Walkers
   3. Patients with Cardiovascular Disorders
   4. Patients with Neurological Disorders
   5. Patients with Pulmonary Disorders
   6. Patients with Musculoskeletal Disorders
   7. Patients with Endocrine Disorders
   8. Patients with Developmental, Behavioral, and Psychiatric Disorders
   9. Patients with Dental Anxiety
   10. Patients with Substance Abuse

CHAPTER REVIEW

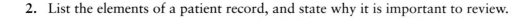

The following is a summary of the chapter. If any of this material is unclear, review it in the textbook again.

The dental assistant has three basic roles: providing technical assistance to the dentist, educating patients and their families, and creating a calm, supportive, environment in which treatment can take place. It is this last role that is the focus of this chapter. Creating an environment in which patient comfort, trust, and calmness thrive is as much an art as a science. It requires that the dental assistant sincerely care for people, enjoy and respect their differences, and seek to find the big and little things that make the dental treatment experience a pleasant one for both patients and team members. The dental assistant who develops a rapport with patients is sincerely missed when not present.

LEARNING ACTIVITIES AND STUDY AIDS

Review the following study aids and/or complete the activities to ensure that you have achieved the learning objectives for this chapter.

1. Explain the process of greeting and seating dental patients.

2. List the elements of a patient record, and state why it is important to review.

3. Describe ways of developing patient rapport.

4. The American Heart Association (AHA) has recently revised the guidelines for administering antibiotics prior to dental treatment. To learn more about these guidelines, go online, find the information, and then write a short summary of these guidelines.

5. Explain the challenges the dental team can face when it comes to dealing with geriatric patients.

6. Conduct research online or using library resources at your school or local library. Look up the following diseases and conditions: sensory impairment, congestive heart failure, hypertension, angina pectoris, endocarditis, anemia, Alzheimer's disease, epilepsy, multiple sclerosis, cerebral palsy, and stroke. Utilizing a separate piece of paper, write a paragraph for each disease/condition. Define each disease or condition; present the signs and symptoms, and the possible treatments available.

7. To further understand patients who have dental anxiety, interview three to five people. If possible, have at least a couple of these individuals indicate to you that they have some anxiety toward going to the dentist. Interview each individual by asking the following questions:

> How do you generally feel about going to the dentist?
>
> Is it something that you look forward to doing? If so, why?
>
> Do you experience any anxiety about going to the dentist? If so, explain.
>
> If you experience anxiety, what types of methods, if any, do you use to reduce the anxiety?
>
> When visiting the dentist, can any anxieties be minimized effectively by the dental team? If so, how is this done?

If negative feelings or fears about the dentist exist, do you know where these originate?

Once all of the individuals have been interviewed, compare and contrast their answers.

Document your information using a separate piece of paper. At the end of your information, provide an analysis of what you discovered in the completion of this activity. Then write a report on your analysis.

8. Differentiate Type I, Type II, and gestational diabetes, and hypo- and hyperthyroidism.

9. Describe the various problems and oral health issues that may arise when a patient abuses alcohol or drugs.

10. Write a short summary of the dental assistant's role in patient care.

MEDICAL TERMINOLOGY REVIEW

Use a dictionary and/or your textbook to define the following terms.

angina pectoris _____

emphysema _____

hypertension _____

hyperthyroidism _____

hypothyroidism _____

mechanical bruxism _____

multiple sclerosis _____

muscular dystrophy _____

phobia _____

pulmonary disorder _____

resorption _____

stroke or cerebrovascular accident _____

xerostomia _____

ABBREVIATIONS

ADA _____

AHA _____

COPD _____

e-PHI _____

HIPAA _____

PHI _____

CRITICAL THINKING

1. Why is dental care for the pregnant patient of concern for the dental assistant, and what considerations may be given during treatment?

2. Why is it important for the dental assistant to establish rapport with patients? What ways enable a dental assistant to be better equipped to establish patient rapport?

3. What are three things a dental assistant can do to ensure patient safety prior to seating a patient?

4. What are some additional preparatory things that can be done in order to expedite patient treatment?

CHAPTER REVIEW TEST

MULTIPLE CHOICE

Circle the letter of the correct answer.

1. Rapport is:
   a. dental alveolar ridge bone loss
   b. the use of complementary body language
   c. loss of muscle function from neurologic injury
   d. a positive working relationship between people

2. The foundation of effective patient rapport includes:
   a. factual information carefully presented
   b. natural kindness and empathy
   c. maintenance of a respectful professional distance
   d. avoidance of all personal topics of conversation

3. Dental law mandates that patient records be:
   a. up-to-date
   b. complete
   c. accurate
   d. a and c
   e. all of the above

4. The dental assistant should periodically audit all of the following for quality assurance purposes EXCEPT:
   a. patient charts
   b. emergency standards
   c. tax records
   d. office policies

5. Which of the following statements is true?
   a. A patient's chart should be bibbed or in a secure area to prevent unauthorized persons from viewing the data.
   b. The first step in preparing the room for a patient is to bring the patient into the room and place the patient napkin.
   c. Electronic protected health information is not held to the same strict privacy standards as information that was written on paper.
   d. The patient should be warned about avoiding any obstacles in the pathway to the treatment room before the assistant begins to escort him/her there.

6. The patient's vital signs should be taken when he/she is:
   a. standing up
   b. sitting down
   c. lying down
   d. either standing or lying down

7. Before a patient enters the operatory, the chair should:
   a. be lowered to about fifteen to eighteen inches from the floor
   b. be positioned so the back is tilted slightly back
   c. have the arm on the patient's entrance side raised
   d. a and c
   e. all of the above

8. A pretreatment rinse can be offered to the patient to freshen his/her mouth and:
   a. remove debris
   b. lower the intraoral microorganism count
   c. create a contrasting color to enhance the dentist's visibility
   d. a and b
   e. b and c

9. A patient napkin should be placed on the patient so that:
   a. the plastic side is down toward the patient's clothing
   b. the larger portion of the napkin is toward the operator
   c. the clip holds the bib securely in place
   d. the patient's clothing or skin is not caught in the clip
   e. all of the above

10. Which of the following may make the pregnant patient more comfortable?
    a. longer appointment times
    b. sitting in a reclined position
    c. lying on her left side
    d. using a papoose board

TRUE/FALSE

Indicate whether the statement is true (T) or false (F).

_____ 1. The best time for treating a pregnant patient is during the first trimester.

_____ 2. Pregnant patients with periodontal disease are at higher risk for preterm and low-birth-weight babies.

_____ 3. Gingival bleeding is normal for a pregnant patient.

_____ 4. It is important for the dental assistant to remove her mask and position herself so her mouth is visible when talking to a hearing-impaired patient.

_____ 5. Visually impaired patients may need additional help understanding what the dental assistant is saying.

_____ 6. Some geriatric patients may need to be kept away from any microwave activity, including microwave technology used to perform dental procedures, because they have an implanted pacemaker.

_____ 7. Increased prevalence of oral disease, the presence of multiple chronic diseases, and increased use of prescription medications may be encountered in the geriatric patient, especially the oldest old, aged eighty-five years and beyond.

_____ 8. Alveolar bone resorption, root caries, and dark, brittle teeth that are susceptible to fracture are most likely to be encountered in the diabetic patient.

_____ 9. Fluoride varnish, prescription fluoride pastes, and fluoride gels in custom trays are used to prevent caries formation in patients with xerostomia.

_____ 10. The handbrake of a wheelchair should be unlocked to permit wheelchair movement when a patient is being transferred from the wheelchair to the dental chair.

FILL IN THE BLANK

Using words from the list below, fill in the blanks to complete the following statements.

bathroom breaks	healthy teeth and gums	not advisable
COPD	heart disease	readily available
epilepsy	hemophilia	upright
expelling	mental	

1. Recent research indicates periodontal diseases can lead to _____, especially in severe cases where the periodontal infection is left untreated.

2. Patients with congestive heart failure may need to sit more _____ in the chair and take more frequent _____.

3. Patients with angina pectoris should have their medication _____ during their dental appointment.

4. The American Heart Association now reports that the best line of defense against contracting endocarditis from an invasive dental procedure is _____.

5. A patient with _____ should receive invasive treatment only after consultation with his/her physician.

6. Alzheimer's disease is characterized by deterioration of _____ abilities.

7. It is _____ to place anything in the mouth of a patient who is having a seizure.

8. Many victims of cerebral palsy also have a seizure disorder termed _____.

9. Asthma patients have difficulty getting air _____ the lungs; emphysema patients have difficulty _____ it.

10. Nitrous oxide and oxygen is not recommended for pain management for patients with _____.

CHAPTER 23
Vital Signs

CHAPTER OUTLINE

Review the Chapter Outline. If any content area is unclear, review that area before beginning the workbook exercises.

    A.   Factors That Affect Vital Signs

    B.   Body Temperature
        1. Methods of Taking Temperature
        2. Normal Values
        3. Types of Thermometers
        4. Reading a Thermometer
        5. Documentation

    C.   Blood Pressure
        1. Blood Pressure Equipment
        2. Blood Pressure Readings
        3. Documentation
        4. Normal Values

    D.   Respiration
        1. Characteristics of Respirations
        2. Taking Respirations
        3. Documentation

CHAPTER REVIEW

The following is a summary of the chapter. If any of this material is unclear, review it in the textbook again.

Vital signs are important clues to the general health of an individual. The signs commonly measured are temperature, blood pressure, pulse, and respiratory rate. Standard sites and methods are used for measuring and recording vital signs. Ranges are used to designate what is normal for each sign because people vary slightly in their normal functioning. The dental assistant must be aware of the factors that can affect vital signs, and know the standard procedure for measuring each sign, the range considered to be normal for the sign, and the correct procedure for recording each measurement taken. Vital signs are commonly taken for every dental patient before treatment begins.

LEARNING ACTIVITIES AND STUDY AIDS

Review the following study aids and/or complete the activities to ensure that you have achieved the learning objectives for this chapter.

1. List and define the four vital signs commonly measured in the dental office.

2. List at least five factors that can temporarily affect a patient's vital signs.

3. State the range of measurements considered normal for each vital sign.

4. Complete the following table by listing eight separate sites where pulse can be taken, and explaining the location of each. Place the three sites dental assistants would be most likely to use in the top three boxes.

Table 23-1

Pulse Site	Location

5. Explain the circumstances that the dental assistant may need to consider when taking a child's temperature.

6. List and define the three standard words used to describe the characteristics of respirations.

7. Complete the table by providing the information on how the measurement obtained should be recorded.

Table 23-2

Measurement Obtained:	Recorded As:

8. Go online to learn more about instruments used to measure temperature. Use each type of thermometer as a graphics search term, then print pictures of the thermometers you find. Study these pictures as you read the material about the different types of thermometers in your chapter so you can relate the directions for clinical use to the configuration of the thermometer. This will be helpful in reviewing for examinations in which questions may be asked about temperature-measuring devices that are less commonly used. Submit your pictures to your instructor for a grade to this exercise.

9. Describe the "white lab coat syndrome," and explain what steps can be taken to address this condition.

10. State why respirations are measured when the patient is unaware this is being done.

MEDICAL TERMINOLOGY REVIEW

Use a dictionary and/or your textbook to define the following terms.

aneroid _____

antecubital _____

axillary _____

brachial _____

bradycardia _____

carotid _____

diaphoresis _____

diastolic _____

expiration _____

hypertensive _____

hypotensive _____

hypothalamus _____

inspiration _____

radial _____

sphygmomanometer _____

stethoscope _____

systolic _____

tachycardia _____

ABBREVIATIONS

BP _____

bpm _____

C _____

F _____

Hg _____

LCD _____

CRITICAL THINKING

1. Why is it important for the sphygmomanometer to fit correctly and be accurately placed? What could be the results of a blood pressure reading if the cuff did not fit correctly?

2. Define respiration, inspiration, and expiration. What are the functions of inspiration and expiration?

3. Why is it important for a dental assistant to know how to take and interpret a patient's vital signs?

CHAPTER REVIEW TEST

MULTIPLE CHOICE

Circle the letter of the correct answer.

1. Blood pressure is:
   a. the throbbing felt in the arteries as a result of the heartbeat
   b. the amount of heat produced by the body
   c. the amount of force against the walls of an artery caused by the blood flow
   d. all of the above

2. The following factors can affect an individual's vital signs:
   a. anxiety
   b. pregnancy
   c. exercise
   d. a and c
   e. all of the above

3. A patient who presents with a fever may have or be:
   a. an infection
   b. exhausted
   c. fearful
   d. a ruptured eardrum

4. This substance formerly enjoyed widespread use in thermometers but is now considered a biohazardous chemical that in some states may not be used or purchased.
   a. gold
   b. silver
   c. mercury
   d. titanium

5. On conventional glass Fahrenheit thermometers, every other long line represents:

a. an odd degree   c. .2 of a degree

b. an even degree   d. .1 of a degree

6. The systolic reading of a blood pressure measurement refers to the:

a. sounds heard when using a stethoscope.

b. regularity of the circulatory blood flow

c. arterial pressure during the heart's relaxation phase

d. arterial pressure during the heart's contraction phase

7. Select the correct documentation for a blood pressure reading of 78 for the diastolic measurement and 118 for the systolic measurement.

a. BP 78/118 bpm irregular, shallow

b. BP 118/78 bpm regular, deep

c. R BP 78/118

d. L BP 118/78

8. It is important that patients not know their respiratory rate is being measured because:

a. the rate changes when patients are aware

b. respiration depths are fragile and difficult to measure

c. the rhythm remains stable regardless of what it normally is

d. awareness changes the accompanying blood pressure reading

9. Individuals who regularly engage in cardiovascular exercise activities:

a. have a consistently higher heart rate

b. have a consistently lower pulse

c. exhibit slower, deeper breathing

d. exhibit faster, shallower breathing

10. Temperatures tend to be _____ in the early part of the day.

a. more variable

b. more consistent

c. higher

d. lower

TRUE/FALSE

Indicate whether the statement is true (T) or false (F).

_____ 1. Ovulation and pregnancy cause the body temperature to rise.

_____ 2. Children have slower pulses.

_____ 3. Body temperature varies slightly in concert with variations in outside weather temperatures.

_____ 4. Shaking a traditional glass thermometer can cause the mercury level to decrease faster.

_____ 5. Temperature-sensitive tape thermometers are placed on the patient's forearm to obtain an accurate reading.

_____ 6. A stethoscope is a device used to amplify blood pressure sounds.

_____ 7. Clothing covering the antecubital area is removed prior to measuring brachial blood pressure to avoid entangling the sphygmomanometer tubes.

_____ 8. Pulse is generally measured for sixty seconds; the result is then multiplied by two to obtain an accurate reading.

_____ 9. Hypertensive patients have low blood pressure readings.

_____ 10. Patients with bradycardia have a slow pulse.

FILL IN THE BLANK

Using words from the list below, fill in the blanks to complete the following statements.

12–20 bpm	Fahrenheit	salt
<120/<85	hypertension	systolic
97°F–99°F	pulse	tympanic
Celsius		

1. The normal respiratory rate for an adult is _____.

2. A patient with a blood pressure reading of 145/95 would be considered to have mild _____.

3. Normal blood pressure values for an adult are _____.

4. The sharp tapping first heard as blood pressure is being measured indicates the _____ measurement.

5. _____ thermometers have lines representing 94°–108° marked in even degree and 0.2° increments.

6. _____ thermometers have lines representing 34°–42° marked in single degree and 0.1° increments.

7. _____ thermometers measure temperature in the ear canal.

8. Normal oral and ear canal temperatures are _____.

9. _____ ingestion increases blood pressure.

10. The throbbing in the arteries as a result of the heartbeat is the _____.

CHAPTER 24
Dental Instruments

CHAPTER OUTLINE

Review the Chapter Outline. If any content area is unclear, review that area before beginning the workbook exercises.

A. Identifying Hand Instruments
   1. Hand Instrument Design
   2. Instrument Classifications
   3. G. V. Black's Instrument Formula
   4. Categories of Dental Instruments
   5. Dental Examination Instruments
   6. Restorative Instruments
   7. Adjunctive Dental Instruments

B. Rotary Equipment
   1. Dental Handpieces
   2. Rotary Cutting Instruments
   3. Dental Burs
   4. Diamond Rotary Instruments
   5. Finishing Rotary Instruments
   6. Abrasive Rotary Instruments
   7. Laboratory Rotary Instruments

C. Instrument Systems
   1. Cassette Systems
   2. Tub and Tray Systems

CHAPTER REVIEW

The following is a summary of the chapter. If any of this material is unclear, review it in the textbook again.

The onset of dental technology continues to expand the variety of dental instruments available for use within each facet of the dental profession. Each hand or rotary instrument available performs a particular function during patient treatment. The basic instruments used in the practice of general dentistry include cutting and noncutting instruments. The two categories of cutting instruments are hand-cutting and rotary. Hand-cutting instruments smooth cavity walls, refine cavity preparations, and remove soft debris. Rotary instruments accomplish the same as hand-cutting but with the use of compressed air and/or water with electronic speed. The high-speed handpiece with a selection of burs is used to remove gross debris; the slow-speed handpiece is used to refine and remove soft debris. The instrument to be used is dictated by the specific treatment procedure. The dental assistant's responsibility is to keep the instruments sterilized, organized, and in pristine working condition. For best time-management and accuracy in restoration outcome, the dental assistant keeps the instrument tray set up in order of instrument use.

LEARNING ACTIVITIES AND STUDY AIDS

Review the following study aids and/or complete the activities to ensure that you have achieved the learning objectives for this chapter.

1. The KaVo Dental high-speed handpiece is equipped with a fiber-optic light. List two advantages of using a fiber-optic handpiece, and how it is maintained.

2. List the six categories of instruments with their function of use classified by Dr. G. V. Black.

3. Compare and contrast hand-cutting instruments and rotary instruments.

4. List an advantage of working with a double-ended dental instrument.

5. How does Dr. G. V. Black's instrument formula help dental assistants identify specific dental instruments?

6. What is the importance of sequential placement of instruments from left to right within the procedure tray?

7. List the instruments used in operative dentistry for cutting or refining cavity preparations for amalgam placement.

8. The dentist uses a spoon excavator to remove soft debris, decay, and dentin from the tooth preparation. Typically the next hand-cutting instrument to be used would be the chisel. How would the dentist use this instrument, and what purpose does the chisel instrument serve?

9. Dental burs are available in a variety of shapes, functions, and sizes. When the dentist desires a specific bur for use within the cavity preparation, he/she will request the bur by its number, and the dental assistant immediately understands what bur is needed using the numbered bur system for a particular function.

   a. Describe the function of the round bur, and provide a 1–6 number range of these burs, beginning with the smallest number.

   b. Describe proper sterilization of dental burs.

c.   Name the three parts of the dental bur, and identify the part that is placed into the turbine of the high-speed handpiece.

10.   Match the word in Column A with the correct definition in Column B by placing the corresponding letter on the line provided.

Table 24-1

Column A	Column B
A. spoon excavator	_____ transports freshly prepared amalgam material to the cavity preparation
B. enamel hatchet	_____ used for condensing and contouring composite resin material
C. chisel	_____ designed to cleave or cut enamel along the lines of enamel rods
D. hoe	_____ used to smooth and polish amalgam restoration and remove scratches left from carving instruments
E. gingival margin trimmer	_____ used with a pulling motion to smooth and shape the floor of a cavity preparation
F. amalgam carrier	_____ its sharp cutting edges are used to shape, form, and cut tooth anatomy into amalgam preparation
G. condenser	_____ operates at 380,000 rpm to 400,000 rpm; used in cavity preparation to remove bulk enamel, dentin, or old restorations
H. carver	_____ double-ended instrument with a spoon- or disk-shaped blade; used to remove debris, decay, and dentin from tooth preparation
I. burnisher	_____ operates at 5,000 rpm to 80,000 rpm; used to remove caries, refine cavity preparation, perform coronal polish, and adjust restorations and acrylics
J. composite resin instrument	_____ modified hatchet that has working ends with opposite curvatures and bevels; used on distal and mesial surface of a restoration

(continued)

(continued)

K. high-speed hand-piece	_____ three varieties: long straight (HP), latch-type (RA), and friction grip (FG)
L. slow-speed hand-piece	_____ used to cleave or split unsupported enamel by dentin along the lines of enamel rods, and smooth and sharpen cavity walls
M. dental bur shank	_____ also called a plugger, used to condense or pack amalgam filling material into the cavity preparation

MEDICAL TERMINOLOGY REVIEW

Use a dictionary and/or your textbook to define the following terms.

12-bladed bur _____

air abrasion _____

amalgam _____

basic setup _____

bevel _____

bin-angle _____

burnisher _____

carriers _____

carvers _____

chisel _____

composite resin instrument _____

condenser _____

contra-angle _____

cotton pliers _____

dental bur _____

dental handpiece _____

diamond bur _____

Dr. G. V. Black _____

enamel hatchet _____

fiber optics _____

friction grip _____

fulcrum _____

gingival margin trimmer _____

G.V. Black's Instrument Formula _____

hand-cutting instrument _____

hatchet _____

high-speed handpiece _____

hoe _____

mandrel _____

mono-angled _____

mouth mirror _____

nib _____

periodontal probe _____

plastic filling instrument _____

prophy angle _____

shank _____

slow- or low-speed handpiece _____

spoon excavator _____

straight attachment _____

triple-angled _____

tub and tray system _____

working end _____

ABBREVIATIONS

F _____

FDA _____

FG _____

HP _____

R _____

RA _____

RPM _____

CRITICAL THINKING

1. How does knowing the names and functions of all dental instruments help the dental assistant accomplish his/her responsibilities?

2. List and describe the three basic parts (components) and functions of each component for every hand instrument. Which portion is the longest? What is the average length of a dental hand instrument? What other information may be found on the handle of an instrument?

3. How is G. V. Black's classification of dental instruments helpful to the dental assistant?

4. What instruments are contained within a BDS (basic dental set up)? What functions do these instruments have?

CHAPTER REVIEW TEST

MULTIPLE CHOICE

Circle the letter of the correct answer.

1. The _____ is **not** part of the dental hand instrument.
   a. flute
   b. handle
   c. shank
   d. working end

2. The three basic components of a dental hand instrument include the handle, _____, and working end.
   a. nib
   b. fiber optics
   c. bin angle
   d. shank

3. The high-speed handpiece uses _____ burs.
   a. latch-type
   b. friction-grip
   c. mandrels and
   d. snap-on

4. A mandrel is used to:

   a. attach finishing and polishing devices to the handpiece
   b. finish the occlusal surface of a restoration
   c. polish the interproximal surface of a restoration
   d. remove soft decay from the cavity preparation

5. A _____ is used primarily to remove decay and/or soft dentin within the cavity preparation.

   a. dental explorer
   b. dental hatchet hand-cutting instrument
   c. dental hoe hand-cutting instrument
   d. dental spoon excavator instrument

6. The _____ formula was developed to standardize the exact size, width, and angulation of an instrument.

   a. manufacturer's number   c. Gold's Black
   b. G. V. Black's   d. scientific number

7. The instrument(s) used to assist in cavity preparation design are:

   a. large and small double-ended amalgam carrier
   b. dental carver
   c. acorn amalgam burnisher
   d. hand-cutting instrument

8. It is important to polish dental amalgam, composite, and gold restorations to improve appearance and longevity of the restoration. This is accomplished by using:

   a. impregnated soft rubber cups, points, wheels, and disks
   b. impregnated fluted dental burs in the high-speed handpiece
   c. the right-angle with the slow-speed and burnisher
   d. the straight slow-speed with a long shank cutting disk

9. The _____ system prevents the dental team from becoming injured by a contaminated sharp instrument during transportation and cleaning.

   a. tub and tray   c. color-coded
   b. cassette system   d. scrub brush

10. The shepherd's hook explorer is identified or referred to as the _____ explorer.

   a. # 17 right-angle   c. # 23 semicircle
   b. # 2 pigtail   d. # 8 long handle

TRUE/FALSE

Indicate whether the statement is true (T) or false (F).

_____ 1. Dental hand instruments have three basic components.

_____ 2. Dr. G. V. White developed the classification of dental instruments.

_____ 3. The periodontal probe is used to probe root contours when exploring for calculus and root roughness.

_____ 4. Condensers, carvers, and burnishers are all instruments used in amalgam restorations.

_____ 5. When placing a composite resin, only noncoated stainless steel instruments are used.

_____ 6. All dental handpieces use air and water as a cooling mechanism.

_____ 7. High-speed handpieces range from 380,000 rpm to 400,000 rpm, and are used for cavity preparations to remove bulk enamel, dentin, or old restorations.

_____ 8. Fiber optics is when the light travels through the fibers, reflecting without heat generating.

_____ 9. All high-speed handpieces should be sterilized in immersion solution.

_____ 10. Another term for "air abrasion" is "microdentistry."

FILL IN THE BLANK

Using words from the list below, fill in the blanks to complete the following statements.

excavator	explorer	working
shank	hoe	Arkansas
air/water syringe	finishing	enamel hatchet
carbide burs	cotton pliers	

1. The _____ end of the handpiece is where burs, stones, and attachments are held.

2. _____ burs have at least twelve blades.

3. The _____ part of the instrument connects the handle to the working end.

4. _____ are used to transport and manipulate various materials. They are available in locking or nonlocking handles.

5. The _____ hand instrument's working end is a thin, sharp point of flexible steel.

6. A(n) _____ cutting instrument is designed to cleave or cut enamel to prepare the walls of a cavity preparation.

7. Dental _____ are used with a pulling motion to smooth and shape the floor and sides of a cavity preparation.

8. When manually sharpening hand-cutting instruments, a _____ sharpening stone is used.

9. Laboratory burs are larger _____ with a normal shank.

10. The _____, which is used to remove carious material, has a cutting edge that is rounded all the way around the periphery of the blade.

CHAPTER 25
Ergonomics

CHAPTER OUTLINE

Review the Chapter Outline. If any content area is unclear, review that area before beginning the workbook exercises.

A. Ergonomics in the Dental Office
   1. Risk Factors

B. Posture
   1. The Neutral Position
   2. Horizontal Reach

C. Injuries Sustained by Dental Assistants
   1. Musculoskeletal Disorders

D. Muscle-Strengthening Exercises

E. Four-Handed Dentistry
   1. Practicing Four-Handed Dentistry

F. Motion Economy

G. Operating Zones

H. The Expanded-Function Dental Assistant
   1. Knowledge and Skills Required of the EFDA

CHAPTER REVIEW

The following is a summary of the chapter. If any of this material is unclear, review it in the textbook again.

Simply put, ergonomics is the science of making things and procedures fit people rather than the other way around. The dental assistant who understands and practices the principles of ergonomics can avoid pain, improve the quality of his/her working life, reduce stress and strain on the members of the dental team, and increase the productivity and profitability of a dental practice. Simple techniques such as maintaining correct working posture and position, using equipment correctly, conserving energy by practicing motion economy, and performing short simple muscle exercises several times a day are the keys. Conversely, a dental assistant who does not put the principles of ergonomics into practice is a strong candidate for the painful musculoskeletal and cumulative trauma disorders that result from the repetitive nature and force of the tasks dental assistants routinely perform.

LEARNING ACTIVITIES AND STUDY AIDS

Review the following study aids and/or complete the activities to ensure that you have achieved the learning objectives for this chapter.

1. List the three major causes of musculoskeletal and cumulative trauma disorders.

2. State the goal of practicing four-handed dentistry.

3. Outline the ergonomic principles on which four-handed dentistry is based.

4. To fully understand the functions that only an expanded-function dental assistant can perform in your state, go online to research your state practice dental act. Write a short paragraph outlining what you learned.

5. Complete the following table by listing each zone, location, and use of the four activity zones used in four-handed dentistry.

Table 25-1

Zone	Location/Side	Use

6. Describe the neutral position.

7. List seven practices that decrease the risk of injury for a dental assistant during daily work activities.

8. Define motion economy, and state why it is practiced.

9. List and define the classes of motion.

10. Define and describe carpal tunnel syndrome.

MEDICAL TERMINOLOGY REVIEW

Use a dictionary and/or your textbook to define the following terms.

assistant's zone _____

carpal tunnel syndrome _____

cumulative trauma disorder _____

ergonomics _____

expanded-function dental assistant _____

four-handed dentistry _____

fulcrum _____

motion economy _____

musculoskeletal disorder _____

operating zone _____

sprain _____

static zone _____

strain _____

transfer zone _____

ABBREVIATIONS

CTD _____

CTS _____

EFDA _____

MSD _____

CRITICAL THINKING

1. How can the overall use of good or bad ergonomics affect the members of the dental care team, as a whole and individually?

2. What are some things a dental assistant can do to prevent musculoskeletal injuries?

3. How does the position of the operatory light affect the operator, patient, and overall procedure?

4. What are some strategies/techniques the dental assistant can use to ensure proper posture when treating a patient?

CHAPTER REVIEW TEST

MULTIPLE CHOICE

Circle the letter of the correct answer.

1. What is the goal of motion economy?
   a. energy conservation
   b. improved vision
   c. increased speed of practice
   d. avoidance of other team members' zones

2. Carpal tunnel syndrome is a common result of:
    a. placing too much force on muscles that grasp a small instrument
    b. using instruments that are too slender and too small
    c. repetitively overusing muscles that extend and flex the wrist
    d. positioning the light such that poor posture is necessary for vision

3. Describe the supine position for a patient.
    a. head is approximately 35° higher than the spine
    b. head rest supports patient's head comfortably
    c. knees are approximately four inches higher than the chin
    d. knees and nose are on the same level

4. The positions of the operator and assistant practicing four-handed dentistry are designed to:
    a. minimize patient discomfort
    b. provide access and visibility
    c. reduce the amount of oral fluid secreted
    d. relax the patient as much as possible

5. The benefits of stretching muscles include increased:
    a. blood flow
    b. flexibility
    c. joint lubrication
    d. a and c
    e. all of the above

6. What type of instrument handle is recommended for use in dental practice?
    a. short and slender
    b. slender and textured
    c. long and large
    d. large and textured

7. The major disadvantage of using ambidextrous gloves is:
    a. poor fit results in the application of uneven pressures on the hand
    b. repetitive hand washing may cause tingling and numbness of the hand
    c. loss of feeling in the fingertips may result in grasping with too much force
    d. a and c
    e. all of the above

8. Pressure on the median nerve causes:
    a. carpal tunnel syndrome
    b. tingling in the thumb and first two fingers
    c. debilitating pain in the elbow
    d. a and b
    e. b and c

9. Daily overuse of certain muscle groups causes:
    a. loss of tissue feeling
    b. tissue fatigue and inflammation
    c. atrophy of the muscle fibers
    d. fiber stretching and softening

10. Instruments, equipment, and supplies should be placed _____ the working dental assistant.
    a. to the side of
    b. in front of
    c. behind
    d. next to

TRUE/FALSE

Indicate whether the statement is true (T) or false (F).

_____ 1. Instrument transfer always takes place above and across the patient's chin.

_____ 2. To practice efficiently, dental team members must stick to practicing only their assigned roles.

_____ 3. Dentists work more efficiently sitting down, but assistants have greater visibility and can operate more efficiently when standing up.

_____ 4. Sprains and strains typically result from overstretching ligaments and muscles.

_____ 5. When practicing four-handed dentistry, the dental assistant's eyes should be at the same level as the operator's eyes.

_____ 6. The dental assistant's torso should be conserved by using it for rotation and twisting to reach for items that are above and behind the assistant.

_____ 7. The amount of force placed on a muscle group can be more harmful than the number of repetitions.

_____ 8. Improper head positioning and poor posture can cause headaches.

_____ 9. To avoid muscle injury, it is important to maintain the same position as long as possible.

_____ 10. The most likely time to feel the pain of carpal tunnel syndrome is early morning.

FILL IN THE BLANK

Using words from the list below, fill in the blanks to complete the following statements.

downward	fist clenches	parallel
elbow	front	shoulder/chest/elbow
ergonomically	hand circles	upward
finger spread	informed	

1. _____ stretches can help loosen muscles in the chest and shoulder area.

2. Extension of the _____ joint helps realign the skeleton.

3. _____ can exercise the wrists.

4. Pressure and tension in the hand can be relieved by _____.

5. A _____ will help to increase circulation in the hand.

6. Dental equipment must be _____ designed to minimize repetitive motion.

7. The patient should always be _____ before the chair is adjusted.

8. When positioning the operating light for work on the maxillary arch, the light is always directed _____ before turning it on, then tilted _____.

9. When serving as an operator, the dental assistant's thighs are positioned _____ to the floor.

10. The _____ edge of the dental assistant's chair should be positioned _____ with the patient's mouth.

CHAPTER 26
Moisture Control

CHAPTER OUTLINE

Review the Chapter Outline. If any content area is unclear, review that area before beginning the workbook exercises.

    A. Oral Evacuation Systems
        1. High-Velocity Evacuator (HVE)
        2. Saliva Ejector—Low-Volume Evacuator (LVE)
        3. Surgical Suction Tips
        4. Air/Water Syringe
        5. Daily Maintenance of the Evacuation System

    B. Rinsing the Oral Cavity
        1. Limited Area Rinsing
        2. Complete Mouth Rinsing

    C. Isolation of the Teeth
        1. Cotton Roll Isolation
        2. Dry Angle Isolation
        3. Dental Dam Isolation

    D. The Dental Dam
        1. Dental Dam Frame
        2. Dental Dam Napkin
        3. Dental Dam Lubricants
        4. Dental Dam Stamp and Template
        5. Dental Dam Punch
        6. Dental Dam Forceps
        7. Dental Dam Clamps
        8. Dental Dam Stabilizing Cord

    E. Dental Dam Placement and Removal

    F. The Quickdam

    G. Special Applications for the Dental Dam

CHAPTER REVIEW

The following is a summary of the chapter. If any of this material is unclear, review it in the textbook again.

Moisture control is an integral part of the operative dental procedure. A knowledgeable chairside dental assistant achieves a clear field of vision for all dental procedures by using the isolation technique required for each procedure. By using the proper hand grasp for the HVE and air/water syringe, the dental assistant is able to quickly maintain isolation and visibility. The dental assistant must keep current on the CDC and OSHA guidelines and recommendations on dental waterline disinfection and biofilm reduction within the dental unit's evacuation system. Keeping biofilm under 200 colony forming units (CFUs) ensures a safe range of biofilm. Many isolation techniques can be used for each procedure. Maintaining a dry field of vision can be accomplished by placing a cotton roll within the muccobuccal fold of the maxillary arch and/or on the lingual side of the mandible and under the tongue. Dri-angle isolation involves the use of a triangular absorbent pad that isolates posterior areas in both the maxillary and mandibular arches over the Stenson's duct of the parotid gland. The dental dam is a thin, stretchable latex material used as a barrier for either a single tooth or a section of teeth. The dental dam allows for the highest level of moisture control for dental procedures. Some advantages are infection control, protection of the patient's oral cavity from contact with debris and infectious material of an infected tooth, protecting the patient from inhaling or ingesting small tooth or dental material, providing better visibility, and increasing dental team efficiency.

LEARNING ACTIVITIES AND STUDY AIDS

Review the following study aids and/or complete the activities to ensure that you have achieved the learning objectives for this chapter.

1. List the instruments to be used for isolation in the endodontic procedure.

2. How does the dental assistant maintain a clear vision of the operating field?

3. Write a description of each hole punch that correlates to the appropriate tooth: Hole size 5, Hole size 4, Hole size 3, Hole size 2, and Hole size 1

4. List some methods of reducing airborne contamination.

5. Using cotton roll isolation, list the areas of the oral cavity where cotton rolls are placed in the mandibular and maxillary.

6. List the equipment needed for rubber dam placement.

7. In the following table, provide the placement of the HVE tip to correlate with the operator position.

Table 26-1

HVE Tip Placement	Operator Position
	Right-handed operator is working on the buccal of any maxillary or mandibular molar
	Operator is working on the facial surface of any maxillary or mandibular anterior tooth
	Operator is working on the left side of the oral cavity
	Operator is working on the lingual surface of any maxillary or mandibular anterior tooth

8. When assisting a right-handed operator, the dental assistant holds the air/water syringe in his/her left hand and the HVE in the right hand. Fill in the blanks below as related to using the air/water syringe at maximum efficiency.
   a. Turn the tip of the air/water syringe in the _____ of the arch, _____ for the maxilla, and _____ for the mandible.
   b. To minimize aerosol, keep a _____ distance between the operative site and the syringe tip.
   c. To thoroughly cleanse the site, place the tip _____ over the opening of the preparation when a cavity preparation is being flushed.
   d. Be assertive in cleansing a site. Place the tip within _____, and press firmly on the buttons to cleanse the area.
   e. Quickly move the syringe tip into the area to be _____, then flush, _____, and move the tip out of the area quickly.

9. List the suggested procedures for daily maintenance of the evacuation system.

10. Compare and contrast "limited area rinsing" and "complete mouth rinsing."

MEDICAL TERMINOLOGY REVIEW

Use a dictionary and/your textbook to define the following terms.

air/water syringe _____

biofilm _____

complete mouth rinse _____

cotton roll isolation _____

dental dam _____

dental dam clamps _____

dental dam forceps _____

dental dam frame _____

dental dam lubricants _____

dental dam napkin _____

dental dam punch _____

dental dam stabilizing cord _____

dental dam stamp and template _____

dry angle _____

high-velocity evacuator (HVE) _____

isolation _____

limited area mouth rinse _____

lingua-fix _____

oral evacuation _____

pen grasp _____

quick dam _____

saliva ejector _____

self-contained system _____

surgical suction tips _____

thumb-nose grasp _____

ABBREVIATIONS

CDC _____

CEJ _____

HVE _____

OSHA _____

PFI _____

CRITICAL THINKING

1. Why is maintaining a clear, dry working field so critical to the success of a procedure?

2. In which areas of the mouth is the pen grasp normally used for holding the HVE suction tip?

3. In which areas of the mouth is the thumb-to-nose grasp normally used when holding the HVE suction tip?

4. How does the saliva ejector differ from the HVE? Which procedures is the saliva ejector best suited for?

CHAPTER REVIEW TEST

MULTIPLE CHOICE

Circle the letter of the correct answer.

1. Which of the following is used to remove small amounts of fluid and debris from the oral cavity?
   a. The salvia ejector
   b. The oral evacuator
   c. The HVE
   d. The air/water syringe

2. Water and debris that is suctioned from the mouth through the evacuator tip (HVE) goes into
   _____
   a. The cuspidor
   b. The filter
   c. The sink
   d. A recycling center

3. Hole size _____ is used for the anchor tooth, which holds the rubber dam clamp
   a. No. 1
   b. No. 3
   c. No. 4
   d. No. 5

4. The HVE handle may be held in a _____ grasp
   a. Reverse pen
   b. Pen
   c. Pen and thumb-to-nose
   d. Modified pen

5. When the operator is working on the facial surface of a maxillary anterior tooth, the HVE should be placed on the _____ of the tooth being worked on.
   a. Facial portion
   b. Buccal portion
   c. Lingual portion
   d. Occlusal portion

6. A limited rinse is one that _____.
   a. Is completed at the beginning of the procedure
   b. Is completed at the end of the procedure
   c. Rinses the whole mouth
   d. Rinses a specific area in the mouth

7. The main function of the saliva ejector is to _____
   a. Remove fluids and liquids from the oral cavity
   b. Remove large pieces of tooth material from the oral cavity
   c. Give the patient something to distract them
   d. Remove medicaments from the oral cavity

8. The microscopic bacteria found in the air/water syringe is called

   a. bacteri
   b. dental
   c. Biofilm
   d. Infectious biofilm

9. The CDC and OSHA recommend specific guidelines for maintaining the evacuation system. They indicate to flush all hoses between patients for _____ with the dental unit water.
   a. One minute
   b. 20–30 second
   c.
   d. 5 seconds

10. When using cotton roll isolation the cotton should be placed close to the _____ within the vestibule or under the tongue.
   a. Salivary gland ducts
   b. Retro-molar pad
   c. Anterior
   d. teeth

TRUE/FALSE

Indicate whether the statement is true (T) or false (F).

_____ 1. The most common size of precut rubber dam material for utilization in the posterior is 6 × 6.

_____ 2. The dental dam instrument used to place holes into the dam material is the forceps.

_____ 3. The dental dam clamp is used for anchoring and stabilizing the dental dam.

_____ 4. Surgical suction tips are all one size, large, to suction small pieces of bone fragments.

_____ 5. When using the Lingua-Fix suction the dental assistant would place the Lingua-Fix into the HVE hose line.

_____ 6. The dental assistant will only use the Lingua-Fix suction with the air/water syringe.

_____ 7. The air/water syringe is primarily used to rinse and dry the oral cavity.

_____ 8. When utilizing the air/water syringe the dental assistant should keep it in their left hand and the HVE in their right hand.

_____ 9. Self contained water reservoirs are used to prevent contaminated biofilm from entering the oral cavity.

_____ 10. A "complete mouth rinse" is preformed at the beginning of the procedure.

FILL IN THE BLANK

Using words from the list below, fill in the blanks to complete the following statements.

Dental Dam	mandibular	aerostation
Cotton roll	frame	Stenson's duct
Maxillary	Isolation	Ostby
Dri-angle	stylus	

1. _____ is the act of keeping a tooth or an area separate or dry.

2. _____ isolation involves the use of tightly formed absorbent pre-shaped cotton.

3. The CDC does not recommend rinsing the oral cavity with the air/water aerated spray do to _____.

4. The dental dam _____ is made or either a durable plastic or metal material.

5. _____ isolation technique involves the use of a triangular absorbent pad.

6. The _____ is a thin stretchable latex or latex-free material used as the highest level of moisture control.

7. The number 4 hole in the dental dam punch is used for _____ molars

8. The _____ frame is a round plastic frame with sharp projections on its outer margin.

9. When using the dri-angle the pad is placed directly over the _____.

10. When punching a hole in the dental dam it is important that the _____ remain positioned directly over the corresponding hole.

CHAPTER 27
Pharmacology

CHAPTER OUTLINE

Review the Chapter Outline. If any content area is unclear, review that area before beginning the workbook exercises.

A. Overview of Drugs

B. Identification and Classification of Drugs

C. Dispensing of Drugs

D. Prescriptions

E. Calls Regarding Patient Medications

F. Drug Reference Materials

G. Drug Administration

H. Controlled Substances Act

I. Classifications of Drugs

J. Antibiotic Prophylaxis

K. Adverse Drug Effects

CHAPTER REVIEW

The following is a summary of the chapter. If any of this material is unclear, review it in the textbook again.

Drugs are used for a variety of reasons, including curing and/or preventing diseases and disorders, and prolonging the life of patients with incurable conditions. Three government agencies deal with the regulation of drugs in the United States: the Food and Drug Administration, Drug Enforcement Administration, and Federal Trade Commission. When researching a drug using the *Physician's Desk Reference* (PDR) manual, the dental assistant should be familiar with prescription drugs' generic and trade names. How drugs are administered depends on how fast or slow the drug takes effect. Understanding this concept prepares the dental assistant in educating patients regarding prescribed drugs. The more knowledgeable the dental assistant is about pharmacokinetics, the better he/she is in communicating matters on adverse drug effects. The American Heart Association (AHA) often updates the standards of antibiotic prophylaxis within dentistry. Frequent access of the AHA Web site for updates on the latest standards of care provides useful information related to the premedication of patients.

LEARNING ACTIVITIES AND STUDY AIDS

Review the following study aids and/or complete the activities to ensure that you have achieved the learning objectives for this chapter.

1. How can alcohol increase the effects of a stimulant?

2. A patient's medical history indicates that the patient has been taking antidepressants for ten years. The patient states that she plans to stop taking the antidepressant when her prescription runs out. The dental assistant documents this information on the chart for the dentist to assess. What is the importance of this information?

3. Using the Internet or materials in your school or local library, research software programs that reference drug information. Find one type of software program, research it, and then on a separate piece of paper write a half-page to one-page report on your findings. Suggested sites include *http://www.healthsquare.com/drugmain.htm*, *http://www.healthatoz.com/healthatoz/Atoz/clients/haz/general/custom/default.jsp*, and *http://www.drugs.com/*

4. To further understand writing and reading prescriptions, write the following information on the blank prescription pad provided. As appropriate, use the common abbreviations seen on prescriptions.

DEA # 1234 Adam Sandler, DDS, 1526 Sunset Strip, Los Angeles, California, 09543

Patient name: Betty Robinson Age: 22 Date: 1-6-08

Address: 8729 Hardwood Ave. Cherry Blossom, California, 09365

Keflex, 10 mg dispense, 20 tablets, take every 8 hours or four times a day for 5 days, until gone. Brand name only, no refills.

```
┌─────────────────────────────────────────────┐
│ DEA#                                          │
│                                               │
│                                               │
│                                               │
│  Patient name: _____  Age: ____ │
│  Address: _____  Date: _____ │
│  _____      │
│                                               │
│  Rx                                           │
│                                               │
│                                               │
│                                               │
│  Refill                                       │
│  Signature                                    │
│                                               │
└─────────────────────────────────────────────┘
```

5. Complete the following table, listing the schedule of the drug and examples of each scheduled drug.

Table 27-1

Schedule	Description	Examples
	Mixtures with limited opiates.	
	Have no current accepted or medical use. Prescriptions are not usually written for these drugs.	
	Does have acceptable medical use. Requires a written prescription and can be renewed or refilled. Routinely used in dental offices.	
	Does have acceptable medical use. Requires a written prescription and can be renewed or refilled. Routinely used in dental offices.	
	Does have acceptable medical use. Requires a written prescription and cannot be renewed or refilled. These drugs can lead to addiction.	

6. When is the use of antibiotic prophylaxis recommended by the American Heart Association (AHA)? On a piece of paper, list the types of individuals who would fall into this category. For more information, go to *http://www.americanheart.org/presenter.jhtml?identifier=4548*

7. What are the four stages that a drug undergoes once it enters the body?

8. List the four classifications of drugs.

9. What bacterium found in the oral cavity concerns the dental healthcare provider, and why?

0. If the pharmacist calls the office regarding a patient's prescription and concerns about the patient's medical history, is it appropriate for the dental assistant to handle this call? Why or why not?

1. Using a PDR or similar information source, look up the drug Plavix to answer the following questions:

   a. What is the generic name?

   b. What is the brand name?

   c. What is it used for?

   d. What medications, if any, interact with Plavix?

   e. What are some side effects?

   f. Overdose information?

   g. Color and size of Plavix?

MEDICAL TERMINOLOGY REVIEW

Use a dictionary and/or your textbook to define the following terms.

Absorption _____

Adverse effect _____

Analgesic _____

body _____

brand names _____

closing _____

distribution _____

drug allergy _____

drug hypersensitivity _____

drug interaction _____

drug monograph _____

ethical drug _____

excretion _____

generic _____

habituation _____

heading _____

inscription _____

metabolism _____

monograph _____

official name _____

parenteral _____

patent drugs _____

pharmacokinetics _____

pharmacology _____

premedication _____

side effect _____

streptococcus viridians _____

subacute bacterial endocarditis _____

sublingual _____

therapeutic effect _____

topically _____

trade name _____

ABBREVIATIONS

CSA _____

DEA _____

FDA _____

FTC _____

OTC _____

PDR _____

SBE _____

CRITICAL THINKING

1. Why is it important to know the difference between a generic name for a drug and the brand name?

2. Why is it important for the dental assistant to have a working knowledge of pharmacology.

3. What role does the dental assistant have in discussing medications with a patient?

CHAPTER REVIEW TEST

MULTIPLE CHOICE

Circle the letter of the correct answer.

1. The abbreviation PDR stands for:
   a. Physician's Dictionary Reference
   b. Physician's Dental Reference
   c. Patient Drug Reference
   d. Physicians Drug Reference

2. An acute allergic reaction that can be life threatening is known as:
   a. acidosis
   b. anaphylaxis
   c. angina
   d. asthmatic attack

3. The part of a prescription where the DEA number is found is called the:
   a. body
   b. closing
   c. heading
   d. beginning

4. The term "patent drugs" refers to drugs purchased:
   a. by a prescription
   b. by a prescription without a DEA number
   c. over the counter
   d. with an approved CDA identification

5. Schedule V drugs are placed in this category:
   a. least dangerous
   b. most addictive
   c. most harmful
   d. least allergic reactions

6. Patients who present with a history of rheumatic fever should be given _____ to dental treatment.
   a. SBE prior
   b. antibiotic prophylaxis prior
   c. antibiotic therapy after
   d. SBE after

7. An allergic reaction is caused by an:
   a. allergen
   b. analgesic
   c. antihistamine
   d. none of the above

8. Directions written on a prescription, "Sig: 1 stat 1 qid til gone" is read:
   a. take one tablet now and one four times a day until all medication is completed
   b. take one tablet now and four tablets a day until all medication is completed
   c. take one tablet now and two tablets a day until all medication is completed
   d. take four tablets now and one a day until all medication is completed

9. The term "drug monograph" refers to:
   a. drug name, strength, and purity only
   b. drug classification schedule only
   c. drug description, name, chemical formula, strength, and purity
   d. drug description and interactions only

10. When referring to the route of administration of a drug, the term "parenteral" refers to:
    a. through tissue
    b. under the tongue
    c. through injection
    d. by mouth

TRUE/FALSE

Indicate whether the statement is true (T) or false (F).

_____ 1. Aspirin is a Schedule I drug.

_____ 2. All drugs must have a registered U.S. patent name.

_____ 3. The dental assistant can call in a prescription over the phone for the patient.

_____ 4. When a patient becomes physically dependent on a drug, it is called "obsession."

_____ 5. The Drug Enforcement Administration and the Federal Trade Commission regulate drugs.

_____ 6. Federal law requires that all prescriptions have a heading, body, and closing.

_____ 7. The term that describes the exact chemical structure of a drug is the "chemical name."

_____ 8. All narcotic prescriptions for a patient can be called in.

_____ 9. Prescriptions do not need to contain Latin abbreviations.

_____ 10. The effect that is desired by taking a drug is called the "therapeutic effect."

FILL IN THE BLANK

Using words from the list below, fill in the blanks to complete the following statements.

prescription	generic	tid
at bedtime	Schedule V	CSA
Schedule I	dose	pharmacokinetics
premedication	orally	

1. The term _____ is used for the amount of drug to be administered.

2. A _____ is a written authorization or order for a drug.

3. _____ is the study of how drugs enter the body, circulate, and exit the body.

4. _____ is the abbreviation for "twice a day."

5. For the slowest rate of absorption, a drug would be taken _____

6. _____ are drugs sold without a brand name and/or trademark.

7. Drugs that are most dangerous and have no recognized medical use are found in _____.

8. The Latin abbreviation "hs" means _____.

9. A patient with an artificial heart valve scheduled for an extraction is given _____ at least one hour prior to the appointment.

10. Depending on the potential for addiction and abuse, a drug is controlled by the _____.

CHAPTER 28
Anesthesia and Pain Control

CHAPTER OUTLINE

Review the Chapter Outline. If any content area is unclear, review that area before beginning the workbook exercises.

A. Local and Topical Anesthetic Agents
   1. Topical Anesthesia
   2. Local Anesthesia
   3. Local Anesthetic Solution
   4. Vasoconstrictor
   5. Duration and Action of Anesthetics

B. Injection Techniques
   1. Local Infiltration
   2. Block Anesthesia
   3. Intraosseous Anesthesia
   4. Periodontal Ligament Injection
   5. Intrapulpal Injection
   6. Computer-Controlled Local Anesthesia Delivery System

C. Local Anesthesia Setup
   1. Tray Setup
   2. Syringes
   3. Passing and Receiving the Syringe
   4. Needles
   5. Cartridges
   6. Loading the Cartridge
   7. Needle Sticks Reporting

D. Complications and Precautions
   1. Paresthesia
   2. Hemotoma
   3. Trismus

E. Electronic Anesthesia

F. Inhalation Sedation
   1. Equipment for Inhalation Sedation
   2. Safety and Precautions
   3. Medical Assessment and Monitoring
   4. N_2O/O_2 Sedation

G. Antianxiety Agents

H. Intravenous Sedation

I. General Anesthesia

J. Documentation of Anesthesia and Pain Control

CHAPTER REVIEW

The following is a summary of the chapter. If any of this material is unclear, review it in the textbook again.

It is common for patients to feel nervous and anxious about dental procedures. To control patient anxieties, medications and/or sedation may be used. The dentist determines the form of anesthesia or combination methods to control pain, depending on the patient and the procedure. The dental assistant is responsible for preparing, transferring, and caring for the anesthetic syringe and accessories. The skilled dental assistant prepares a long needle for a mandibular block, a short needle for an infiltration, nonepinephrine for patients with heart conditions, and must know when to use nitrous oxide inhalation on appropriate patients. The dental assistant must abide by the laws of Occupation Safety Health Association (OSHA) and Material Safety Data Sheets and Hazardous Waste procedures. Data collection and documentation must be clear, accurate, and detailed with preoperative and postoperative vital signs, tidal volume (inhalation sedation), time when anesthesia began and ended, type and quantity of anesthetic agent used, number of cartridges used, peak concentration administered, patient recovery time, and any adverse reactions or patient complaints.

LEARNING ACTIVITIES AND STUDY AIDS

Review the following study aids and/or complete the activities to ensure that you have achieved the learning objectives for this chapter.

1. The dentist begins a mandibular block injection and sees blood in the carpule when they aspirate. What should the dentist do next?

2. What is the first part of the anesthetic syringe that the dental assistant disassembles postoperative, and why?

3. After seating the patient, the dental assistant reviews the patient's medical history and notices that the patient is now taking an aspirin daily. What would be the next question the dental assistant would ask?

4. The dental assistant prepares the anesthetic syringe for an infiltration injection. Prior to transferring the syringe to the dentist, the dental assistant checks the needle tip. What is the purpose of checking the needle tip, and why is this important?

5. What are the various ways that topical anesthesia can be applied?

6. In the following table, match the term in Column A with its definition in Column B.

Table 28-1

Column A	Column B
A. local infiltration	_____ injection into a nerve bundle to enable diffusion to a wider area
B. field block anesthesia or regional anesthesia	_____ injection at the site of mental foramen
C. inferior alveolar nerve block	_____ injection directly into the tissue site
D. incisive nerve block	_____ injection anesthetic into the incisive papilla
E. nasopalatine nerve block	_____ injected around the nerve endings
F. maxillary nerve block	_____ given directly into the spongy bone for a single tooth or multiple teeth in the same quadrant
G. intraosseaus	_____ injection at the height of the mucobuccal fold above the distal of the maxillary second molar

7. Provide the names of each part of the aspirating syringe in the following figure.

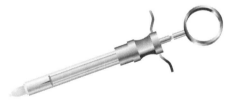

Figure 28-1

8. List the tray setup for local anesthesia.

9. OSHA requires that engineering and work practice controls be used within the dental practice to eliminate or minimize exposure to bloodborne pathogens. Define "engineering controls" and "work practice controls," and provide examples of each.

10. The dentist begins treatment on a patient and notices he/she is going into anaphylactic shock. The first step the dentist takes is to stop treatment immediately. What steps do the dentist and/or dental assistant take after stopping the treatment?

11. What is a Trieger test, and what does it assess?

MEDICAL TERMINOLOGY REVIEW

Use a dictionary and/or your textbook to define the following terms.

air embolism _____

amide anesthetic _____

analgesic _____

anesthetic _____

anxiety _____

aspirate _____

block anesthesia _____

duration _____

ester anesthetic _____

hematoma _____

induction _____

infiltration _____

intrapulpal injection _____

intravenous sedation _____

lumen _____

microair abrasion _____

pain _____

paresthesia _____

periodontal ligament injection _____

sedatives _____

titration _____

topical anesthetic _____

trismus _____

vasoconstrictor _____

wand _____

ABBREVIATIONS

ADACSA _____

GAD _____

IASP _____

IV _____

LASER _____

N_2O/O_2 _____

N_2O _____

OPIM _____

OSHA _____

pm _____

PSI _____

RA _____

CRITICAL THINKING

1. When a dental assistant places topical anesthetic prior to a local anesthesia injection, why is it important to know the length of time before the anesthetic reaches maximum effectiveness?

2. What forms of topical anesthetics are available? What are some of the more commonly used topical anesthetics? If you had a patient who suffered from a severe gag reflex while you were taking radiographs, what method might be considered to alleviate the gag reflex?

3. What are vasoconstrictors? Why are they added to local anesthesia? What is the most common vasoconstrictor added to local anesthesia? Why must the dental assistant be able to determine the type and amount of vasoconstrictor contained within a local anesthetic?

4. What are the three methods/techniques primarily used for administering local anesthesia? What areas of the mouth are these techniques for? Why is it important for the dental assistant to be able to anticipate the method of local anesthesia to be used for each procedure?

CHAPTER REVIEW TEST

MULTIPLE CHOICE

Circle the letter of the correct answer.

1. The injection method that deposits anesthesia near larger terminal nerve branches is:

   a. computerized
   b. a block injection
   c. local
   d. infiltration

2. A long needle would be used for what type of injection?

   a. mental
   b. infiltration
   c. infraorbital
   d. incisive

3. The physiological state characterized by emotions is called:

   a. anxiety
   b. analgesic stress
   c. apprehension
   d. rapid heart beat

4. An option available for providing painless or controlled pain without the use of a dental handpiece (drill) would be:

   a. laser dentistry
   b. dental etchant acid
   c. macro air abrasion
   d. water therapy

5. _____ is the type of anesthetic placed prior to injecting the gingiva.

   a. Numbing anesthesia
   b. Oral anesthesia
   c. Sedative anesthesia
   d. Topical anesthesia

6. The most common type of syringe used today is:

   a. the nonaspirating syringe
   b. the aspirating syringe
   c. the computerized syringe
   d. laser therapy

7. When the dental assistant passes the syringe, he/she holds the _____ in place as he/she places the thumb ring over the dentist's thumb.

   a. needle shield
   b. barrier cover
   c. cartridge cover
   d. needle cover

8. _____ is the sensation of feeling numb.

   a. Paresthesia
   b. Anesthesia
   c. Analgesia
   d. Sedation

9. When the dental assistant disassembles the used syringe, he/she first removes the _____ to provide an air vent.

   a. needle
   b. carpule
   c. needle cover first
   d. none of the above

10. When stocking cartridges onto shelves, it is most important to place them in order of the:

    a. expiration date
    b. label color
    c. size of the cartridge box
    d. alphabet

TRUE/FALSE

Indicate whether the statement is true (T) or false (F).

_____ 1. The harpoon is a thumb-powered piston pump on the dental syringe.

_____ 2. The first evidence of local anesthetic toxicity involves the nervous system.

_____ 3. Record-keeping standards require all dental offices to maintain strict guidelines for patients' charts.

_____ 4. Prior to placement of a local anesthetic, the dental assistant should explain the feeling of paresthesia.

_____ 5. Engineering controls are the use of sharps disposal and self-sheathing needles.

_____ 6. Hemotoma is permanent damage to the blood vessel around an injection site.

_____ 7. An OSHA 300 log is completed yearly.

_____ 8. Workplace practice controls are the measures that reduce the risk of exposure, such as eliminating the two-handed scoop technique.

_____ 9. To use inhalation sedation (laughing gas), the dentist must be specially trained.

_____ 10. If the doctor injects a patient where an infection is present, the doctor will need to use more anesthetic.

FILL IN THE BLANK

Using words from the list below, fill in the blanks to complete the following statements.

OSHA 300	lower	weighed
green	air embolism	N_2O
mental nerve block	IV scavenging	scoop
blue		

1. The term _____ is a medical condition wherein air bubbles are caught into the blood stream.

2. A _____ system is used to capture excess N_2O.

3. It is not recommended to use _____ on patients with either bowel obstructions or middle ear disturbances.

4. Nitrous oxide sedation will _____ the pain threshold without the loss of consciousness.

5. The injection _____ is used for anesthesia in the mandibular quadrant.

6. A _____ form is filled out when a used needle stick occurs.

7. The one-handed _____ technique is a safe technique to recap the anesthesia needle.

8. The national color to recognize oxygen tanks is _____.

9. To determine _____ dosage calculation, the patient must be _____.

10. Oral surgeons and periodontists with intensive anesthesia training and operation experience can perform _____ sedation.

CHAPTER 29
Dental Radiography

CHAPTER OUTLINE

Review the Chapter Outline. If any content area is unclear, review that area before beginning the workbook exercises.

A. Discovery of X-Radiation
    1. Pioneers of Dental Radiography
    2. History of the Cathode Tube

B. Radiation Physics
    1. Atomic Structure
    2. Ionization
    3. Electromagnetic Radiation

C. The Dental X-ray Unit
    1. The Control Panel
    2. The Extension Arm
    3. The Tube Head
    4. The X-ray Tube
        a. Cathode
        b. Anode

D. The Production of X-rays
    1. Types of Radiation

E. Radiation Effects
    1. Somatic and Genetic Effects
    2. Radiation Effects on Critical Organs

F. Radiation Measurement
    1. Maximum Permissible Dose

G. Radiation Safety
    1. Patient Protection
    2. Operator Protection

H. Controlling Radiation
    1. Controlling Factors
        a. mA, kVp, Exposure Time

I. Radiation Image Characteristics
    1. Density
    2. Contrast

CHAPTER REVIEW

The following is a summary of the chapter. If any of this material is unclear, review it in the textbook again.

Dental radiography is the process of producing, mounting, and diagnosing images obtained through the controlled use of ionizing radiation. Radiographs enable the dentist to visualize structures and tissues that cannot be seen on clinical inspection. Dental assistants complete nearly all of the radiograph production and mounting in a dental office. Excessive radiation exposure can cause tissue injury. Safety measures must be taken to protect the patient and operator from unnecessary exposure. The dental assistant's knowledge and skill in radiograph production is essential to the proper functioning of a dental practice and to the protection of patient and personnel health.

LEARNING ACTIVITIES AND STUDY AIDS

Review the following study aids and/or complete the activities to ensure that you have achieved the learning objectives for this chapter.

1. List the three conditions necessary to the production of radiation, and state how each is met in the dental x-ray machine.

2. Explain the basic parts of the dental x-ray machine, and the process of dental x-ray production. If more room for your information is required, utilize a separate sheet of paper.

3. Define primary, secondary, scatter, and leakage radiation.

4. State the means by which radiation damages cells.

5. Differentiate somatic and genetic effects, and radioresistant and radiosensitive tissues, then provide examples of each.

6. List and define the units of radiation measurement in the traditional and international systems.

7. Define ALARA, and state why its practice is important.

8. Differentiate MPD and MAD, and state how each is calculated.

9. List and define the means of controlling radiation that are inherent in x-ray machine design and operation.

10. Discuss the means of controlling radiation exposure through film choice, manipulation of exposure factors, and operator technique.

11. List the means of patient and operator protection that are used while radiographs are being exposed.

12. Discuss density and contrast as they relate to radiograph quality.

MEDICAL TERMINOLOGY REVIEW

Use a dictionary and/or your textbook to define the following terms.

ALARA concept _____

anode _____

atom _____

cathode _____

contrast _____

density _____

electron _____

frequency _____

impulse _____

ion _____

ionization _____

ionizing radiation _____

kilovoltage peak _____

milliampere _____

nucleus _____

photon _____

primary radiation _____

proton _____

radiograph _____

radiolucent _____

radioresistant _____

radiosensitive _____

scatter radiation _____

secondary radiation _____

thermionic emission _____

tungsten target _____

wavelength _____

x-radiation _____

ABBREVIATIONS

ALARA _____

C/kg _____

Gy _____

kVp _____

mA _____

MAD _____

MPD _____

PID _____

R _____

rad _____

rem _____

Sv _____

XPC-I _____

XPC-II _____

CRITICAL THINKING

1. What is ionizing radiation, and what does it do to human cells?

2. Why should dental assistants be concerned with the effects of ionizing radiation for their patients? For themselves?

3. What are the three types of radiation found within the dental office? Which type poses the greatest risk of dangers to the patient, and why?

4. What is the primary method available for the dental assistant to use when taking x-rays that can greatly reduce the risk of retakes and unnecessary radiation exposure?

CHAPTER REVIEW TEST

MULTIPLE CHOICE

Circle the letter of the correct answer.

1. The first dentist in the United States to expose dental radiographs on a live patient was:

    a. W. J. Morton
    b. Otto Walkoff
    c. Wilhelm Conrad Roentgen
    d. C. Edmund Kells

2. Energy results when matter is:

    a. gained
    b. lost
    c. changed
    d. none of the above

3. An ion is created when an atom:

    a. gains an electron
    b. loses an electron
    c. maintains a balance between electrons and protons
    d. a and b
    e. b and c

4. Photons are:
   a. units of light energy
   b. measures of radiation exposure
   c. positive electrodes
   d. radiation beams that have been scattered

5. The characteristics of electromagnetic waves include _____, which is the distance between the high points of the waves; _____, which is the number of waves that pass a fixed point in a given period of time; and _____, which is the height of the waves.
   a. frequency; amplitude; wavelength
   b. wavelength; frequency; amplitude
   c. amplitude; wavelength; frequency
   d. amplitude; frequency; wavelength

6. Radiation beam force, or penetrating power, is controlled by the _____ setting.
   a. mA   c. kVp
   b. exposure meter   d. timer

7. Which type of PID is preferred because it better limits the size of the primary beam as the beam exits the tube head?
   a. collimator   c. round
   b. filter   d. rectangular

8. The area inside the machine where the electrons are converted to x-rays is the:
   a. cathode   c. filament
   b. copper stem   d. focal spot

9. Radiosensitive tissues and organs include:
   a. reproductive, blood, and young bone cells   d. a and c
   b. the lining of the mouth and thyroid gland   e. all of the above
   c. the lens of the eye and bone marrow

10. A person must be _____ years of age to work with radiation.
    a. 16   c. 21
    b. 18   d. 25

TRUE/FALSE

Indicate whether the statement is true (T) or false (F).

_____ 1. The MPD of radiation for occupationally exposed personnel is eight rem per year.

_____ 2. Collimation must restrict the size of the primary beam to 2.75 inches in diameter.

_____ 3. Aluminum filtration is used to increase the penetrating power of a weak radiation beam.

_____ 4. As the speed of a film increases, the amount of radiation required to produce a diagnostically acceptable film increases proportionally.

_____ 5. When a radiograph is being exposed, the operator should stand at least six feet away from the tube head or behind a lead barrier.

_____ 6. It is acceptable for a dental assistant to hold radiographic film in position in the mouth for children, the elderly, and disabled patients.

_____ 7. The amount of radiation produced is called "amperage."

_____ 8. The dental assistant should wear a film badge whenever he/she may be exposed to radiation.

_____ 9. Increasing exposure time increases the contrast on a radiograph.

_____ 10. If a film has low contrast it means many shades of gray are present.

FILL IN THE BLANK

Using words from the list below, fill in the blanks to complete the following statements.

cathode	larger	Roentgen
children	light	secondary
focal spot	pregnant women	sievert
inefficient	primary	

1. The _____ produces electrons.

2. The area where electrons are converted to photons is the _____.

3. Dental x-ray production is a very _____ process because 99.8% of the energy of the electron stream is converted to heat, and 0.2% is converted to radiation.

4. This physicist discovered radiation: _____.

5. _____ radiation is the most dangerous to the operator.

6. _____ radiation is directed toward the object of interest and travels in straight lines until it collides with matter.

7. Irradiation of a _____ area increases the vulnerability of the tissues to damage.

8. Radiopaque structures appear _____ on a finished film.

9. These two groups are especially sensitive to the effects of radiation: _____ and _____.

10. A _____ is a measure of the dose of radiation to which the tissues were exposed.

CHAPTER 30

Dental Film and Processing Radiographs

CHAPTER OUTLINE

Review the Chapter Outline. If any content area is unclear, review that area before beginning the workbook exercises.

A. Dental Film Holders
  1. Types of Dental Film Holders
  2. Beam Alignment Devices

B. Dental X-ray Film
  1. Film Packet
  2. Film Composition
  3. Latent Image

C. Film Types
  1. Intraoral Film
  2. Extraoral Film
  3. Duplicating Film

D. Film Storage

E. Film Speed

F. Film Processing
  1. The Darkroom
  2. Five Steps in Film Processing
  3. Composition of Processing Chemicals
    a. Manual Processing
    b. Automatic Processing
  4. Processing Errors

G. Legal Considerations in Dental Radiography
  1. Equipment Regulations
  2. Certification Requirements

H. Quality Assurance in Dental Radiography
  1. Quality Assurance for Dental Equipment

I. Infection Control in Dental Radiography
  1. Film Holding and Alignment Devices
  2. Handling Exposed Film

CHAPTER REVIEW

The following is a summary of the chapter. If any of this material is unclear, review it in the textbook again.

Exposing, processing, and mounting dental radiographs are important duties of the dental assistant. A finished radiograph must be diagnostically acceptable. A sound understanding of the technical aspects of film selection and storage, film and beam alignment devices, darkroom preparation and care, film processing, quality control measures, infection control during radiographic procedures, and trouble-shooting errors is the first step toward production of a diagnostically acceptable radiograph. Film may be intraoral, extraoral, or duplicating. It is also available in several different sizes, each of which is used for specific types of procedures. Patient exposure must be as low as is reasonably achievable (ALARA). Film, exposure aids, radiographic equipment, and the darkroom must be maintained in excellent operating condition. Infection control protocols must be developed and followed. The dental assistant's radiographic knowledge and skill are essential components of smooth functioning in a dental practice.

LEARNING AND STUDY AIDS

Review the following study aids and/or complete the activities to ensure that you have achieved the learning objectives for this chapter.

1. List and describe the available types of film holders.

2. List the components of a dental film packet, and state the function of each.

3. List the three types of film used in dental radiography, and relate each to its function.

4. Complete the following table, indicating the use of each size of intraoral film.

Table 30-1

Size	Uses
0	
1	
2	
3	
4	

5. Discuss the five steps in film processing, and explain why each is completed.

6. Make two large flash cards. On one side of the first card, write "Manual Processing Steps," and then list them on the other side. Repeat these steps on the second flash card for automatic processing. Making flash cards is a helpful exercise because you can use these as a study tool while in school and then later as a reference card in the workplace. Turn your flash cards into your instructor to receive a grade for this activity.

7. In your own words, describe film processing.

8. Complete the following table by listing the function of the components of developer and fixer solutions.

Table 30-2

Ingredient	Chemical(s)	Functions
Developer agent	Hydroquinone	
	Elon	
Preservative	Sodium sulfite	
Accelerator	Sodium carbonate	
Restrainer	Potassium bromide	
Fixer agent	Sodium thiosulfate, ammonium thiosulfate	
Preservative	Sodium sulfite	
Hardening agent	Potassium alum	
Acidifier	Acetic acid, sulfuric acid	

9. List the tasks of a sound quality control protocol.

10. State the two aims of all quality control procedures in a dental office.

MEDICAL TERMINOLOGY REVIEW

Use a dictionary and/or your textbook to define the following terms.

automatic processor _____

beam alignment device _____

cassette _____

cephalometric radiograph _____

duplicating film _____

emulsion _____

film _____

film holder _____

film processing _____

film speed _____

intensifying screen _____

intraoral film _____

latent image _____

occlusal radiograph _____

panoramic film _____

radiograph _____

ALARA _____

; _____

PID _____

KCP _____

CRITICAL THINKING

1. Why should the dental assistant know the components that comprise an intraoral film packet? List each component, and describe what each portion is for or what it does.

2. When thinking about the composition of dental x-ray film, what component stores the energy necessary to create an image on the film?

3. Describe the five different types of intraoral dental film, and their uses. If a patient complains of pain underneath the tongue and a very slow or limited salivary flow from this area, which of these types of films might be exposed in order to determine the cause of the patient's complaint?

CHAPTER REVIEW TEST

MULTIPLE CHOICE

Circle the letter of the correct answer.

1. Which component of the film packet is a hazardous material that is recycled rather than thrown away?
    a. outer covering
    b. lead foil
    c. emulsion
    d. black paper

2. Which TWO principles should be observed when loading film onto racks for manual processing?
    a. load from the top down
    b. load from the bottom up
    c. load from the center out in both directions
    d. load alternating sides

3. What prevents overlapping of films when loading the automatic processor?
    a. load slowly
    b. reduce track running speed
    c. use smaller size film
    d. all of the above

4. The recommended developing time when processing films manually is _____ minutes at _____ degrees Fahrenheit.
    a. 1; 84
    b. $2^1/_2$; 76
    c. $4^1/_2$; 68
    d. $6^1/_4$; 54

5. Reusable film holding devices are classified as semicritical instruments that must be:
    a. wiped with a disinfectant
    b. soaked in disinfectant solution
    c. autoclaved
    d. thrown away after three uses

6. When testing the automatic processor, a developed film that appears _____ indicates the processor is working properly.
    a. clear and dry
    b. dark and wet
    c. clear and wet
    d. dark and dry

7. Daily preparation for use of manual processing tanks includes all of the following EXCEPT:
    a. solutions in the developer and fixer tanks must be stirred
    b. developer and fixer solution levels must be checked
    c. solutions must be replenished if levels are low
    d. water for the water bath must be turned on
    e. timer and safelight accuracy must be checked

8. If film integrity has been maintained, the quality control film that is processed when a new box of film is opened should appear:
    a. slightly gray with some clear areas
    b. very dark throughout
    c. clear all over with a light blue tint
    d. slightly foggy with patches of yellow

9. Automated processing is faster because:
   a. time is not lost on the rinsing and washing steps
   b. the films are moved forward at an even speed
   c. loading film onto automated processor film holders is faster
   d. the chemicals used are formulated for use at higher temperatures

10. Duplicating film differs from radiographic film because it:
    a. has emulsion on only one side
    b. is one inch smaller in size
    c. is packaged in individual packets
    d. has larger silver halide crystals

TRUE/FALSE

Indicate whether the statement is true (T) or false (F).

_____ 1. A daylight loader enables intraoral film loading outside the darkroom.

_____ 2. The American Dental Association recommends the use of D speed film.

_____ 3. Adult bitewings are ordinarily taken with size 2 film.

_____ 4. Panoramic film is used to produce a radiograph that shows a full facial profile.

_____ 5. A latent image is an invisible image on the film after it has been exposed to radiation but before it has been processed.

_____ 6. Anterior and posterior XCP film holder/beam alignment devices are interchangeable if the aiming ring is turned over.

_____ 7. The primary benefit of using a film holder is that it provides beam alignment assistance to the dental assistant.

_____ 8. The emulsion on a radiographic film increases the film's sensitivity to radiation.

_____ 9. Beam alignment devices are used to position the PID accurately.

_____ 10. The black paper that is in a film packet protects the film from contamination with moisture.

FILL IN THE BLANK

Using words from the list below, fill in the blanks to complete the following statements.

one	increase fixing time	four to six
oxidation	sixty	replenish developing solution
certification	stricter	establish more appropriate storage
conditions	training	handle only the edges of film
white spots on the finished film		

1. The tank lid must be in place when the tanks are not in use to prevent _____ of the developer and fixer solutions.

2. The darkroom counter must be kept clean and free of chemicals to prevent _____.

3. Automated processing requires approximately _____ minutes to complete, whereas manual processing requires approximately _____ minutes.

4. When state or local laws or regulations differ from federal mandates, the _____ law or regulation applies.

5. Individuals who operate ionizing radiation equipment must receive _____ and _____.

6. If a developed film is too light, this correction may need to be made: _____.

7. If yellowish brown stains appear on a developed film, this correction may need to be made: _____.

8. If a black fingerprint mark appears on a developed film, this correction needs to be made: _____.

9. If fog appears on a developed film, this correction may need to be made: _____.

10. Adult anterior films and posterior bitewings for children are exposed using size _____ film.

CHAPTER 31
Intraoral Radiographic Procedures

CHAPTER OUTLINE

Review the Chapter Outline. If any content area is unclear, review that area before beginning the workbook exercises.

A. Intraoral X-ray Techniques
   1. Full Mouth Survey

B. Common Vertical and Horizontal Errors
   1. Patient Preparation for Intraoral Radiographs
   2. Principles for Intraoral Radiography
   3. The Gag Reflex
   4. Pediatric Patients

C. Technical Errors in Intraoral Radiography
   1. Errors of Angulation and Centering of the PID
   2. Film and Digital Receptor Placement Errors

D. Mounting Intraoral Radiographs
   1. Labial and Lingual Mounting
   2. Anatomic Landmarks
   3. Intraoral Radiograph Mounting Procedure
   4. Radiograph Storage

CHAPTER REVIEW

The following is a summary of the chapter. If any of this material is unclear, review it in the textbook again.

Intraoral radiographs are an essential diagnostic tool for the dentist. To be useful, the images on a radiograph must be accurate and readable. Correct patient, film, and beam positioning provide the accuracy; correct kVp, MA, and exposure settings provide the readability. There are two basic intraoral exposure techniques: paralleling and bisecting. Paralleling is the more accurate technique and is recommended by the American Academy of Oral and Maxillofacial Radiology. The bitewing (interproximal) and mandibular occlusal techniques are variations of paralleling. The maxillary occlusal technique is a variation of bisecting. All of the techniques have advantages for certain diagnostic needs, and it is the dentist's professional decision as to what would be most useful for a specific patient. The dental assistant must become proficient in all of the techniques in order to expose films as needed for each patient.

LEARNING ACTIVITIES AND STUDY AIDS

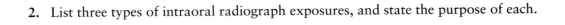

Review the following study aids and/or complete the activities to ensure that you have achieved the learning objectives for this chapter.

1. Discuss patient preparation prior to radiograph exposure.

2. List three types of intraoral radiograph exposures, and state the purpose of each.

3. Outline the steps in exposing radiographs using the paralleling and bisecting techniques. Feel free to utilize an additional piece of paper if more space for your information is needed.

4. Describe the protocol for exposing bitewing radiographs.

5. Explain the procedure and patient positioning necessary for correct exposure of occlusal radiographs.

6. Describe methods of managing patients with special needs: edentulous patients, pediatric patients, and patients with a hypersensitive gag reflex. Utilize an additional sheet of paper if needed for your information.

7. Describe techniques for managing patients with physical and mental disabilities. Utilize an additional piece of paper if more space is required for your information.

8. On a separate piece of paper, make a chart listing ten types of errors in radiograph production, and identify a means of correcting each.

9. Explain the protocol for mounting radiographs.

10. List the necessary documentation information that is needed for each radiograph or series of radiographs.

MEDICAL TERMINOLOGY REVIEW

Use a dictionary and/or your textbook to define the following terms.

ala _____

bisecting angle technique _____

bitewing radiograph _____

cone cut _____

elongation _____

foreshortening _____

horizontal angulation _____

interproximal _____

long axis of the tooth _____

overlapping _____

paralleling technique _____

periapical radiograph _____

perpendicular _____

position indicator device _____

radiograph _____

tragus _____

vertical angulation _____

ABBREVIATIONS

ALARA _____

BAI _____

CMS _____

CMX _____

FMS _____

FMX _____

MPD _____

PID _____

XCP _____

CRITICAL THINKING

1. What are the differences between the two main types of radiography used within dentistry? Describe these techniques. Why does the dental assistant need to know these differences?

2. What types of x-rays are used when practicing extraoral radiography? If you were a dental assistant working in an oral surgeon's office, which type of extraoral x-ray might you expose most often? What if you were working in an orthodontist's office?

3. When positioning the PID horizontally for an intraoral x-ray, what is the "best rule of thumb" to follow?

4. What are the five guiding principles to be followed during intraoral radiography? Describe each one.

CHAPTER REVIEW TEST

MULTIPLE CHOICE

Circle the letter of the correct answer.

1. The purpose of intraoral radiography is to view:
   a. relatively large areas of a single jaw
   b. individual teeth and their supporting structures
   c. both jaws in a single radiograph
   d. the patient's profile including both soft and hard tissue

2. Describe the long axis of a tooth.
   a. horizontal line parallel to the cervical line and perpendicular to the root apex
   b. vertical line extending from the highest cusp tip to the root apex
   c. imaginary lengthwise line that divides the tooth in half
   d. a and b
   e. b and c

3. This device is used to correctly align the central ray in relation to the tooth and film.
   a. PID
   b. film holder
   c. glass envelope
   d. tungsten target

4. Select the error that occurs from improper horizontal beam alignment.
   a. foreshortening
   b. double image
   c. overlapping
   d. elongation

5. When a paralleled FMX is being exposed for a typical adult patient, size _____ film is used for the anterior teeth, and size _____ film is used for the bitewings and posterior teeth.
   a. 0; 1
   b. 1; 2
   c. 2; 3
   d. 3; 4

6. Necessary documentation that must be recorded for every radiograph or series of radiographs includes:
   a. type of radiograph exposed, exposure factors used, and patient's name
   b. exposure technique used, dates radiographs were exposed and mounted, and patient's name
   c. patient's, operator's, and dentist's names, and the date the radiographs were processed
   d. patient's name and the date the radiographs were exposed

7. The dental assistant should inspect the patient's mouth prior to exposing a radiograph to determine if any of these conditions are present.
   a. shallow palate
   b. bony protrusions
   c. small mouth
   d. all of the above

8. The dental assistant never slides radiographic film into position, particularly in the maxillary posterior areas, because doing so may:
   a. cause the palatal tissues to bleed
   b. irritate the patient's muscles
   c. activate the patient's gag reflex
   d. cause the patient to bite down

9. Before beginning an intraoral radiography procedure, the dental assistant must ensure that the:
   a. patient is covered with a lead apron and thyroid collar
   b. exposure button and kVp dial or button are working correctly
   c. film is the speed recommended by the American Academy of Oral and Maxillofacial Radiology
   d. patient's occlusal plane is perpendicular to the floor

10. When an XCP paralleling instrument is assembled correctly, the bite block should be the locator ring.
    a. adjacent to
    b. protruding above
    c. protruding below
    d. centered in

TRUE/FALSE

Indicate whether the statement is true (T) or false (F).

_____ 1. The dot on a film packet is always positioned toward the occlusal or incisal surface of the tooth.

_____ 2. A cone cut occurs when the central beam is not positioned perpendicular to the film.

_____ 3. Bitewings are used primarily for diagnosis of caries and observation of early periodontal disease.

_____ 4. Vertical angulation for exposure of bitewings is approximately +25 degrees.

_____ 5. When exposing radiographs of the maxillary arch, the patient should be positioned upright so the occlusal plane is parallel, and the midsagittal plane is perpendicular, to the floor.

_____ 6. The most effective technique for obtaining a radiograph when the patient is uncomfortable is distraction.

_____ 7. It is not necessary for the caregiver of a patient with a disability to wear a lead apron when holding a film in the patient's mouth because the radiation beam is directed toward the patient rather than the caregiver.

_____ 8. Federal laws require dentists to ensure that their services are equally accessible to disabled and nondisabled persons.

_____ 9. All periapical radiographs should be taken on edentulous patients using the paralleling technique.

_____ 10. When radiographs are mounted using the lingual system, the films will appear as if the person viewing the radiographs is looking at the patient from outside the mouth.

FILL IN THE BLANK

Using words from the list below, fill in the blanks to complete the following statements.

bending	elongation	MA
blurred	exposure time	not exposed
cone cut	foreshortening	radiopaque
double image	herringbone pattern	

1. Insufficient vertical angulation causes _____ of the image.

2. Placing the film packet in the mouth backwards causes a _____ to appear on the image.

3. When part of the film isn't exposed, the image is _____.

4. Excessive vertical angulation causes _____ of the image.

5. When a film is exposed more than once, a _____ appears.

6. If the patient moves while the film is being exposed, the resulting image will be _____.

7. If no image appears after processing, the film was _____.

8. Artifacts on films appear as _____ objects.

9. An excessively dark radiograph may have been caused by excessive _____ or too high an setting.

10. A dark line across the corner of a radiograph is often caused by _____ the film.

CHAPTER 32

Extraoral and Digital Radiographic Procedures

CHAPTER OUTLINE

Review the Chapter Outline. If any content area is unclear, review that area before beginning the workbook exercises.

   A. Panoramic Radiography
      1. Panoramic Image Receptors
      2. Panoramic Radiograph Positioning
      3. Common Panoramic Technical Errors

   B. Other Extraoral Radiography
      1. Cephalometric Skull View
      2. Towne's Skull View
      3. Water's Skull View
      4. Additional Extraoral Radiograph Techniques

   C. Digital Radiography
      1. Direct Sensors
      2. Phosphor Plate Technology
      3. Digital Scanners
      4. Extraoral Digital Radiography

CHAPTER REVIEW

The following is a summary of the chapter. If any of this material is unclear, review it in the textbook again.

Extraoral radiographic techniques are used to portray large views: the jaws, skull, large areas of soft tissue, or extraoral bony structures such as sinuses, parts of the mandible, the temporomandibular joint, facial bones, or bones of the orbit. Exposures can be made using conventional radiographic techniques or newer digital imaging methods. When film is used, film sizes are large, and a cassette is used to position the film extraorally. Some types of extraoral film are exposed by light emitted by intensifying screens in the cassette when they are exposed to radiation. Film loading and positioning, and patient preparation and positioning, are critical to technique success. Digital imaging methods use a sensor or phosphor plate rather than film, greatly reduce radiation exposure to patients, do not require the use of hazardous chemicals for processing, and provide unparalleled flexibility in image manipulation, storage, printing, and transfer.

LEARNING ACTIVITIES AND STUDY AIDS

Review the following study aids and/or complete the activities to ensure that you have achieved the learning objectives for this chapter.

1. Differentiate panoramic and cephalometric radiographs.

2. Describe how film is loaded into a cassette for an extraoral radiograph.

3. Discuss how to prepare a patient for extraoral and digital radiograph exposure.

4. List and locate four anatomical planes used to position the patient for a panoramic radiograph.

5. List, describe, and state a means of correcting four common extraoral radiograph technique errors.

6. Differentiate cephalometric, Towne's view, and Water's view of extraoral radiographs.

7. List and define three methods used to create digital radiographs.

8. Explain how a direct scanner is used in digital radiography.

9. Describe how direct sensors are cleaned and disinfected following use.

10. Discuss technique modifications for children, the elderly, and edentulous patients.

MEDICAL TERMINOLOGY REVIEW

Use a dictionary and/or your textbook to define the following terms.

ala-tragus line _____

anteroposterior plane _____

artifact _____

canthomeatal line _____

cassette _____

cephalometric radiograph _____

computerized tomography _____

edentulous _____

extraoral radiograph _____

Frankfort plane _____

intensifying screen _____

kilovoltage _____

lateral _____

magnetic resonance imaging _____

midsagittal plane _____

milliamperage _____

panoramic radiography _____

ABBREVIATIONS

AP _____

APS _____

CCD _____

CMOS _____

CT _____

kVp _____

mA _____

MRI _____

PA _____

PSP _____

TMJ _____

CRITICAL THINKING

1. What are some patient factors to consider when taking extraoral radiographs?

2. What are the advantages and disadvantages of digital radiography over traditional radiography?

3. When thinking about the silver halide crystals used on traditional film, what component does digital film posses that is similar to these crystals, and how is the energy stored on a digital film?

CHAPTER REVIEW TEST

MULTIPLE CHOICE

Circle the letter of the correct answer.

1. Who is responsible for all aspects of safe radiation exposure in the dental office?
   a. dental assistant
   b. office manager
   c. dental hygienist
   d. dentist

2. An intensifying screen is used in extraoral radiography procedures to:
   a. convert x-ray energy into light energy
   b. protect film from exposure to light
   c. hold and position film extraorally
   d. create a latent image on a plate

3. What extraoral technique rotates the x-ray beam and film in opposite directions during exposure to obtain an image?
   a. digital
   b. cephalometric
   c. panoramic
   d. magnetic resonance imaging

4. The Frankfort plane is a horizontal line extending from the:
   a. wing of the nose to the outer ear opening
   b. upper margin of the ear to the lower margin of the orbit
   c. top of the head to the middle of the chin
   d. contact area between the lateral incisor and canine forward and backward

5. When positioning a panoramic patient, the individual should be asked to remove the following:
   a. jewelry
   b. glasses
   c. dentures
   d. all of the above

6. Milliamperage refers to the:
   a. penetrating power of the electron beam
   b. reduced setting necessary for child patients
   c. artifact created when earrings are not removed
   d. amount of radiation produced

7. A light pale radiograph has this problem:
   a. patient's head is tilted
   b. film is crooked in cassette
   c. too little exposure
   d. too much exposure

8. Cephalometric radiographs are used to:
   a. measure facial relationships
   b. predict growth patterns
   c. both a and b
   d. none of the above

9. After use, a direct sensor should be:
   a. autoclaved
   b. soaked in disinfecting solution
   c. wiped with a disinfectant wipe
   d. covered with a clean plastic barrier

10. Direct digital scanning is presently used for:
    a. exposing periapical radiographs
    b. digitizing existing radiographs
    c. copying bitewing radiographs
    d. processing panoramic radiographs

TRUE/FALSE

Indicate whether the statement is true (T) or false (F).

_____ 1. A phosphor plate is used to store a latent image that is then digitized using a special drum and laser scanner.

_____ 2. Exposure time should be increased for an edentulous patient.

_____ 3. The plane of occlusion is parallel to the midsagittal plane.

_____ 4. Panoramic film is light sensitive.

_____ 5. Although busy, a dental assistant must take the time to explain to an extraoral radiography patient the purpose and operation of the equipment.

_____ 6. Extraoral radiographs are used to aid and confirm diagnoses.

_____ 7. Towne's skull view is exposed by directing the beam toward the posterior of the skull when the occlusal plane is perpendicular to the floor.

_____ 8. Water's skull view is especially useful for evaluating facial fractures, including fractures of the maxilla.

_____ 9. Computer tomography creates extraoral images by scanning layers of the body and sending the resulting digital data to a computer monitor.

_____ 10. Radiation to the patient is reduced approximately 30%–40% when digital radiography is used.

FILL IN THE BLANK

Using words from the list below, fill in the blanks to complete the following statements.

antistatic	one-fourth	spine
digital	patient movement	the patient is too far back
direct sensors	radiation sensitive	the patient is too far forward
kVp		

1. _____ capture an image directly.

2. Phosphor plates used in digital image capture are _____.

3. This type of radiograph can be stored, sent electronically, or printed for use in a patient's record: _____.

4. This setting controls the penetrating power of the radiation beam: _____

5. The problem when anterior teeth appear blurred and too wide on a panoramic radiograph is _____.

6. If the premolars on a panoramic film are overlapped and the anteriors are blurred and too narrow, the problem is _____.

7. Radiation exposure should be reduced by _____ for children and the elderly.

8. Film cassettes and screens should be cleaned using cleaning and _____ solutions.

9. A pyramid-shaped opacity that appears on a panoramic radiograph is likely an image of the _____.

10. The most common reason for blurriness of an extraoral film is _____.

CHAPTER 33
Restorative and Esthetic Dental Materials

CHAPTER OUTLINE

Review the Chapter Outline. If any content area is unclear, review that area before beginning the workbook exercises.

    A.   Standardization of Dental Materials

    B.   Properties of Dental Materials

    C.   Restorations

    D.   Direct Restorations

    E.   Indirect Restorations

CHAPTER REVIEW

The following is a summary of the chapter. If any of this material is unclear, review it in the textbook again.

A dental assistant must have a basic understanding of the properties of dental materials, and how they hold up in the oral cavity environment. Having a basic understanding of mechanical and thermal properties, and the effects of these properties intraorally, helps to ensure a successful restoration. The dental assistant presents verbal and written postoperative instructions to the patient, explaining the importance of avoiding extreme temperatures for the first 24 hours. This allows for comfort during the expansion and contraction period of the material within the restoration until completely set. The type of restorative material selected depends on the tooth structure and location of the restoration. In using a composite resin, a macrofilled resin is best used in the posterior for strength, whereas a microfilled resin is best suited for an anterior restoration. A microfilled resin allows a higher polish, smoothness, and better esthetics. Temporary restorative materials include intermediate restorative (IRM) and provisional restorative materials. IRM is a direct restorative material mixed chairside and placed directly into the cavity preparation; a provisional is indirect, and fabricated outside the mouth. The dental assistant is responsible for understanding dental material manipulation, shelf life, and purpose of use.

292

© 2009 Pearson Education, Inc

LEARNING ACTIVITES AND STUDY AIDS

Review the following study aids and/or complete the activities to ensure that you have achieved the learning objectives for this chapter.

1. Triturate a double spill capsule of dental alloy (amalgam) for five seconds more than recommended. Triturate a double spill capsule of dental alloy (amalgam) for five seconds less than recommended. In both situations, take note of how the alloy appears. On a piece of paper, document the appearance and feel of each alloy as each scenario is completed.

2. Place a small dab of light cure composite resin on a coated tablet, and expose it to the dental operatory light for one hour. Write a short description of what happens to the composite resin.

3. The dentist has prepared tooth #30 for a full crown and places a temporary restoration until the permanent crown is cemented. The patient loses the temporary crown after two days. Explain what the gingiva and crown preparation will look like when the patient comes in for the permanent restoration.

4. List five advantages of placing composite restorations:

   a.

   b.

   c.

   d.

   e.

5. To further understand the standardization of dental materials, conduct research on the Internet and/or by using materials from your school or local library. Information on this topic can be found on the Web sites for the following organizations: National Institute of Standards and Technology (NIST), National Institute of Dental Research (NIDR), National Institute of Health (NIH), and the American Dental Association (ADA). On a separate piece of paper, write a one-page report on your findings.

6. Dental materials are made from various properties. Describe clearly each of the following properties: mechanical, thermal, electrical, solubility, and application property.

7. The safety of dental amalgam is under constant review by the scientific community, and since the 1990s the FDA has kept a watchful eye on this issue. To read more on this topic, visit the following Web sites and then on a separate piece of paper write a short paper describing what you learned: *http://www.fda.gov/cdrh/consumer/amalgams.html* and *http://www.fda.gov/cdrh/meetings/090606-summary.html*.

8. When placing a composite resin in a posterior tooth, explain what size filler particles the dentist would choose, and why.

9. In the following table, match the term in Column A with its definition in Column B.

Table 33-1

Column A	Column B
A. a provisional restorative material	_____ hard, used for inlays, crowns, three-quarter crowns, and bridge abutments
B. solubility	_____ to maintain the position of a prepared tooth, as well as the surrounding teeth, until permanent cementation
C. type III alloy	_____ floor of the cavity preparation is wider than the opening of the preparation
D. undercut	_____ the measurement of how much a material will dissolve in a liquid

10. List the postoperative instructions that should be given to a patient after restorative treatment.

11. Explain how amalgam materials differ from composite materials in structure and tooth preparation requirements.

MEDICAL TERMINOLOGY REVIEW

Use a dictionary and/or your textbook to define the following terms.

adhesion _____

alloy _____

amalgam _____

BIS-GMA _____

bonding _____

ceramics _____

chemical retention _____

composite resin _____

compressive stress _____

cured _____

curing _____

curing light _____

direct restoration _____

filler _____

flow _____

galvanic _____

glass ionomer _____

indirect restoration _____

inlay _____

IRM _____

macrofiller _____

malleability _____

matrix _____

mechanical properties _____

microleakage _____

onlay _____

palladium _____

platinum _____

retention _____

shear stress _____

smear layer _____

solubility _____

tensile stress _____

thermal properties _____

triturate _____

viscosity _____

zirconium oxide _____

ABBREVIATIONS

ADA _____

Ag _____

Au _____

FDI _____

IRM _____

NIDR _____

NIH _____

NIST _____

Pd _____

Pt _____

WHO _____

CRITICAL THINKING

1. What criteria must be met for new dental materials to be approved by the ADA? Why is the approval important?

2. What is the term given to all dental material regarding placement into a human? What other steps or procedures must a material go through in order to be considered safe?

3. What is the difference between an amalgam and an alloy? Can you name some dental materials that meet this definition?

4. Is mercury considered liquid or metal? Does this substance have any health concerns? Is mercury used in abundance in dentistry?

CHAPTER REVIEW TEST

MULTIPLE CHOICE

Circle the letter of the correct answer.

1. The ability of a material to withstand compressive stresses without fracturing is called:
   a. malleability
   b. ductility
   c. palliative
   d. viscosity

2. The _____ is responsible for researching dental materials for their safety, efficiency, and economical benefit for the public.
   a. NIDR
   b. ADA
   c. CDC
   d. NIST

3. _____ change within the dental amalgam is important to understand for expansion and contraction within the cavity preparation.
   a. The mechanical
   b. The thermal
   c. The environmental
   d. The electrical property

4. Recurrent caries is caused by _____, allowing for bacteria to grow between the tooth and restoration.
   a. microleakage
   b. bacterial leakage
   c. chemical leakage
   d. physical changes

5. _____ is a surface discoloration that occurs over time and can be polished away.
   a. Palladium
   b. Corrosion
   c. Tarnish
   d. Smear layer

6. For a dental material to be successful, it needs to exhibit certain properties at time of placement, called:
   a. thermal properties
   b. application properties
   c. preventative properties
   d. mechanical properties

7. The ability to easily flow over small, irregular surfaces is known as:
   a. flow ability
   b. adhesion
   c. wetting
   d. viscosity

8. The dentist places mechanical retention within the cavity preparation known as:
   a. overcuts
   b. cut away
   c. retention stability
   d. undercuts

9. When two dental materials are held together and create retention, it is called:
   a. bonding retention
   b. chemical retention
   c. mechanical retention
   d. amalgam retention

10. For an amalgam restoration to become completely set or cured takes:
    a. 24 hours
    b. 12 hours
    c. 2 hours
    d. 4 hours

TRUE/FALSE

Indicate whether the statement is true (T) or false (F).

_____ 1. The dental assistant must mix dental amalgam in an amalgamator or triturator.

_____ 2. The light used in curing lights is either tungsten or halogen.

_____ 3. Fillers are rock-like particles that add color to the composite resin.

_____ 4. The dental assistant places the mixed amalgam onto the dental tray prior to placement in the cavity preparation.

_____ 5. Three major components to a composite resin are: inorganic fillers, organic resin matrix, and coupling agent.

_____ 6. The smear layer is achieved by placing acid etchant within the cavity preparation.

_____ 7. The macrofill composites are placed primarily in the anterior of the mouth

_____ 8. The dentist must condense the amalgam within the cavity preparation to release excess mercury.

_____ 9. Trituration is the mechanical means of combining dental alloy and mercury.

_____ 10. The most attractive feature of glass ionomers is that they release fluoride into the tooth structure.

FILL IN THE BLANK

Using words from the list below, fill in the blanks to complete the following statements.

cure	provisional	resin
zirconium	oxide	polymerization
palladium	fillers	glass ionomer
indirect	direct	ceramics

1. The noble metals mixed with gold for dental indirect restorations are _____, platinum, and silver.

2. _____ are extremely hard, heat- and corrosive-resistant material that is clay fired.

3. A very promising dental restorative material that is strong, esthetic, and biocompatible with the posterior of the mouth is _____.

4. The _____ restoration is necessary to protect the prepared tooth or teeth and soft tissue until final restoration is permanently placed.

5. Castings that are created by a laboratory technician to be cemented or bonded into a cavity restoration are called _____.

6. When blended with an alloy, the _____ and metal create a very strong wear-resistant dental material.

7. The ionomer that releases fluoride is called a _____ ionomer.

8. Composite resins can be polished once _____ has occurred.

9. White light within the dental operatory can cause resin bonding material to _____ prematurely.

10. Rock-like particles called _____ are added to composite resin for strength.

CHAPTER 34

Dental Liners, Bases, and Bonding Systems

CHAPTER OUTLINE

Review the Chapter Outline. If any content area is unclear, review that area before beginning the workbook exercises.

CHAPTER REVIEW

The following is a summary of the chapter. If any of this material is unclear, review it in the textbook again.

Intermediary materials are placed between moderately deep to deep cavity preparations and final restorative materials. Intermediary materials include liners, bases, cements, varnishes, and sealers. All are placed to protect the tooth and pulp in some way, or to decrease patient sensitivity. Which specific material is chosen depends on how far the cavity preparation extends into the dentin, how close the preparation is to the pulp, and how much tooth structure remains. Liners are placed to seal tooth structure in the deepest part of the preparation and may also provide pulp sedation, promote the formation of secondary dentin, or exert a bacteriostatic effect. Bases are placed to provide insulation, sedation, or protection from mechanical forces. Cements can be used as bases and liners, and to lute restorations to teeth. Varnishes seal the cut dentin tubules. Sealers seal or block open dentin tubules, thereby decreasing dentin hypersensitivity and protecting tubules from microleakage and migration of metallic ions.

LEARNING ACTIVITIES AND STUDY AIDS

Review the following study aids and/or complete the activities to ensure that you have achieved the learning objectives for this chapter.

1. Fill in the following table by providing the types of stimuli that may cause tooth sensitivity, and an example of each.

Table 34-1

Type of Stimuli	Example

2. Differentiate a cavity liner, cavity varnish, dentin sealer, and dental base.

3. Identify the materials used to accomplish each of the following tasks.

Table 34-2

Task	Material
Lining	
Pulp sedation	
Sealing dentinal tubules	
Basing	
Bonding	

4. Discuss how and why dentin sealers are used.

5. Describe how and why a base is placed.

6. List the reasons why a cavity liner is placed.

7. Explain the etching process, and state why it is used in bonding.

8. Differentiate and describe enamel and dentin bonding.

9. List the types of restorations under which copal varnishes cannot be used.

10. Describe means of preventing or lessening dentinal hypersensitivity.

MEDICAL TERMINOLOGY REVIEW

Use a dictionary and/or your textbook to define the following terms.

acid etchant _____

desensitizer _____

desiccate _____

eugenol _____

exothermic _____

hypersensitivity _____

luting agent _____

microleakage _____

micromechanical _____

retention _____

sedative _____

smear layer _____

traumatic occlusion _____

ABBREVIATIONS

ZOE _____

CRITICAL THINKING

1. What is the purpose of placing a liner or base? If you were treating a patient who required the use of a base underneath an amalgam restoration, what would the reason for this be?

2. If during a dental procedure the dentist deemed it necessary to place a base, how would you explain this to your patient?

3. What are the safety/patient treatment guidelines that should be followed when applying acid etchant?

CHAPTER REVIEW TEST

MULTIPLE CHOICE

Circle the letter of the correct answer.

1. Describe the dental assistant's role in dentin bonding.
   a. prepare the materials for each step
   b. keep the area dry and free of debris
   c. maintain patient comfort
   d. all of the above

2. Intermediary material selection is determined by the:
   a. preparation site
   b. degree of tooth involvement
   c. physical structure and function of the tooth
   d. b and c

3. It may take _____ for the sensitivity of a tooth to quiet down following restoration placement.
   a. days
   b. weeks
   c. months
   d. b and c

4. Microleakage refers to:
   a. entrance of fluid and dissolved substances into the area between a tooth and a restoration
   b. process of sedating a tooth that has been or is experiencing hypersensitivity
   c. micromechanical bonding of the tooth, intermediary material, and final restorative material
   d. release of supplementary materials into the dental and oral environment

5. Calcium hydroxide is placed to:
   a. promote the growth of secondary dentin
   b. stop the growth of bacteria under the restoration
   c. etch the tooth surface
   d. a and b

6. The only intermediary material that is used as a sedative base is:
   a. zinc phosphate
   b. zinc oxide and eugenol
   c. polycarboxylate
   d. glass ionomer

7. Varnishes are used to protect the tooth from:
   a. shrinkage of restorative material
   b. blockage of the dentin tubules
   c. moisture
   d. biting forces

8. If a sealer is to be used on a tooth, the tooth must be clean and:
   a. dry
   b. moist
   c. desiccated
   d. wet

9. Polycarboxylate is best used as a(n):
   a. sedative base
   b. insulating base
   c. liner
   d. luting agent

10. Resin and glass ionomer liners are commonly used because:
    a. the process for their application is simple and quick
    b. research indicates they have better longevity
    c. they bond to dentin and restorative materials
    d. expanded-function dental assistants are allowed to place them

TRUE/FALSE

Indicate whether the statement is true (T) or false (F).

_____ 1. A liner must be placed between the cavity preparation and a zinc phosphate base to protect the pulp from acid.

_____ 2. Dental bonding agents, adhesives, and bonding resins all refer to the same category of materials.

_____ 3. The material of choice for repairing fractured teeth is varnish.

_____ 4. Phosphoric acid is the active ingredient in etchant material.

_____ 5. The smear layer in a cavity preparation forms as a response to glass ionomer placement.

_____ 6. Sealants and orthodontic brackets are bonded to enamel.

_____ 7. Having a knowledge and skills base allows the dental assistant to anticipate the dentist's next step.

_____ 8. Supplementary material placement follows restorative material placement.

_____ 9. Recent research indicates salivary contamination may actually help sealant and bonding agent adherence.

_____ 10. Calcium glass ionomer is used as a dentin sealer, liner, and restorative material.

FILL IN THE BLANK

Using words from the list below, fill in the blanks to complete the following statements.

acid	eugenol	increase retention
cements	fluoride releasing varnish	removed
copal varnish	glutaraldehyde	resin
desensitizer		

1. This material should not be applied directly to the pulp because it contains impurities and is an irritant: _____.

2. This material should not be used under resin or composite restorations because it contains an organic solvent: _____.

3. This material is used for reducing hypersensitivity in cervical areas: _____.

4. This material is used instead of varnish to seal cut dentin tubules and reduce sensitivity: _____.

5. This material blocks the dentin tubules, thereby preventing the fluid movement in the tubules that causes pain: _____.

6. All of these materials have similar insulating and thermal conductivity characteristics: _____.

7. This type of bonding material bonds to the tooth mechanically: _____.

8. The purpose of bonding a restorative material to the tooth is to _____.

9. The smear layer in a cavity preparation is _____ to establish micromechanical retention.

10. This material must not come in contact with soft tissue or adjacent tooth surfaces during an enamel bonding procedure: _____.

CHAPTER 35
Dental Cements

CHAPTER OUTLINE

Review the Chapter Outline. If any content area is unclear, review that area before beginning the workbook exercises.

    A. Classification of Dental Cements

    B. Types of Cements
        1. Zinc Oxide Eugenol Cement
        2. Zinc Phosphate Cement
        3. Polycarboxylate Cement
        4. Glass Ionomer Cement
        5. Composite Resin Cement

    C. Removing Excess Cement

CHAPTER REVIEW

The following is a summary of the chapter. If any of this material is unclear, review it in the textbook again.

Dental cements are materials used for luting, basing or bonding, and restorations. Each cement has distinctive properties that make it useful for some applications but not for others. Characteristics of importance include acidity, setting time, fluoride release, strength, solubility, and ability to form a thin film. Cements are technique sensitive. For excellent results, the dental assistant must store, proportion, mix, and use cements in accordance with the manufacturer's directions. Many states permit dental assistants to remove excess cement provided they have adequate knowledge and training in the area.

LEARNING ACTIVITIES AND STUDY AIDS

Review the following study aids and/or complete the activities to ensure that you have achieved the learning objectives for this chapter.

1. In the following table, list each type of cement along with its uses.

Table 35-1

Cement	Uses

2. Differentiate temporary, permanent, high-strength, and low-strength cements.

3. List six factors that impact cement selection.

4. Provide the common uses of the following cements.

Table 35-2

Cement	Usual Uses
Zinc oxide eugenol	
Zinc phosphate	
Polycarboxylate	
Glass ionomer	
Composite resin	

5. Discuss why cements are technique sensitive.

6. List the instruments and supplies needed for mixing any cement.

7. Outline the procedure for removing excess cement.

8. State why a liner or sealer is used to protect the pulp prior to placing zinc phosphate cement.

9. Discuss what needs to be done to prepare a tooth for placement of composite resin cement.

10. Identify the cement that releases fluoride into nearby tissue after it has set.

MEDICAL TERMINOLOGY REVIEW

Use a dictionary and/or your textbook to define the following terms.

base _____

chemical cured _____

eugenol _____

exothermic reaction _____

grit _____

homogenous _____

light cured _____

liner _____

luting agent _____

solubility _____

ABBREVIATIONS

ADA _____

ISO _____

ZOE _____

CRITICAL THINKING

1. Why is the difference between temporary and permanent cements of concern to the dental assistant?

2. Can a base or liner material be used as temporary cement? Explain

3. Which cement has to be mixed over a wide area to dissipate heat? What harm could come from using this cement if a liner were not placed between the cement and the patient's tooth?

CHAPTER REVIEW TEST

MULTIPLE CHOICE

Circle the letter of the correct answer.

1. Although this cement is acid, it is soothing to the pulp.
   a. composite resin
   b. polycarboxylate
   c. zinc oxide eugenol
   d. zinc phosphate

2. Although this cement is often used for temporary applications, this form of it is used for permanent cementation of cast metal restorations.
   a. Type I
   b. Type II
   c. Type III
   d. Type IV

3. This cement is quite acidic, so the tooth must be protected with a liner or sealer before it is placed.
   a. glass ionomer
   b. polycarboxylate
   c. zinc phosphate
   d. a and c

4. This cement must be mixed on a glass slab to cool it and slow its setting time.
   a. zinc phosphate
   b. glass ionomer
   c. composite resin
   d. zinc polycarboxylate

5. The tooth must be clean, dry, etched, and bonded before this cement is applied.
   a. composite resin
   b. glass ionomer
   c. zinc oxide eugenol
   d. polycarboxylate

6. This cement releases fluoride into nearby tissues after it sets.
   a. composite resin
   b. polycarboxylate
   c. zinc oxide eugenol
   d. glass ionomer

7. This cement **chemically** bonds to tooth structure.
   a. composite resin
   b. polycarboxylate
   c. zinc oxide eugenol
   d. zinc phosphate

8. This type of cement bonds chemically and mechanically to enamel, dentin, and metal.
   a. composite resin
   b. glass ionomer
   c. zinc oxide eugenol
   d. zinc phosphate

9. The liquid for zinc oxide eugenol cement is:
   a. polyacrylic acid
   b. water
   c. phosphoric acid
   d. oil of cloves

10. All cements should be _____ in color and consistency when correctly mixed.
    a. wet
    b. dull
    c. glossy
    d. homogenous

TRUE/FALSE

Indicate whether the statement is true (T) or false (F).

_____ 1. Zinc phosphate cement should always be mixed with an autoclavable nylon spatula.

_____ 2. The finishing touch to removal of excess cement is flossing of the interproximal spaces to ensure all cement has been removed.

_____ 3. When the dentist has placed the crown being cemented in position on the tooth, the dental assistant should transfer a cotton roll for the patient to bite on.

_____ 4. After the major portion of the excess cement has been removed, the dental assistant should use dental floss to open and examine the gingival crevice.

_____ 5. The test for completion of mixing zinc oxide eugenol for a temporary restoration is that the material can be rolled into a small ball.

_____ 6. Glass ionomer is commonly used as a liner in esthetic restorations.

_____ 7. Many cements can be mixed on an oiled paper pad to save clean-up time.

_____ 8. Mixing zinc phosphate in increments enables heating of the mix to the correct temperature for placement.

_____ 9. The patient who has had a crown cemented must be taught the importance of keeping the margins of the crown clean in order to avoid developing caries underneath.

_____ 10. Most children easily understand words such as crown and cement as they are used in relation to dental procedures.

FILL IN THE BLANK

Using words from the list below, fill in the blanks to complete the following statements.

one-inch string	lengths	shiny	completely
low	skill	glass ionomer	luting
spatula	glossy	putty	zinc phosphate
high			

1. Temporary cements may be of _____ strength but permanent cements must have _____ strength.

2. The dental assistant's confidence and _____ help to allay patients' fears.

3. _____ consistency is similar to that of a small dough ball.

4. _____ cements are used as bases or liners.

5. To ensure correct consistency of a zinc phosphate insulating base, the dental assistant checks to see that the mixed material can form a _____.

6. Orthodontic brackets may be luted in position with _____ or _____.

7. When a two-paste system is used for preparing cement, equal _____ of the base and catalyst pastes are used.

8. The inside of a crown should be filled by scraping the material off the _____ along the margin of the crown.

9. The dental assistant should ensure that the cement _____ covers the inside walls of the crown before transferring it to the dentist for cementation.

10. Polycarboxylate cements should be thick and have a _____, _____ surface when mixing is complete.

CHAPTER 36
Impression Materials

CHAPTER OUTLINE

Review the Chapter Outline. If any content area is unclear, review that area before beginning the workbook exercises.

    A. Types of Impressions

    B. Impression Materials

    C. Hydrocolloid Impression Materials

    D. Elastomeric Impression Materials

    E. Impression Trays

CHAPTER REVIEW

The following is a summary of the chapter. If any of this material is unclear, review it in the textbook again

Various impression materials are available for all dental impressions. The selection of material is based on the procedure to be performed and the dimensional stability, tear strength, elastic recovery, and wettability of the material. All impressions provide a negative into which gypsum material is poured and a positive case is made. Gypsum productions have a variety of uses, such as prosthetic devices like crowns, bridges, veneers, implants, partial dentures, and complete dentures. Impression materials are either hydrophilic, meaning works well in a moist environment, or hydrophobic, meaning an aversion for water. Each impression material has properties indicated for specific purposes to ensure obtainable results. Once placed in the patient's oral cavity as a sol impression, it converts to a gel through a thermal or chemical process. The impression tray selection can be disposable, stock, custom, triple, or dual arch with regard to material used. There are two types of hydrocolloid impression material: reversible, which can change from a sol to a gel and back to a sol; and irreversible, which can change from a sol to a gel. Operator problem-solving impression techniques can produce highly accurate impressions. It is best to recognize impression detail, avoiding voids, tearing, and air bubbles. The operator must be sure to properly load and seat the impression tray and know how long it takes the material to set prior to removing it from the patient's mouth. Perfection cannot be achieved every time, but with proper attention to detail and practice, the dental assistant will achieve the experience and skills necessary to accomplish successful impressions.

LEARNING ACTIVITIES AND STUDY AIDS

Review the following study aids and/or complete the activities to ensure that you have achieved the learning objectives for this chapter.

1. Mix a bowl of alginate with very warm water. Explain what happens to the alginate when mixed, and the setting time. Mix a bowl of alginate with very cold water. Explain what happens to the alginate when mixed, and the setting time.

2. Take either a maxillary or mandibular alginate impression on a manikin and/or typodont. Let the impression sit out on the counter uncovered for four hours. Explain how the alginate looked after four hours.

3. Take either a maxillary or mandibular alginate impression on a manikin and/or typodont. Wrap it in a wet paper towel, than place into a plastic zip lock bag, and leave to be poured for the next day. Explain how the alginate looked after 24 hours.

4. Mix together the base and catalyst of an elastomeric impression material. Explain how long it takes for the polymerization process to complete, and the cause of polymerization.

5. Identify the compartments of the following reversible hydrocolloid conditioning unit:

    a. First compartment is known as the _____

       Used to change the hydrocolloid from a _____ to a _____

       The temperature is _____

    b. Second compartment is known as the _____

       Used for _____ up to eight hours

       The temperature is _____

    c. Third compartment is known as the _____

       Used to _____ the temperature of the material

       The temperature is _____

6. In the following table, match the letter in Column A with the definition in Column B.

Table 36-1

Column A	Column B
A. alginate impression material	_____ impression material supplied in tubes and heated in a conditioning unit
B. polyether impression material	_____ used for orthodontic models, opposing models, bleaching trays, mouthguards, custom trays, and occlusal splints

C. glutaraldehyde	_____ impression should be removed quickly to minimize tear strength and permanent deformation; should be done immediately to prevent dimensional change
D. silicone impression materials	_____ setting time is 8–12 minutes; only custom tray with adhesive should be used for removable and fixed prosthodontic impressions; good reproduction of detail; poor dimensional stability
E. polysiloxane/vinylpolysiloxane (VPS)	_____ used for crown and bridge restoration and bite registrations; available in three viscosities; custom or stock tray with adhesive; provides dimensional stability, highly accurate detail, and good wettability
F. bite registration	_____ Condensation Type I, Curing Type II; light, medium, and heavy body; very high viscosity putty material
G. agar	_____ not recommended for disinfecting alginate impressions
H. polysulfide impression materials	_____ accomplished with wax, zinc oxide eugenol paste, acrylic, polyether, and vinylpolysiloxane materials; determines accurate occlusal relationship
I. reversible hydrocolloids	_____ also called addition reaction silicone; most dimensionally stable; available in low-, medium-, and high-viscosity (most commonly used) consistencies; expensive; latex glove powder inhibits setting of the material

7. Number the following steps to indicate which step would come first, second, third, etc.

   Steps to Achieve an Alginate Impression

   _____ Dip the supplied scoop lightly into the powder until the scoop is full. Do not pack the scoop. Tap the scoop against the rim to insure a full measure without voids. Scrape any excess off with a spatula to achieve a level scoop.

   _____ Use a wet finger to smooth the alginate surface, eliminate any air pockets trapped near the surface, and remove any excess material from posterior areas. Ask the patient to relax and take a deep breath through his/her nose, and to keep breathing through the nose during the entire procedure.

_____ Insert the filled tray into the mouth. Use the side of the tray to push one side of the cheek and a finger on the other side, and slide it into the mouth. For an impression of the mandibular arch, ask the patient to lift his/her tongue as the tray is inserted. Press the tray gently into position centered over the arch, placing the posterior portion first to form a seal so the material flows forward and not down the throat.

_____ For two scoops, add 2/3 measurement of room-temperature water. For each three scoops of powder, add one full measure of water. Cooler water retards setting and warmer water accelerates setting.

_____ Tumble the container to gently fluff the powder. Explain the procedure to the patient.

_____ Empty two scoops of powder into a clean, dry mixing bowl for a mandibular impression, and three scoops of powder for a maxillary impression.

_____ Check for and remove any residual material from the mouth, between the teeth, or from around the patient's face.

_____ Rinse the impression thoroughly under running water. Spray with disinfectant solution, wrap in a wet paper towel, and place in a labeled plastic bag before pouring.

_____ Once the material is set, gently break the seal by moving the tray up and down or using the side of a finger at the periphery. Snap the tray loose from the arch and remove the impression from the patient's mouth, protecting the opposite arch with a finger.

_____ Push firmly up when seating the maxillary tray, and press firmly down when seating the mandibular tray. Hold the seated tray immovable for one minute or until the alginate is no longer sticky.

_____ Mix the water and powder carefully until all the powder is wet. Once all the powder is incorporated, continue to spatulate in a vigorous fashion. Do not whip or stir the alginate material. The spatula should be flattened using pressure against the bowl to reduce incorporating air. Spatulate regular-set material for one minute, and fast-set material for **45 seconds**.

_____ Select and/or prepare a suitable impression tray. Try the mandibular and maxillary trays in the patient's mouth to ensure proper fit and comfort.

_____ Once the alginate appears homogenous and creamy without lumps, apply it into the tray. Load the mandibular tray from the lingual sides, and use the flat side of the blade to condense the material firmly in the tray. Place the majority of the alginate in the anterior portion of the tray.

8. Using the following table, list five advantages and five disadvantages of reversible hydrocolloids.

Table 36-2

Advantages	Disadvantages

9. When taking an elastomeric bite registration, the cheek should be retracted enough to expose _____ to be sure the correct relationship of the bite is recorded.

10. Explain the three ways of recording a putty-wash impression.

MEDICAL TERMINOLOGY REVIEW

Use a dictionary and/or your textbook to define the following terms.

agar _____

alginate _____

aqueous hydrocolloids _____

bite registration _____

cast model _____

crenula _____

gel _____

hydrocolloid _____

hydrophilic _____

hydrophobic _____

imbibition _____

impression _____

monophasic _____

nonaqueous elastomers _____

periphery _____

polyether impression _____

polymerization _____

polysiloxane or vinylpolysiloxane (VPS) _____

sol _____

syneresis _____

tori _____

viscosity _____

wettability _____

ABBREVIATIONS

EPA _____

CRITICAL THINKING

1. What is the difference between a cast model and an impression of a patient's mouth?

2. What is the difference in purpose between a preliminary impression and a final impression?

3. What is the difference between wettability and viscosity? Why is it important to have materials with low viscosity?

4. What are three of the most important requirements of an impression material? What advantages do these properties give to the material?

CHAPTER REVIEW TEST

MULTIPLE CHOICE

Circle the letter of the correct answer.

1. The _____ Association sets the standards and specific requirements for the safety and effectiveness of dental products.
   a. Food and Drug
   b. American Dental Assistants
   c. American Dental Hygiene
   d. American Dental

2. Primary impressions are used for:
   a. study models
   b. full crowns
   c. indirect restorations
   d. implants

3. A(n) _____ is a method of replicating a patient's mouth normal occlusion.
   a. rubber base impression
   b. alginate impression
   c. bite registration
   d. gypsum model

4. Impressions that are _____ work well with wetting and a moist environment.
   a. hydrophilic
   b. hydroplastic
   c. hydrophobic
   d. hyperphysical

5. For an accurate impression, a low _____ material is best to use in the gingival sulcus.
   a. agar
   b. strength
   c. viscosity
   d. hydrocolloid impression

6. The types of "elastic" impression material used in dentistry are polysulphide, polyether, silicone, and: _____.
   a. compounds
   b. zinc oxide eugenol
   c. wax
   d. polysiloxane

7. A triple tray is used to take an impression of the tooth or teeth being worked on and the _____ simultaneously.
   a. soft tissue anatomy
   b. patient's occlusion
   c. temporary restoration
   d. implant

8. The folds of tissue connecting the cheeks and lips to the alveolar mucosa is the: _____.
   a. frenula
   b. tori
   c. buccal fold
   d. vestibule

9. The first compartment within the conditioning unit for a reversible hydrocolloid impression should be set at _____ degrees Fahrenheit.
   a. 185
   b. 200
   c. 212
   d. 250

10. Some disadvantages of reversible hydrocolloid impressions are: difficult to disinfect, _____, and high cost of equipment.
    a. bitter taste
    b. low temperature resistant
    c. staining
    d. low tear strength

TRUE/FALSE

Indicate whether the statement is true (T) or false (F).

_____ 1. Working time is defined as the time it takes the dental laboratory to fabricate a full cast crown.

_____ 2. Tear strength and elastic recovery means that the material will retain its shape and form when removed from the mouth.

_____ 3. Another term for "triple tray" is "dual arch."

_____ 4. Syneresis is an advantage of using hydrocolloid impression material.

_____ 5. Imbibition is the process of contracting and shrinking.

_____ 6. Wetting is the capacity of a material to flow over a surface and capture all irregularities.

_____ 7. Alginate is an irreversible hydrocolloid material.

_____ 8. Dental alginate can last over 48 hours without being poured in a gypsum product.

_____ 9. Setting time is the transitional time that plastic properties permit molding of the area.

_____ 10. To disinfect an alginate impression, the dental assistant should spray it with a glutaraldehyde.

FILL IN THE BLANK

Using words from the list below, fill in the blanks to complete the following statements.

alginate	bite registration	sol
working time	tori	monophasic
gel	hydrophobic	periphery
agar	custom	

1. A viscous liquid where particles become attached, forming a loose network, is called _____.

2. Medium viscosity is also called _____ because it is versatile for tray or syringe application.

3. The _____, or the outer border portion of a tray surface, should not distort soft tissue.

4. _____ materials are used to record and simulate how the patient's arches occlude.

5. A(n) _____ impression cannot be converted back to its original state.

6. Mandibular _____ are located bilaterally on the lingual sides of the arch in the premolar area, and are more pronounced in some patients.

7. A(n) _____ impression is said to have an aversion for water and with less wetting ability.

8. The length of time required to mix a material is called _____.

9. When a colloid becomes viscous, thickened, and hardened into an elastic solid, it is said to be a _____.

10. A(n) _____ impression tray can be trimmed with a dental acrylic bur.

CHAPTER 37
Laboratory Materials and Procedures

CHAPTER OUTLINE

Review the Chapter Outline. If any content area is unclear, review that area before beginning the workbook exercises.

A. Safety in the Dental Laboratory

B. Infection Control in the Dental Laboratory

C. Preparing Impressions

D. Dental Laboratory Equipment

E. Equipment Requiring Heat Sources

F. Vacuum Former

G. Articulators and Face Bows

H. Dental Lathe

I. Mixing Bowls

J. Vibrator

K. Model Trimmer

L. Dental Laboratory

M. Diagnostic Cast Models

N. Gypsum Materials

O. Plaster

P. Stone

Q. Die Stone

R. Pouring Dental Models

S. Trimming Dental Models

T. Custom Impression Trays

U. Visible Light Cure

V. Acrylic

W. Thermoplastic

X. Dental Waxes

Y. Compound

CHAPTER REVIEW

The following is a summary of the chapter. If any of this material is unclear, review it in the textbook again.

The chairside dental assistant must be knowledgeable in chairside functions and dental laboratory procedures. Dental assistants who possess a good understanding of safety, infection control, and restoration/prosthetic fabrication in the dental laboratory are an asset to the dental practice and profession. The OSHA Bloodborne Pathogens Standard provides employee and patient safety within the dental laboratory. Adherence to each part of the standard minimizes injury and cross-contamination. The dental laboratory equipment must be maintained routinely and kept in good working order for all laboratory procedures to be completed on a timely bases. The dental assistant must read all the manufacturer's directions on procedure, maintenance, and usage. There are several types of gypsum materials. Dental stone is strong and used widely for working models. Stone is available in pink and yellow (buff). Typically, pink stone is used for fabrication of dental die(s) and buff for removal appliances. Dental plaster is a weaker product that is used primarily for diagnostic models, articulating models, and attaching casts. Custom impression trays are made in the dental office and used with carrier impression material for a more accurate impression. Custom tray design is based on the purpose of the tray and specification needed by the dentist.

LEARNING ACTIVITES AND STUDY AIDS

Review the following study aids and/or complete the activities to ensure that you have achieved the learning objectives for this chapter.

1. List the twelve OSHA bloodborne pathogen standards to be followed in a dental laboratory environment.

2. Fill in the blanks with the best answer:

   The recommended ratio of sodium hypochlorite for disinfecting hydrocolloid and vinylpolysiloxane impressions is _____; other hospital-grade disinfectants such as _____ and _____ can also be used.

3. Complete the following table by listing the disinfecting methods for each impression material.

Table 37-1

Impression material	Disinfecting methods
Alginate	
Polysulfide	
Silicone	
Polyether	
Vinylpolysiloxane	
Reversible hydrocolloid	
Compound	

4. Write in order the steps of fabricating a mouthguard using a vacuum former.

5. Define "centric occlusion."

6. List the steps for "general care" of the model trimmer.

7. In the following table, match the material/process in Column A with the correct description in Column B.

Table 37-2

Column A	Column B
A. dihydrate	_____ half water and half calcium sulfate
B. calcination	_____ rough, irregular, and porous
C. hemihydrate	_____ setting process that gives off heat
D. plaster powder particles	_____ strongest of all gypsum materials
E. stone powder particles	_____ manufacturing process whereby gypsum is converted to Plaster of Paris and artificial stone
F. die stone	_____ fairly smooth, somewhat regular in size, and dense
G. exothermic reaction	_____ a substance consisting of two parts water to one part calcium sulfate

8. List the characteristics of dental stone and dental plaster.

9. Describe the Two-Step Pour Method, Boxed Pour Method, and Inverted Pour Method.

10. In the following table, match the type of wax in Column A with the description in Column B.

Table 37-4

Column A	Column B
a. Baseplate wax	_____ usually green and coated with a water-soluble adhesive on one side; used for registering occlusal contacts on teeth
b. Bite registration wax	_____ red or colorless; comes in rope form; extremely pliable and tacky at room temperature; used on the periphery of impression trays to extend the tray or to make it a more comfortable fit for the patient
c. Indicator wax	_____ made of beeswax, paraffin, and resin; color is orange, darker shades of blue, red, and violet; useful in holding broken parts of a denture together during repair
d. Stick wax	_____ has metal incorporated into the wax; U-shaped wafer; used to record the occlusal relationship between a patient's opposing arches and proper articulation of the maxillary and mandibular models
e. Utility wax	_____ used to block out undercuts on cast models and for bite registration; simulates the vertical dimension of teeth during denture and partial denture fabrication

MEDICAL TERMINOLOGY REVIEW

Use a dictionary and/or your textbook to define the following terms.

anatomic portion _____

articulator _____

aseptic _____

calcination _____

centric occlusion _____

compound _____

die stone _____

exothermic _____

facebow _____

gypsum _____

hemihydrate _____

lathe _____

model trimmer _____

prostheses _____

unit dose concept _____

vacuum former _____

vibrator _____

ABBREVIATIONS

OSHA _____

CRITICAL THINKING

1. How does a dental assistant use his/her knowledge and skills of laboratory materials in his/her job?

2. As a dental assistant, what procedures is one responsible to follow under OSHA's Bloodborne Pathogen Standards?

3. Why is it important to maintain excellent infection control procedures in the laboratory? Whose responsibility is it to ensure that proper infection control procedures are followed?

CHAPTER REVIEW TEST

MULTIPLE CHOICE

Circle the letter of the correct answer.

1. The _____ is a device designed to reproduce the movements of a patient's mandibular arch in proper centric occlusion to the maxillary arch.

   a. articulator
   b. facebow
   c. lathe
   d. vacuum former

2. The rag wheel will be _____ by the dental assistant between patients.

   a. disinfected
   b. sterilized
   c. sprayed with alcohol
   d. dried

3. The anatomic portion of a cast model includes the teeth and:

   a. base
   b. oral structure
   c. retro molar pad
   d. tongue

4. When fabricating a mouthguard, the dental assistant heats plastic material within the forming machine. The dental assistant will pull the frame of the unit down over the cast when the plastic begins to sag between _____ and _____ inches.

a. 2 and 2½

b. 1 and 2

c. ½ and 1

b. 1 and 1½

5. An impression material carrier for a more accurate impression is a:

a. stock tray

b. rim lock tray

c. custom tray

d. triple tray

6. To disinfect hydrocolloid and vinylpolysiloxane impressions, they should be soaked by spraying a(n) _____ disinfectant.

a. hospital

b. over-the-counter

c. alcohol-base

d. low-grade

7. When fabricating a mouthguard, splint for temporary crowns, or nightguards, a _____ is used for rapid fabrication.

a. butane burner

b. vacuum former

c. bunsen burner

d. alcohol torch

8. A dental assistant should wear _____ when there is a potential risk of exposure to pathogens.

a. EPPs

b. PPEs

c. nitrile gloves

d. rubber gloves

9. Wax made from beeswax, paraffin, and resin is called:

a. sticky wax

b. bite registration wax

c. baseplate wax

d. indicator wax

10. Utility wax is red or colorless, comes in rope form, and is used on the _____ of impression trays.

a. anterior portion

b. lingual portion

c. periphery

d. posterior

TRUE/FALSE

Indicate whether the statement is true (T) or false (F).

_____ 1. After the dental assistant has used the laboratory wax spatula, the instrument does not need to be disinfected or sterilized.

_____ 2. Antimicrobial impression material should be used to reduce bioburden and infectious agents in the impression.

_____ 3. The ideal centric occlusion is when the mesial lingual cusps of the maxillary first molar occlude in the central fossa of the mandibular premolar.

_____ 4. The **unit dose concept** prevents the contamination of bulk supplies.

_____ 5. A substance consisting of two parts water to one part calcium sulfate is hemihydrate.

_____ 6. A dental assistant should wait 48 hours prior to separating a gypsum cast from the impression.

_____ 7. Disposable impression trays should be used for only one patient and then discarded.

_____ 8. All dental mixing bowls must be hard and rigid to push the material against the sides of the bowl.

_____ 9. Plaster of Paris is an artificial stone.

_____ 10. When working in the dental laboratory, proper ventilation equipment should be used.

FILL IN THE BLANK

Using words from the list below, fill in the blanks to complete the following statements.

lathe	model trimmer	polyether
vibrator	dihydrate	facebow
vacuum former	prostheses	final
mixing bowl	initial	

1. A dental _____ is an artificial replacement for teeth and other oral structures.

2. _____ is obtained by avoiding any contamination of disease-producing microorganisms.

3. The _____ set for artificial stone is 45 minutes.

4. The _____ is used with water to trim and contour gypsum cast models.

5. The _____ of the articulator is used to record the relationship of the maxillary arch to the horizontal axis rotation of the mandible.

6. _____ impressions cannot be immersed in a disinfectant solution because they are hydrophilic and will distort when placed in liquid solutions.

7. For rapid fabrication of custom trays, mouthguards, splints, and nightguards, a dental assistant will use the _____

8. A _____ is a substance consisting of two parts water to one part calcium sulfate.

9. The dental _____ increases the density of the gypsum product by eliminating air bubbles.

10. The _____ is a rotary machine used for grinding, finishing, and polishing in the dental laboratory.

CHAPTER 38
General Dentistry

CHAPTER OUTLINE

Review the Chapter Outline. If any content area is unclear, review that area before beginning the workbook exercises.

    A.   Cavity Preparation

    B.   Restorations

    C.   Class I Restorations

    D.   Class II Restorations

    E.   Class III and IV Restorations

    F.   Class V and VI Restorations

    G.   Veneers

    H.   Tooth Whitening

CHAPTER REVIEW

The following is a summary of the chapter. If any of this material is unclear, review it in the textbook again.

The most common procedures in general restorative dentistry are the standard Class I–VI restorations, developed by G. V. Black in the late 1880s. Amalgam or composite resin is used in Class I, II, and V; however, esthetics is required in the anterior teeth. Class III, IV, and VI require the use of composite resin to match the natural tooth. The onset of cosmetic dentistry has grown over the last twenty years, and technology has offered a more perfected result. Today, in-office and at-home professional teeth-whitening products are available for the patient who wants whiter teeth. Cosmetic or esthetic dentistry has also gone one step further to improve a patient's dental appearance: the dental veneer, an extremely close resemblance to a natural tooth. A dental assistant must be cognoscente of manufacturer directions and the shelf life of all dental materials and products used within the practice he/she works.

LEARNING ACTIVITES AND STUDY AIDS

Review the following study aids and/or complete the activities to ensure that you have achieved the learning objectives for this chapter.

1. List the objectives of cavity preparation.

2. In the following table, match the class in column A with the definition in column B by placing the appropriate letter in the blank.

    Table 38-1

Column A	Column B
A. Class I	_____ involves the proximal surfaces in the posterior teeth (MO)
B. Class II	_____ found on the gingival third of the facial or lingual surfaces (F)
C. Class III	_____ found on pits and fissures of the posterior teeth (O)
D. Class IV	_____ found on the occlusal cusp height of the posterior teeth
E. Class V	_____ two-surface, three-surface, or multi-surface of the posterior teeth
F. Class VI	_____ involves the proximal surfaces and the anterior teeth (ML)

3. List three primary reasons to whiten teeth.

4. Write the four indications for esthetic dentistry.

5. Fill in the blanks in the following sentences:

   a. The process of cavity preparation is divided into two stages, the initial preparation and the final preparation. The initial stage is to create the _____, by extending the preparation in all directions to sound enamel supported by healthy dentin and obtain a sound pulpal floor.

   b. The _____ is then placed within a cavity preparation to mechanically lock the restorative material and prevent dislodging.

   c. The final phase of the cavity preparation includes removal of _____ and/or old restorative material, and placement of _____ grooves and notches to help prevent the restorative material from dislodging.

6. Provide the type of Class II restoration for the following abbreviations.

   Table 38-2

MO _____	MOD _____
DO _____	DOB _____
MOL _____	

7. Write the type of matrix system that would be used in the following procedures:

   _____ to restore an ML on tooth #8.

   _____ to restore an MOD on tooth #15.

8. Explain the difference in steps for assisting with a Class II composite restoration versus a Class II amalgam restoration.

9. List the areas that are particularly susceptible to Class I and Class II caries.

10. Explain what a dental assistant should do if the new restoration breaks during the final carving and polishing.

MEDICAL TERMINOLOGY REVIEW

Use a dictionary and/or your textbook to define the following terms.

axial wall _____

bonding _____

cavity _____

cavity wall _____

Class I _____

Class II _____

Class III _____

Class IV _____

Class V _____

Class VI _____

diastema _____

esthetic dentistry _____

line angle _____

operative dentistry _____

outline form _____

pulpal wall _____

restoration _____

restorative dentistry _____

retention form _____

veneer _____

whitening _____

ABBREVIATIONS

DO _____

EDDA _____

EFDA _____

IML _____

ML _____

MOD _____

CRITICAL THINKING

1. What are the differences between restorative dentistry and esthetic dentistry?

2. Why is it important for a dental assistant to understand the difference between restorative and esthetic dentistry?

3. During chairside dentistry, there are nine steps that are the responsibility of the dental assistant. List these nine steps, and explain why they are important to a smooth work flow during patient treatment.

CHAPTER REVIEW TEST

MULTIPLE CHOICE

Circle the letter of the correct answer.

1. A Class III restoration involves _____ surfaces of the tooth.

   a. occlusal
   b. pit and fissure
   c. smooth
   d. proximal

2. _____ is the process of conservatively removing defective tooth structure and leaving healthy tooth structure to support the restoration.

   a. Restorative dentistry
   b. Cavity preparation
   c. Operative dentistry
   d. Cavity form

3. The _____ form is the first step during the initial stage of cavity preparation.

   a. outline
   b. line angle
   c. retention
   d. resistance

4. General dentistry or _____ dentistry is the art and science of diagnosis and treatment of defective teeth.

   a. endodontic
   b. operative
   c. restorative
   d. esthetic

5. A dental assistant can determine what type of restorative material will be used by the _____ or cavity preparation.

   a. scheduled time
   b. dental assistant's memory
   c. cavity classification
   d. location of the treated tooth

6. Tooth areas susceptible to Class I caries are _____, buccal, and lingual pits and fissures.

   a. occlusal
   b. mesial
   c. distal
   d. meiso-occlusal

7. The dentist uses a caries _____ following the preparation of the outline form.

   a. removing instrument
   b. indicator dye
   c. dissolving solution
   d. excavator hand instrument

8. When restoring a Class II amalgam, the dentist will place a(n) _____ to replace the missing wall.

   a. rubber dam
   b. wooden wedge
   c. matrix band
   d. ion crown

9. How many surfaces are involved in a Class III?

   a. one
   b. two
   c. three
   d. four

10. The dentist will evaluate the occlusion with _____ following placement.

    a. carbon paper
    b. copy paper
    c. tissue paper
    d. articulating paper

TRUE/FALSE

Indicate whether the statement is true (T) or false (F).

_____ 1. Dr. G. V. Black created the basis of cavity preparation and restoration.

_____ 2. Extensive retention grooves are placed in all cavity preparations.

_____ 3. Class I caries can be found only in the anterior of the mouth.

_____ 4. A diastema can be found between the maxillary central incisors.

_____ 5. The two stages in cavity preparation are the initial and final preparation.

_____ 6. Teeth cannot be overwhitened.

_____ 7. Retention grooves are placed during the final phase of cavity preparation.

_____ 8. A vacuum former is used to fabricate a tooth-whitening tray.

_____ 9. One step to in-office tooth whitening is to isolate the gingival.

_____ 10. A line angle is a junction of three surfaces in a cavity preparation.

FILL IN THE BLANK

Using words from the list below, fill in the blanks to complete the following statements.

mylar	veneer	whitening
Class I	resistance	sensitivity
composite resin	block out	disto-occlusal
Tofflemire	at-home	

1. Caries found at the lingual fossa of tooth #8 is a _____ cavity.

2. The abbreviation DO stands for _____.

3. In the initial cavity preparation, _____ form will be cut into the cavity preparation.

4. The matrix system used interproximal of an anterior tooth is a _____, to which a tooth-colored resin material will be placed.

5. The patient may experience tooth _____ after using a whitening solution.

6. The process of brightening stained or discolored teeth is considered tooth _____.

7. The dental assistant will fabricate a custom-whitening tray by placing _____ material on the facial surface of each tooth within the model.

8. A _____ is a thin layer of tooth-colored composite resin that is made in the laboratory and applied to the facial surface of a tooth.

9. Classes III, IV, and VI require the use of _____ to match the natural tooth structure.

10. Two methods to obtain a whiter smile are in-office and _____ professional whitening products.

CHAPTER 39
Matrix Systems for Restorative Dentistry

CHAPTER OUTLINE

Review the Chapter Outline. If any content area is unclear, review that area before beginning the workbook exercises.

    A. Posterior Matrix Systems
        1. Tofflemire Retainer
        2. Matrix Bands
        3. Wedges

    B. Anterior Matrix Systems

    C. Alternative Matrix Systems
        1. Automatrix System
        2. Sectional Matrices
        3. Anterior and Cervical Matrix Bands
        4. Other Matrix Systems for Primary Teeth

CHAPTER REVIEW

The following is a summary of the chapter. If any of this material is unclear, review it in the textbook again.

Matrix systems are essentially properly shaped retaining walls that confine, contour, and smooth the surface of soft restorative materials in a cavity preparation until they harden. Several systems are available. Which system is selected depends on the location and size of the cavity preparation, the type of restorative material to be used, the operator's preference, and whether the restoration is placed in a primary or permanent tooth. Assembly and placement of matrix systems require attention to detail because the final restoration must recreate the missing tooth anatomy and proximal contact precisely. Several states permit a dental assistant or EFDA to place and remove matrices.

LEARNING ACTIVITIES AND STUDY AIDS

Review the following study aids and/or complete the activities to ensure that you have achieved the learning objectives for this chapter.

1. List four tasks a matrix system must accomplish.

2. To learn more about Dr. G. V. Black's cavity classification system, find one article online or using resources from the school or local library. On a separate piece of paper, write a one-page summary on your findings and what you learned. Be sure to cite your resources.

3. Differentiate a matrix retainer and band.

4. Describe the purpose and process of contouring a matrix band.

5. State why the thickness of a matrix band is important.

6. Discuss why a wedge is used in a matrix system.

7. List two undesirable results on a finished restoration when a wedge that was too small or too large was used as part of the matrix system.

8. State why transparent materials are used for anterior matrix bands.

9. Discuss why special pediatric retainers are needed for use in the Tofflemire matrix system.

10. List the matrix systems used for pediatric patients.

MEDICAL TERMINOLOGY REVIEW

Use a dictionary and/or your textbook to define the following terms.

automatrix _____

celluloid _____

matrix _____

retainer _____

tension ring _____

wedge _____

ABBREVIATIONS

EFDA _____

CRITICAL THINKING

1. Explain what matrices are, and why it is important for the chairside dental assistant to know which matrix will be used.

2. Why would one type of matrices be used for posterior teeth when another type might be used for anterior teeth?

3. How can the dental assistant differentiate between the various types of matrices?

CHAPTER REVIEW TEST

MULTIPLE CHOICE

Circle the letter of the correct answer.

1. All of the following are functions of a wedge in a matrix system EXCEPT:
   a. isolate the preparation
   b. contour the restorative material at the gingival edge
   c. permit light curing of the restorative material
   d. secure the matrix band to the tooth

2. When a t-band is used, the free end is placed toward the:
   a. mesial
   b. distal
   c. buccal
   d. lingual

3. For what class of cavity preparation is a spot welded band used?
   a. I
   b. II
   c. III
   d. IV
   e. V

4. A sectional matrix is retained by a:
   a. wedge
   b. floss ligature
   c. mylar strip
   d. tension ring

5. This motion should be used to remove a matrix band from a newly placed restoration.
   a. single pull
   b. rapid slide to the lingual
   c. gentle rocking
   d. any of the above

6. This matrix system requires the use of a retainer.
   a. Tofflemire
   b. t-band
   c. mylar strip
   d. automatrix

7. A thicker universal matrix band provides more:
   a. smoothing
   b. contouring
   c. flexibility
   d. rigidity

8. Select ALL of the following items that are disposable.
   a. Tofflemire matrix band
   b. Tofflemire matrix retainer
   c. wedge
   d. anterior strip matrix

9. Using a wedge that is too small may result in the creation of:
   a. cupping
   b. excessive tension
   c. patient discomfort
   d. an overhang

10. The smaller loop of a Tofflemire band must be placed toward this area of a tooth.
    a. facial
    b. lingual
    c. occlusal
    d. cervical

TRUE/FALSE

Indicate whether the statement is true (T) or false (F).

_____ 1. The flat side of a wedge should be placed toward the gingiva.

_____ 2. Contouring a matrix band thins it in the interproximal contact area.

_____ 3. Any sharp instrument edge can be used to contour a matrix band.

_____ 4. A wedge may be triangular or curved to an anatomical shape.

_____ 5. A contra-angle Tofflemire retainer is used when the buccal surface is not available.

_____ 6. An extension band is used in a Tofflemire retainer when a more apically positioned gingival wall increases the height of the preparation.

_____ 7. All states allow dental assistants to place and remove matrix systems.

_____ 8. A Tofflemire matrix should be assembled and placed on the tray setup immediately before its placement on the tooth.

_____ 9. A matrix retainer serves to secure the matrix band to the tooth.

_____ 10. The automatrix system alone does not require the use of a retainer.

FILL IN THE BLANK

Using words from the list below, fill in the blanks to complete the following statements.

check contacts	locking device	place wedge
contour band	long knob	short knob
contour gingival area	open folded band loop	spindle
head		

For Questions 1–5, select the part of the Tofflemire retainer that completes the listed task.

1. lock the band into place: _____

2. change the size of the loop: _____

3. position the band for best access: _____

4. screw into the locking device: _____

5. contain a diagonal slot to hold the ends of the band: _____

For Questions 6–10, indicate the use of each item in a matrix placement procedure.

6. burnisher: _____

7. mirror handle: _____

8. wedge: _____

9. floss: _____

10. cotton pliers: _____

CHAPTER 40

Fixed Prosthodontics

CHAPTER OUTLINE

Review the Chapter Outline. If any content area is unclear, review that area before beginning the workbook exercises.

A. Treatment Planning

B. Indirect Restorations
   1. Inlays and Onlays
   2. Veneers
   3. Crowns
   4. Fixed Partial Denture or Bridge
   5. Implants

C. Overview of a Crown Procedure
   1. Shade Selection
   2. Preparation
   3. Retention for Crowns
   4. Tissue Management
   5. Final Impression and Bite Registration
   6. Provisional
   7. Cementation Appointment

D. Overview of a Bridge Procedure
   1. Preparation
   2. Framework Try-in
   3. Cementation Appointment

E. Machined Restorations

F. Patient Instructions

G. Role of the Dental Laboratory Technician
   1. Laboratory Prescription

CHAPTER REVIEW

The following is a summary of the chapter. If any of this material is unclear, review it in the textbook again.

Patients who lose teeth must replace them if they are to maintain good oral health, because missing teeth can cause difficulty in chewing properly, drifting of adjacent teeth, supraeruption of opposing teeth, and caries and periodontal disease of nearby teeth that are both difficult to keep clean and subject to abnormal biting forces because they are out of position. Furthermore, patients may desire a tooth or tooth surface replacement for esthetic reasons. Fixed prostheses are one option for replacements. There are a variety of types: inlays, onlays, veneers, crowns, fixed partial dentures (bridges), and implants. After collecting historical, clinical, radiographic, and photographic data, the dentist will recommend a particular type based on the patient's needs and conditions. Two to three appointments are generally required to complete the prosthesis the patient selects. State laws vary regarding which of the procedures the dental assistant may perform. It is important for the dental assistant to check the state dental laws, rules, and regulations to learn what is legal.

LEARNING ACTIVITIES AND STUDY AIDS

Review the following study aids and/or complete the activities to ensure that you have achieved the learning objectives for this chapter.

1. Define fixed prosthodontics.

2. Make a series of flash cards that have the name and purpose of a type of fixed prosthesis on one side, and a colored picture of that type of restoration on the other. Go online to find the pictures. Good places to start are dental laboratory, education, or individual dentist sites, as for example, *http://www.tischlerdental.com*, *http://www.dental-picture-show.com*, or *http://www.drtooth.hu*. Remember to click on Images in the search engine so you will get pictures rather than words. You can print the pictures you locate, then cut them out and paste them onto your flash cards so you will have a ready reference guide when you are preparing for externship or studying for course or DANB exams. Turn your flash cards into your instructor to receive a grade for your efforts.

3. State why a dentist would recommend a crown rather than a veneer, or a veneer rather than a crown.

4. On a separate piece of paper, make a table listing the indications and contraindications for a fixed prosthesis, then state who makes the final choice of the type of prosthesis to be placed.

5. Explain the procedural steps in a crown preparation appointment. Use an additonal piece of paper, if more space is required for your information.

6. Discuss different methods of tissue management, why tissue management is important, and what can happen if the tissue is not managed well. Use an additonal piece of paper, if more space is required for your information.

7. Describe the role of the dental laboratory technician in a fixed prosthetic procedure.

8. Discuss how ceramic blocks are fashioned into crowns, and state the advantage of this procedure for patients. Then go online, click Images, and go to *http://www.feistdental.com* or *http://www. advantage-dental.com* to see a photo of the milling process in action. Next, go to *http://www. orangevilledental.com* to see a picture of a CAD/CAM machine. You can print these pictures for a ready reference when you are preparing for externship or studying for course or DANB exams.

9. Differentiate core build-ups and retention pins, and state the purpose of each.

10. List patient care instructions for a fixed prosthesis.

MEDICAL TERMINOLOGY REVIEW

Use a dictionary and/or your textbook to define the following terms.

abutment _____

articulator _____

cast post _____

core _____

crown _____

die _____

fixed partial denture _____

implant _____

inlay _____

investment material _____

Maryland bridge _____

master cast _____

milled restoration _____

onlay _____

opaquer _____

pontic _____

porcelain-fused-to-metal crown (PFM) _____

prosthesis _____

prosthodontist _____

veneer _____

ABBREVIATIONS

CAD _____

CAM _____

CEREC _____

PFM _____

CRITICAL THINKING

1. What are the responsibilities of the dental assistant when a patient first presents to the dental office for prosthetic work?

2. What are the indications and contraindications for choosing to place a fixed prosthetic appliance into a patient's mouth?

3. If your patient has a dark-colored completed preparation, yet the patient's other teeth are lighter in color, how might you as the dental assistant "lighten" the completed prosthetic restoration to be placed?

CHAPTER REVIEW TEST

MULTIPLE CHOICE

Circle the letter of the correct answer.

1. The dental specialty pertaining to the restoration and replacement of teeth is:
   a. pathology
   b. periodontics
   c. prosthodontics
   d. pediatrics

2. Regardless of the state in which the dental assistant is working, this duty is always reserved for the dentist.
   a. examination
   b. radiography
   c. photography
   d. impressions for diagnostic models

3. All of the following are indications for a fixed prosthesis EXCEPT:
   a. healthy supporting tissue
   b. good oral hygiene
   c. missing teeth are in the same quadrant
   d. good abutment teeth are not available

4. An inlay is a:
   a. Class II restoration that does not involve the cusps
   b. Class III restoration that involves the incisal angle
   c. Class IV indirect restoration
   d. Class V restoration that is bonded in position

5. The strongest material for the construction of inlays and onlays is:
   a. gold
   b. silver
   c. milled ceramic
   d. cast porcelain

6. The most accurate shade for a fixed prosthesis can be identified using a:
   a. shade guide
   b. series of complementary shade guides
   c. digital shade meter
   d. stump shade

7. This type of cement should be used when cementing a porcelain veneer.
   a. bonded
   b. transparent
   c. zinc-based
   d. opaquer

8. When more retention is desired to make crown placement feasible, the dentist completes this procedure:
   a. post and core placement
   b. placement of retention pins
   c. core build-up
   d. a or c
   e. any of the above

9. When a tooth has a healthy buccal or lingual wall but the remaining walls are damaged, this type of prosthesis would likely be the treatment of choice.
   a. fixed partial denture
   b. onlay
   c. inlay
   d. three-quarter crown
   e. full crown

10. The units of a fixed bridge each pertain to a:
    a. missing tooth
    b. prepared tooth
    c. missing tooth wall
    d. tooth
    e. a and b

TRUE/FALSE

Indicate whether the statement is true (T) or false (F).

_____ 1. A Maryland bridge is used only to replace a missing anterior tooth.

_____ 2. An implant is placed within the jaw bone to provide support for a prosthesis.

_____ 3. The second appointment for a fixed prosthesis involves shade selection, preparation of the tooth structure and the provisional restoration, and try-in of the final restoration.

_____ 4. The shape of a preparation margin is determined by the shape of the bur the dentist uses to cut it.

_____ 5. Placement of a post and core recreates the lost tooth structure of the anatomic crown of a vital tooth.

_____ 6. The most popular material for core build-ups is amalgam because of its strength and esthetics.

_____ 7. Liquids such as blood and sulcus fluid at the margin of the preparation must be controlled in order to obtain an accurate impression.

_____ 8. A good way for the dental assistant to determine the length of retraction cord to cut is to wrap it around the thumb and index finger and cut the cord to this length.

_____ 9. The general reason for impression failure is poor tissue management.

_____ 10. If the provisional restoration for a fixed prosthesis comes off prior to the final cementation appointment, the patient can function well in that condition until the fixed prosthesis arrives.

FILL IN THE BLANK

Using words from the list below, fill in the blanks to complete the following statements.

full crown	periodontal irritation	provisional restoration
implant	pontic	try-in
inlay	post and core	veneer
onlay		

1. A fixed prosthesis that replaces all, or nearly all, of the tooth crown is termed a _____.

2. A thin layer of esthetic material placed on the facial surface of a tooth to improve its esthetics is termed a _____.

3. A temporary restoration that maintains the form and function of a prepared tooth until the permanent fixed prosthesis arrives is a termed a _____.

4. A Class II indirect restoration that involves one or more cusps is termed a(n) _____.

5. A screw-like support surgically inserted into the jaw bone to anchor a prosthetic superstructure is termed a(n) _____.

6. Each missing tooth in a fixed partial denture is replaced with a _____.

7. A Class II indirect restoration that does not involve the cusps is termed a(n) _____.

8. A _____ is placed in a tooth that has been treated endodontically and will receive a crown.

9. The dental assistant may place the final restoration for _____.

10. Excess cement that flows out around the margins of a fixed restoration must be removed to prevent _____.

CHAPTER 41
Provisional Coverage

CHAPTER OUTLINE

Review the Chapter Outline. If any content area is unclear, review that area before beginning the workbook exercises.

   A. Criteria for Provisional Fabrication
      1. Mechanical Criteria
      2. Biological Criteria
      3. Aesthetic Criteria

   B. Types of Provisional Coverage
      1. Provisional Restoration Methods
      2. Direct Technique
      3. Indirect Technique
      4. Custom Provisional Coverage
      5. Preformed Polycarbonate Crown
      6. Celluloid Provisional
      7. Aluminum Crowns

   C. Provisional Restoration Materials
      1. Methacrylate
      2. Bis-Acryl Composite
      3. Bis-GMA Composite

CHAPTER REVIEW

The following is a summary of the chapter. If any of this material is unclear, review it in the textbook again.

Temporary restorations are referred to as provisional coverage. Such coverage maintains the form, function, comfort, and sometimes the esthetics of the natural teeth while permanent restorations are being constructed. The dental assistant fabricates the majority of temporary restorations in many dental offices. A choice of materials and techniques is available. All of the materials used for provisional coverage are forms of plastic except aluminum shell crowns. Provisional coverage may be fabricated in the mouth, on a model, or through the use of preformed crowns or customized techniques. The finished temporary must meet mechanical, biological, and esthetic criteria. A temporary restoration is cemented in position with temporary cement. It is extremely important for the dental assistant to teach the patient proper home care of the finished restoration.

LEARNING ACTIVITES AND STUDY AIDS

Review the following study aids and/or complete the activities to ensure that you have achieved the learning objectives for this chapter.

1. Discuss the importance of provisional restorations.

2. List the different types of provisional restorations.

3. Differentiate direct, indirect, custom, and preformed crown techniques for the fabrication of provisional restorations.

4. Define the term **stent**, and state how a stent is used during temporary restoration fabrication.

5. List the mechanical criteria for a satisfactory provisional restoration.

6. Discuss biological responses to well- and poorly constructed provisional restorations.

7. Define contour, contact, margin, and embrasure form.

8. State why excellent margin adaptation is necessary for successful provisional coverage.

9. Describe relining a preformed crown.

10. State the uses of the different types of preformed crowns.

MEDICAL TERMINOLOGY REVIEW

Use a dictionary and/or your textbook to define the following terms.

aesthetics _____

contour _____

dual curing _____

embrasure _____

exothermic _____

fabricate _____

flash _____

malleable _____

margin _____

polymerization _____

provisional _____

self-curing _____

stent _____

ABBREVIATIONS
None used in this chapter.

CRITICAL THINKING

1. What is the purpose of a provisional restoration? What other terms can be used to identify a provisional restoration?

2. What are the requirements of a provisional restoration? Why must all of these requirements be met?

3. If a dental assistant fabricates a provisional crown and the margins of the crown do not cover the prepared tooth completely, what might the patient experience, and how can this be corrected?

CHAPTER REVIEW TEST

MULTIPLE CHOICE

Circle the letter of the correct answer.

1. Provisional restorations are placed to accomplish all of the following EXCEPT:
   a. protect the prepared tooth
   b. allow for healing of the soft tissue
   c. maintain proper relationship of the contacts between the teeth
   d. maintain proper salivary flow

2. Provisional restorations may be in service for:
   a. days to weeks
   b. days to months
   c. weeks to months
   d. any of the above

3. What type of cement is used to retain a provisional restoration in position in the mouth?
   a. high strength
   b. low acid
   c. temporary
   d. permanent

4. The margin of a provisional restoration must be in this relationship with the margin of the prepared tooth.
   a. flush
   b. extended slightly below the gingiva
   c. slightly short of the gingiva
   d. flashed

5. Factors affecting the durability of a provisional restoration include:
   a. strength of the material selected
   b. esthetics of the material selected
   c. design of the restoration
   d. a and c
   e. all of the above

6. When a patient clenches or grinds his/her teeth, it may be necessary to _____ the provisional restoration.
   a. repeatedly polish
   b. reinforce
   c. double cure
   d. shorten

7. To prevent sensitivity to heat and cold:
   a. the contacts of a provisional restoration must be properly contoured
   b. the margin of a provisional restoration must extend just to the gingiva but not beyond
   c. a base material should be placed before the temporary is cemented in position
   d. materials that set with an exothermic reaction must not be used for restoration fabrication

8. Pulp damage from heat generated during material setting may be lessened by using _____ materials.
   a. self-cure
   b. light-cure
   c. dual-cure
   d. chemical-cure

9. What is a stent?
   a. pattern or mold
   b. material that cures especially rapidly
   c. contact on a fixed temporary bridge
   d. preformed crown

10. An advantage of using the indirect technique for provisional restoration fabrication is:
    a. less time is required for the dental assistant and dentist
    b. the dental assistant can prepare the tooth on the model
    c. the restoration is ready when the patient comes in for the preparation
    d. more heat is released during tooth preparation

TRUE/FALSE

Indicate whether the statement is true (T) or false (F).

_____ 1. Flash is excess material that does not belong to the proper shape of the provisional restoration.

_____ 2. Provisional restorations are trimmed to final shape with rotary instruments.

_____ 3. The celluloid matrix of a preformed crown is removed prior to cementing the restoration to the tooth.

_____ 4. Polycarbonate-preformed crowns are available only in posterior tooth shapes.

_____ 5. An advantage of methacrylate provisional restoration materials is their very low shrinkage during setting.

_____ 6. An advantage of Bis-Acryl composite (Bis-Acryl resin) material is its lower temperature during polymerization.

_____ 7. The health of the tissues surrounding a provisional restoration in the mouth is determined primarily by the material chosen for its construction.

_____ 8. Even a well-made provisional restoration does not fit the mouth as well as a permanent restoration.

_____ 9. A provisional restoration should be removed from the mouth each night to allow the tissues to breathe.

_____ 10. Any tooth drifting due to improper contacts on a provisional restoration may cause the permanent restoration to not fit properly.

FILL IN THE BLANK

Using words from the list below, fill in the blanks to complete the following statements.

air	extrusion	polymerization
burs	impression	preformed crown
contacts	inflammation	scissors
disks	little time	stain
drifting	low cost	water

1. A temporary restoration that extends beyond the preparation margin will irritate the tissue and cause _____.

2. Adequate occlusal relationships between a temporary restoration and its opposing teeth will prevent _____ and _____ of the teeth.

3. Food impaction between the teeth is prevented through correctly contoured _____.

4. If a restoration is not well polished, some provisional restoration materials may _____.

5. A _____ may be used as a stent for fabricating a customized provisional crown.

6. An alginate or polyvinyl _____ is used to initiate direct provisional restoration fabrication.

7. Initial trimming of a provisional restoration can be done with _____; final trimming must be done with _____ and _____.

8. Provisional restoration materials set by _____.

9. _____ and _____ are advantages of the direct fabrication technique.

10. _____ or _____ can be used to cool the teeth during a direct fabrication procedure.

CHAPTER 42
Removable Prosthodontics

CHAPTER OUTLINE

Review the Chapter Outline. If any content area is unclear, review that area before beginning the workbook exercises.

A. History of Removable Prosthetics
B. Factors Influencing the Choice of a Removable Prosthesis
C. The Removable Partial Denture
D. The Complete (Full) Denture
E. Immediate Dentures
F. Overdentures
G. Denture Relining

CHAPTER REVIEW

The following is a summary of the chapter. If any of this material is unclear, review it in the textbook again.

Removable prostheses are artificial replacements for natural teeth and other oral structures that can be readily removed from the mouth for cleaning. There are three main types: a partial denture replaces some of the teeth in an arch; a full denture replaces all of them; and an overdenture is a full or partial denture that is supported by implants, retained tooth roots, or remaining teeth. Replacement of missing teeth is critical to maintaining the positions of the teeth in the arch. Wearing any type of denture is a learned skill. Dental assistants help patients learn to wear dentures successfully by reinforcing positive attitudes about dentures; providing careful, complete, and personalized patient education; and responding to denture-related requests whenever possible.

LEARNING ACTIVITIES AND STUDY AIDS

Review the following study aids and/or complete the activities to ensure that you have achieved the learning objectives for this chapter.

1. Explain the instructions that should be given to patients to ensure proper care of the prosthetic.

2. Differentiate partial dentures, full dentures, overdentures, and immediate dentures.

3. List at least three types of support for partial dentures and two for full dentures.

4. Define a unit and a pontic.

5. Discuss why a removable prosthesis could be the treatment of choice for a particular patient.

6. Provide the information as required to complete the following table.

Table 42-1

Advantages of partial or full dentures	Disadvantages of partial or full dentures

7. Make two flash cards. On one side of the first card list the components of a partial denture; on the other side describe each component. Repeat the process on the second card for a full denture. Submit your cards to your instructor for a grade. These cards can be useful tools when studying.

8. List the factors that need to be examined prior to a patient receiving a removable partial denture.

9. List the proper home care procedures for a denture.

10. Differentiate denture repair, relining, and tissue conditioning procedures.

MEDICAL TERMINOLOGY REVIEW

Use a dictionary and/or your textbook to define the following terms.

abutment _____

alloy _____

alveoloplasty _____

appliance _____

clasp _____

complete denture _____

conditioning _____

denture base _____

edentulous _____

flipper _____

immediate denture _____

overdenture _____

pontic _____

prosthesis _____

reline _____

rest _____

unit _____

wax try-in _____

CRITICAL THINKING

1. Why is patient education so important when dealing with a patient who will be receiving removable prosthetic appliances?

2. What is the dental assistant's role in assisting a patient with removable oral prostheses?

3. State and describe the six rules for a patient to follow after receiving complete dentures. Why is this care so important to the wearer of dentures?

CHAPTER REVIEW TEST

MULTIPLE CHOICE

Circle the letter of the correct answer.

1. Factors that may suggest a partial denture should be the treatment of choice are:
   a. lack of abutment teeth distally
   b. patient's overall health condition
   c. cost of a fixed prosthesis
   d. a and c
   e. all of the above

2. Removable prostheses prevent _____ of teeth.
   a. extrusion and drifting
   b. drifting and decay
   c. decay and rotation
   d. rotation and extrusion

3. What oral hygiene aid is used to clean under a pontic?
   a. toothbrush
   b. mouth rinse
   c. floss threader
   d. periodontal tip

4. What type of prosthesis snaps into position and is then securely held to the tissue?
   a. full denture
   b. partial denture
   c. immediate denture
   d. overdenture

5. What is the major factor influencing whether a patient will successfully learn to wear a denture?
   a. financial considerations
   b. patient's attitude
   c. quality of dentist's impression
   d. lab technician's skill in denture construction

6. Which type of removable prosthesis maintains the space formerly occupied by a lost primary tooth until a new tooth erupts?
   a. flipper
   b. immediate denture
   c. full denture
   d. fixed bridge

7. What type of support does a partial denture clasp provide?
   a. vertical
   b. extrusion
   c. horizontal
   d. intrusion

8. The objectives of the wax try-in appointment are to ensure the finished denture will fit correctly and to establish the bite.
   a. true
   b. false
   c. more information is needed to answer this question

9. Assuming their oral and general health conditions permit, edentulous patients can elect to have one of these types of prosthesis.
   a. flipper
   b. immediate denture
   c. partial denture
   d. traditional complete denture
   e. b and d

10. What provides the main support for any type of removable denture?
   a. mucosa
   b. alveolar bone
   c. design of the prosthesis
   d. muscle action

TRUE/FALSE

Indicate whether the statement is true (T) or false (F).

_____ 1. A denture patient should be provided with a tissue for privacy when the denture must be removed.

_____ 2. Resorption of the alveolar ridge occurs in denture wearers over time from pressures the denture places on the bone.

_____ 3. Dental assistants should be good listeners when serving denture patients.

_____ 4. Only the dentist can sign a laboratory prescription.

_____ 5. A maxillary complete denture is held in position by suction.

_____ 6. Patients should not be fitted with a denture until they are at least 45 years old.

_____ 7. Porcelain denture teeth are preferred to acrylic teeth because they do not clack or cause alveolar bone resorption.

_____ 8. The patient with advanced periodontal disease and extensive bone loss is a good candidate for an overdenture.

_____ 9. The natural appearance of a denture is enhanced by dimpling and scoring the denture base.

_____ 10. The initial appointment for a denture patient is a consultation appointment.

FILL IN THE BLANK

Using words from the list below, fill in the blanks to complete the following statements.

abutment	home care procedures	occlusion
acrylic resin	immediate	patient
consultation	metal	shortens
disinfect	no	

1. _____ placement of a denture following surgery _____ both healing time and time to relining.

2. A partial denture is supported internally by a(n) _____ framework.

3. _____ became the dominant material for dentures a little over a century ago and remains the most popular material today.

4. The _____ should initial any change in the health history.

5. Financial arrangements are discussed with the patient at the _____ appointment.

6. A(n) _____ tooth provides support for a partial denture.

7. Edentulous patients have _____ natural teeth.

8. A partial denture is designed to replace missing teeth, evenly distribute the pressures on the abutment teeth, and reestablish correct _____.

9. It is necessary to _____ any denture before it is sent to the laboratory for processing.

10. At the delivery appointment for a full or partial denture, it is imperative that the dental assistant educate the patient regarding _____.

CHAPTER 43
Dental Implants

CHAPTER OUTLINE

Review the Chapter Outline. If any content area is unclear, review that area before beginning the workbook exercises.

    A.   The Dental Implant Patient

    B.   Types of Implants

    C.   Preparation for Implantation

    D.   Dental Implant Maintenance

    E.   The Future of Implants

CHAPTER REVIEW

The following is a summary of the chapter. If any of this material is unclear, review it in the textbook again.

Dental implants are a technologically advanced, modern form of dental treatment. They replace the roots of natural teeth that either never developed or were removed. The majority of implants are made of titanium, a relatively inert metal, and inserted directly into or on the bone. Different types of implants—subperiosteal, endosteal, transosteal, and mini—are available to meet different patient needs. Implant patients are selected carefully and then fully educated regarding the risks, benefits, and procedures of implant placement and maintenance. Dental assistants play wide-ranging roles in implant patient examination, education, care, and maintenance, as well as providing clinical assistance to the dentist and patient during placement and assessment procedures.

LEARNING ACTIVITIES AND STUDY AIDS

Review the following study aids and/or complete the activities to ensure that you have achieved the learning objectives for this chapter.

1. List the components of the process used to select an implant patient.

2. Suppose that during the medical history review you notice that the implant candidate uses a drug such as Aredia or Zometa (both examples of bisphosphonates). Explain why this information is important to bring to the attention of the doctor.

3. List the factors that contribute to implant success.

4. Future trends in implantology are limitless. Using resources found online or at your school or local library, research the various techniques currently used for implants. On a separate piece of paper, write a one-page report on your findings. Be sure to cite your resources.

5. Discuss the role of informed consent in implant therapy. Explain what the dental assistant's role is in obtaining informed consent from a patient prior to implant.

6. List the contraindications to implant therapy.

7. On one side of a flash card list the types of implants currently available. On the other side describe each type. Use this flash card to assist you in studying the information.

8. List the major uses of the different types of implants.

9. Differentiate one-step and two-step implant placement.

10. List the general items needed on a surgical setup for implant surgery.

MEDICAL TERMINOLOGY REVIEW

Use a dictionary and/or your textbook to define the following terms.

aesthetic _____

armamentarium _____

bisphosphonates _____

bruxism _____

endosteal _____

hex _____

implant _____

loading _____

mucoperiosteal _____

osseointegration _____

osteonecrosis _____

Paget's disease _____

subperiosteal _____

surgical stent _____

transosteal _____

ABBREVIATIONS

CT _____

OSHA _____

CRITICAL THINKING

1. Why is it important for the dental assistant to consider the patient's attitude, as well as emotional and psychological profile, when discussing implants?

2. Why is the patient's willingness or ability to provide good oral home care for himself/herself of concern to the dental assistant? How might one discover if good home care is being practiced?

3. When advising a patient of the proper instruments to use when cleaning his/her implants, what type would you as the dental assistant advise, and why?

CHAPTER REVIEW TEST

MULTIPLE CHOICE

Circle the letter of the correct answer.

1. These TWO types of patients may not be suitable for implant therapy.
   a. very young patients with incomplete bone formation
   b. patients who want their implant placement and loading to occur on the same day
   c. patients who have been wearing loose-fitting dentures
   d. elderly patients with advanced bone resorption

2. The keys to implant success that are the responsibility of the dental assistant are:
   a. obtain informed consent and complete treatment in a reasonable time period
   b. provide professional homecare instructions and follow-up care
   c. obtain a thorough psychological profile and clear financial arrangements
   d. provide treatment to otherwise healthy patients and check progress frequently

3. Advantages of using one-step surgery for implant placement and loading include all of the following EXCEPT:
   a. preservation of crestal bone
   b. receipt of an immediate esthetic restoration
   c. increased chair time
   d. ability to load a denture on the implant the same day

4. This procedure is NOT recommended during the initial healing phases of implant therapy.
   a. mechanical plaque removal
   b. eating a soft diet
   c. antibiotic therapy
   d. rest

5. Implant patients who use an oral irrigator should be instructed to direct the spray:
   a. horizontally
   b. vertically
   c. toward the buccal surface
   d. toward the lingual surface

6. This procedure is essential to implant success.
   a. rinsing with saline solution
   b. polishing with fluoridated dentifrice
   c. use of sharp scalers on the implant surface
   d. practicing meticulous oral hygiene

7. Patients with the most severe resorption of the mandibular ridge are the most likely candidates for a(n) _____ implant.
   a. endosteal
   b. transosteal
   c. mini
   d. subperiosteal

8. Mini implants were designed specifically to treat:
   a. badly resorbed alveolar ridges
   b. routine tooth replacements
   c. denture instability
   d. areas with inadequate space for an implant

9. The function of a surgical stent in implant therapy is to:
   a. provide a model for retreatment if failure should occur
   b. demonstrate brushing and flossing using the new system
   c. allow the patient to practice speaking with the new implant
   d. aid in placing the implant in exact position

10. Osseointegration is:
    a. placement of the implant under the periosteum
    b. provision of a wound dressing made of iodine gel
    c. fusion of an implant to the bone
    d. topping an implant with a prosthetic abutment

TRUE/FALSE

Indicate whether the statement is true (T) or false (F).

_____ 1. Bisphosphonate therapy may trigger osteonecrosis following surgery.

_____ 2. A patient having limited ability to cope with psychological stress should not be accepted for implant therapy.

_____ 3. Extraoral radiographs or a CT scan may be requested as part of the examination process for a proposed implant patient.

_____ 4. Implant therapy is considered only for patients with sufficient bone to retain a full denture.

_____ 5. Bone must have adequate density if it is to be used to support an implant.

_____ 6. Bruxism and other oral habits are common indicators for implant therapy.

_____ 7. Subperiosteal implants are essentially staples that are placed in the mandible to replace tooth roots.

_____ 8. In two-step implant therapy, the implant and hex are placed during two different surgeries.

_____ 9. When endosteal implants are placed with two-step surgeries, a healing period of one to three weeks is required between the two procedures to enable osseointegration to occur.

_____ 10. Implants may be shaped like a blade, framework, or screw.

FILL IN THE BLANK

Using words from the list below, fill in the blanks to complete the following statements.

90%	occlusal	single
are	one	standard of care
financial investment	plastic	titanium
is not	psychological	

1. All brushes and instruments used for implant maintenance must be made of _____ graphite, Teflon, or nylon.

2. Toothbrushes and other oral hygiene aids for cleaning implant prostheses should be angled toward the _____ surface to avoid irritation and damage.

3. The current focus of implant therapy is the placement of a(n) _____ implant in _____ appointment.

4. The most important benefits of implant therapy are likely _____.

5. Single tooth implant therapy is successful in about _____ of cases.

6. Routine recall visits _____ necessary for the patient with an implant.

7. The majority of implants are constructed of _____.

8. Use of chlorhexadine antimicrobial mouthrinse therapy _____ necessary but may be desirable for an implant patient.

9. A substantial commitment of time, patience, and _____ is required of the implant patient.

10. The _____ in implant therapy is what any reasonably prudent person of similar knowledge and skill would do in similar circumstances.

CHAPTER 44

Endodontic Procedures

CHAPTER OUTLINE

Review the Chapter Outline. If any content area is unclear, review that area before beginning the workbook exercises.

A. Causes of Pulpal Damage

B. Symptoms of Pulpal Damage
   1. Reversible Pulpitis
   2. Irreversible Pulpitis
   3. Pulpal Necrosis
   4. Periapical Abscess

C. Endodontic Diagnosis
   1. Radiographs
   2. Percussion
   3. Palpation
   4. Mobility
   5. Cold Test
   6. Heat Test
   7. Electric Pulp Tester
   8. Anesthetic Test

D. Endodontic Procedures
   1. Access Opening
   2. Shaping and Filing
   3. Obturation
   4. Final Restoration

E. Instruments and Accessories
   1. Dental Dam
   2. Endodontic Explorer
   3. Endodontic Spoon Excavator
   4. Broaches
   5. Reamers
   6. Files
   7. Endodontic Measuring Devices
   8. Bead Sterilizer
   9. Paper Points
   10. Lentuolo Spiral
   11. Endodontic Spreader
   12. Endodontic Condenser
   13. Gates Glidden Burs
   14. Peeso Reamers
   15. Apex Finder
   16. Endodontic Handpiece

F.   Medicaments and Dental Materials in Endodontics
G.   Overview of Endodontic Treatment
H.   Surgical Endodontics
1.   Apicoectomy
2.   Retrograde Filling
3.   Root Amputation
4.   Lasers, Endodontic Microscopes, and Ultrasonics

CHAPTER REVIEW

The following is a summary of the chapter. If any of this material is unclear, review it in the textbook again

Endodontic therapy is used to treat diseased or injured teeth that cannot be helped using restorative techniques. Infection from the spread of microorganisms in dental caries is the most common cause of pulpa disease, and mechanical trauma is the most common cause of injury. The goal of endodontic therapy is to save the tooth. The treatment procedure selected depends on the extent of the infection or injury, whether or not the pulp is vital, and for young patients, the degree of root development. If the tooth cannot be saved, the only alternative is extraction. The dental assistant assists in many ways during endodontic procedures: patient education; exposure and processing of radiographs; preparation of instruments, equipment, and supplies; operatory set-up and clean-up, extensive assistance during the procedure itself; and attention to the patient's comfort.

LEARNING ACTIVITIES AND STUDY AIDS

Review the following study aids and/or complete the activities to ensure that you have achieved the learning objectives for this chapter.

1.   List the causes of pulpal damage.

2.   Discuss the signs and symptoms of pulpal damage.

3. List and define the tests used as aids to establishing an endodontic diagnosis.

4. State the uses of radiographs in an endodontic procedure.

5. Describe the steps in a nonsurgical endodontic procedure. Utilize an additional piece of paper if more space is required for your information.

6. Explain how and why surgical endodontic procedures are performed. Utilize an additional piece of paper if more space is required for your information.

7. In the following table, list the functions of each type of equipment or supply used in endodontic procedures.

Table 44-1

Instrument or supply	Function
Dental dam	
Endodontic explorer	
Endodonic spoon excavator	
Broaches	
Reamers	
Files	
Stops	
Endodontic measuring gauges	
Bead sterilizer	
Paper points	
Lentuolo spiral	
Endodontic spreader	
Endodontic condenser	
Glick 1	

Gates-Glidden burs	
Peeso reamers	
Apex finder	
Phenol Iodine Formocresol Antibiotics	
Sodium hypochlorite Hydrogen peroxide	
Zinc oxide eugenol Calcium hydroxide Glass ionomer	
Gutta percha	

8. Differentiate reversible pulpitis, irreversible pulpitis, pulpal necrosis, periapical abscess, fistula, and cellulitis.

9. Explain why it is important for a dental assistant to keep the tooth undergoing endodontic procedures clean and cool.

10. Differentiate a pulpotomy, pulpectomy, direct pulp capping, and indirect pulp capping.

MEDICAL TERMINOLOGY REVIEW

Use a dictionary and/or your textbook to define the following terms.

abscess _____

apexogenesis _____

apicoectomy _____

debridement _____

endodontics _____

extirpation _____

exudate _____

fistula _____

irreversible pulpitis _____

necrotic pulp _____

obturate _____

percussion _____

periapical _____

periradicular _____

pulpitis _____

resorption _____

reversible pulpitis _____

ABBREVIATIONS

EBA _____

I & D _____

IRM _____

MTA _____

RC _____

CRITICAL THINKING

1. What causes the pulp of a tooth to be damaged? Why is it important for a dental assistant to know these causes?

2. What is the most valuable diagnostic tool for use before, during, and after an endodontic procedure?

3. What are some other tests used to diagnose a tooth that may need endodontic treatment?

4. What are the differences between a pulpotomy and a pulpectomy?

CHAPTER REVIEW TEST

MULTIPLE CHOICE

Circle the letter of the correct answer.

1. The overriding goal of endodontics is to:
   a. retain the natural tooth in the arch
   b. prevent microbial reinfection of the pulp
   c. arrest bone resorption from periapical infection
   d. seal the root canals of an infected tooth

2. The TWO results of microbial invasion of the pulp are:
   a. patient discomfort
   b. infection
   c. inflammation
   d. both b and c

3. Which of the following is a sign of reversible pulpitis?
   a. periapical abscess has formed
   b. decay is extensive
   c. pulp is vital
   d. pain is absent

4. Excruciating pain from a tooth is the result of:
   a. fistula drainage
   b. fluid and gas pressure within the tooth
   c. inflammation of the facial cellular spaces
   d. bone resorption

5. The most valuable diagnostic aid for the dentist who is seeking to establish an endodontic diagnosis is
   a. heat test
   b. cold test
   c. mobility test
   d. radiograph

6. If the pulp is inflamed, the patient will experience a lingering sensation in response to:
   a. cold
   b. heat
   c. percussion
   d. a and b
   e. b and c

7. If the patient does not experience any discomfort when heat is applied, the pulp is:
   a. reversibly inflamed
   b. irreversibly inflamed
   c. necrotic
   d. infected

8. The tooth must be _____ and have _____ to begin an electrical pulp test
   a. clean and dry; toothpaste applied
   b. moist; an electrode applied
   c. nonvital; no response to heat or cold
   d. necrotic; no inflammation

9. The material most commonly used to obturate the root canal space is:
   a. amalgam
   b. creosote
   c. sodium hypochlorite
   d. gutta percha

10. The master point the dentist uses to begin the root canal filling process is:
   a. the width and length of the initial broach used
   b. the width and length of the last file used
   c. measured to the working length of the canal
   d. measured to the radiographic length of the canal

TRUE/FALSE

Indicate whether the statement is true (T) or false (F).

_____ 1. Temporary restorations effectively prevent contamination for approximately 18 months.

_____ 2. An endodontically treated tooth will need a crown as a final restoration to guard against future fracture.

_____ 3. As soon as a root canal is filled, it must be completely cleaned.

_____ 4. The dental assistant should order carbon steel files because they are stronger than stainless steel.

_____ 5. The dental assistant should prepare a slow-speed handpiece with a latch-type angle if a Lentuolo spiral will be used.

_____ 6. Zinc oxide eugenol, calcium hydroxide, and glass ionomer are used for root canal sealing and cementing.

_____ 7. Apicoectomy and retrograde filling procedures are performed when nonsurgical root canal procedures have failed.

_____ 8. Amputation of an infected root is indicated when other roots of the tooth are treatable.

_____ 9. A disadvantage of laser treatment is that the patient usually requires more anesthesia to be comfortable.

_____ 10. Sometimes the patient exhibits no obvious signs and symptoms, even though pulpal damage has occurred.

FILL IN THE BLANK

Using words from the list below, fill in the blanks to complete the following statements.

apex finder	Lentuolo spiral	radiograph
broaches	paper points	reamers
dental dam	Peeso reamer	stops
endodontic spreader		

1. This single-ended endodontic instrument with a long, pointed tip is used during the obturation phase of therapy to spread filling materials horizontally and create space for additional gutta percha points: _____.

2. These endodontic supplies are used to dry moist root canals following debridement or irrigation: _____.

3. These endodontic supplies are placed on reamers, files, and broaches to mark the length of a root canal:_____.

4. These barbed endodontic instruments are used during the debridement phase of therapy to remove infected pulp tissue from within a pulp canal: _____.

5. This endodontic supply isolates the tooth being treated, maintains a sterile operating field, prevents small instruments and supplies from being swallowed, and improves the general efficiency of treatment: _____.

6. This diagnostic aid provides vital information throughout the endodontic therapy diagnosis and treatment process: _____.

7. These endodontic instruments enlarge the root canal following pulp debridement: _____.

8. This endodontic instrument is used to place sealer, cement, or medication in a root canal before the gutta percha filling is placed: _____.

9. This instrument is used to remove a portion of the gutta percha filling in a root canal to prepare a treated tooth for placement of a post: _____.

10. This diagnostic aid helps in locating the root apex, especially when the root is curved: _____.

CHAPTER 45
Periodontal Procedures

CHAPTER OUTLINE

Review the Chapter Outline. If any content area is unclear, review that area before beginning the workbook exercises.

A. The Periodontal Practice

B. The Professional Examination
   1. Biofilm
   2. Calculus
   3. Gingival Appearance
   4. Periodontal Probing Depths
   5. Tooth Mobility
   6. Suppuration
   7. Furcation Involvement
   8. Recession
   9. Width of Attached Gingiva
   10. Occlusion
   11. Radiographic Evaluation

C. Periodontal Instruments
   1. Periodontal Probe
   2. Naber's Probe
   3. Explorers
   4. Scalers
      a. Sickle Scalers
      b. Hoe Scalers
      c. Chisel Scalers
      d. File Scalers

D. Curettes
   1. Universal Curettes
   2. Area-Specific Curettes
      a. Extended Shank Gracey Curettes
      b. Miniature Gracey Curettes
   3. Sonic and Ultrasonic Instruments
   4. Scalpel
   5. Periodontal Knives
      a. Orban Interdental Knives
      b. Kirkland Knife
   6. Pocket Markers
   7. Hemostats
   8. Tissue Forceps
   9. Needle Holders
   10. Rongeurs
   11. Periodontal Scissors
   12. Periosteal Elevators

E.   Nonsurgical Periodontal Treatment
F.   Surgical Periodontal Treatment
    1.   Procedures for Treatment of Periodontal Defects
    2.   Procedures for Gaining Access
    3.   Procedures for Treatment of Osseous Defects
    4.   Surgical Procedures for Regeneration of the Periodontium
        a.   Bone Grafting
        b.   Guided Tissue Regeneration
    5.   Crown Lengthening Surgery
    6.   Periodontal Dressing
G.   Lasers in Periodontics
    1.   Advantages of Laser Surgery
    2.   Laser Safety

CHAPTER REVIEW

The following is a summary of the chapter. If any of this material is unclear, review it in the textbook again.

Periodontal procedures are performed to return the supporting tissues of the teeth to health. Once health is attained, the patient and periodontal team work together to maintain it. Treatment begins with a thorough examination of the historical, systemic, and local factors that are affecting the periodontium. Systemic factors are then controlled or reduced as much as possible, and local factors are eliminated. This in turn reduces the bacterial load, providing an improved environment for periodontal function. Dental hygienists provide patient education and nonsurgical treatment services such as examination, mechanical debridement, and chemical therapy. The periodontist diagnoses periodontal conditions, directs the team, and provides surgical services. The dental assistant assists the dentist and dental hygienist with all phases of periodontal therapy, provides patient education, and ensures patient comfort.

LEARNING ACTIVITIES AND STUDY AIDS

Review the following study aids and/or complete the activities to ensure that you have achieved the learning objectives for this chapter.

1. Define biofilm, calculus, probing depth, tooth mobility, suppuration, furcation involvement, recession, and width of attached gingiva.

2. List the components of the periodontal examination.

3. List and state the function of the three types of instruments used for periodontal examination.

4. Differentiate hand scalers and curettes, and sonic and ultrasonic instruments.

5. State the advantage of using area-specific curettes.

6. Describe the rationale for nonsurgical periodontal treatment.

7. Utilizing a separate piece of paper, create a table listing the different periodontal surgery procedures, and state why each is performed.

8. Explain why and how a periodontal dressing is placed.

9. Explain the procedures for which the FDA has approved laser treatment.

0. Describe patients for whom gingivectomy may be the treatment of choice.

MEDICAL TERMINOLOGY REVIEW

se a dictionary and/or your textbook to define the following terms.

ofilm _____

lculus _____

udate _____

enectomy _____

rcation involvement _____

ngivectomy _____

ngivitis _____

ngivoplasty _____

eriodontal debridement _____

eriodontal pocket _____

eriodontal probe _____

eriodontitis _____

cession _____

ot planing _____

aling _____

BBREVIATIONS

EJ _____

)A _____

CL _____

)O _____

SPT _____

CRITICAL THINKING

1. Why is it important for a dental assistant to have a thorough knowledge of periodontal disease and the many procedures that may be involved in treatment of this disease?

2. When performing an oral examination, what important changes in the tissue should be noted in the patient record, and why?

3. When a periodontist or hygienist is probing periodontal pocketing around each tooth, what is the responsibility of the dental assistant? What is considered to be a normal depth, and how would you explain this to a patient?

CHAPTER REVIEW TEST

MULTIPLE CHOICE

Circle the letter of the correct answer.

1. Characteristics of healthy alveolar bone include all of the following EXCEPT:
   a. the alveolar bone crest is $1 - 1\frac{1}{2}$ mm closer to the apex than the CEJ
   b. the level of horizontal bone should be parallel to an imaginary line from the CEJ on one tooth to the CEJ on an adjacent tooth
   c. bone along the proximal surface should be $2 - 3$ mm apical to the CEJ
   d. both a and b

2. Which type of bitewing radiographs is preferred for periodontal evaluation?
   a. horizontal bitewings
   b. vertical bitewings
   c. bitewings are not used for periodontal evaluation
   d. both a and b

3. All of the following must be maintained for periodontal instruments EXCEPT:
   a. sterility
   b. sharpness
   c. flexibility
   d. blade angulation

4. Pocket depth is measured from the:
   a. base of the pocket to the gingival margin
   b. farthest buccal movement to the farthest lingual movement
   c. cementoenamel junction to the gingival margin
   d. base of the pocket to the mucogingival junction

5. _____ is the measurement of movement of the tooth in the socket.
   a. Tooth mobility
   b. Probing
   c. Furcation
   d. Scaling

6. All of the following are risks of undergoing periodontal treatment EXCEPT:
   a. heightened sensitivity to cold
   b. postoperative discomfort
   c. swelling
   d. teeth appear shortened

7. Gingivectomy may be the treatment of choice for patients taking drugs such as phenytoin, cyclosporine, or calcium channel blockers that cause gingival:
   a. recession
   b. enlargement
   c. clefting
   d. blunting

8. Osteoplasty and ostectomy are undertaken to:
   a. create a healthier, shallower sulcus
   b. develop more active sites of polymorphonuclear leukocyte formation
   c. establish a physiologic alveolar form for the gingival tissue to follow
   d. reduce the time required to complete gingival healing

9. _____ is a type of graft material that is taken from the body of the patient so it is not rejected as foreign tissue.
   a. Xenograft
   b. Allograft
   c. Autograft
   d. Alloplast

10. Guided tissue regeneration uses _____ to control the healing rates of selected cells in different locations.

   a. repeated surgeries
   b. narrow spectrum antibiotics
   c. chemotherapy
   d. membrane placement

TRUE/FALSE

Indicate whether the statement is true (T) or false (F).

_____ 1. Smoking is a risk factor for periodontal disease.

_____ 2. The first therapeutic task for the patient–periodontal team is to develop an appropriate home care regimen.

_____ 3. Periodontal probing depths must be measured and recorded at each visit.

_____ 4. Dentists in general practice typically refer all periodontics cases to a periodontist.

_____ 5. The surgery site for a graft must be well brushed each day to reduce the bacterial load.

_____ 6. The advantage of an allograft is that it comes from a human donor other than the patient.

_____ 7. Bleeding on probing indicates the presence of inflammation; suppuration in a periodontal pocket indicates the presence of infection.

_____ 8. It is no longer recommended that disclosing solution be part of a plaque assessment regimen.

_____ 9. Recession may be a result of trauma, rapid tooth movement, extensive restorative treatment, or periodontitis.

_____ 10. On a radiograph, healthy alveolar bone should be parallel to an imaginary line drawn from the CEJ to the apex.

FILL IN THE BLANK

Using words from the list below, fill in the blanks to complete the following statements.

file scaler	periosteal elevator	sickle scaler
Gracey curette	pocket marker	ultrasonic scaler
Naber's probe	rongeurs	universal curette
periodontal probe		

Select the instrument of choice for each procedure listed below.

1. Locate and assess the degree of furcation involvement: _____.
2. Measure pocket depth: _____.
3. Provide easier, area-specific access for debridement of periodontal pockets: _____.
4. Use vibrations and water for machine removal of tenacious calculus: _____.
5. Make minute perforations in the gingival tissue: _____..
6. Nip bone fragments and shape soft tissue: _____.
7. Retract soft tissue away from the bone: _____.
8. Remove supragingival calculus: _____.
9. Remove overhangs from restorations: _____.
10. Remove subgingival calculus from any area of the mouth: _____.

CHAPTER 46
Oral Surgery Procedures

CHAPTER OUTLINE

Review the Chapter Outline. If any content area is unclear, review that area before beginning the workbook exercises.

A. Indications for Oral and Maxillofacial Surgery
B. The Oral Surgeon
C. The Dental Surgical Assistant
   1. Ethical and Legal Ramifications
D. The Surgical Setting
E. Specialized Instruments and Accessories
   1. Bone Files
   2. Dressing Pliers
   3. Elevators
   4. Forceps
   5. Hemostat and Needle Holder
   6. Mouth Props and Mouth Gag
   7. Operating Light
   8. Retractors
   9. Rongeurs
   10. Root Tip Picks
   11. Scalpels/Surgical Blades and Blade Removal Device
   12. Scissors
   13. Surgical Aspirator
   14. Surgical Burs
   15. Surgical Chisels and Mallet
   16. Surgical Curettes
   17. Surgical Preset Trays
   18. Suture Needles and Materials
F. Surgical Asepsis
   1. Care and Sterilization of Surgical Instruments
   2. Surgical Scrub and Handwashing
G. Surgical Preparation
   1. Medical and Dental History
   2. Intra- and Extraoral Examination
   3. Vital Signs
   4. Radiographs
   5. Informed Consent
   6. Preoperative Instructions
   7. Patient Preparation
   8. Pain Control in Oral Surgery

CHAPTER REVIEW

The following is a summary of the chapter. If any of this material is unclear, review it in the textbook again.

Oral surgery is the specialty in dentistry that includes the diagnosis and treatment of diseases, injuries, and defects of the oral and maxillofacial region. Oral and maxillofacial surgery may be completed in an office or hospital setting. The surgical dental assistant has special roles to play in patient assessment and monitoring, education, securing informed consent, preparing patients for surgery, assisting the dentist and other surgical team members as needed during treatment procedures, caring for the patient following surgery, and providing patient reassurance, understanding, and comfort. Appropriate methods of pain control is a consideration for each patient. Medication may be prescribed before or after the surgery, and the dentist or another team member may administer local anesthesia, general sedation, or general anesthesia as the procedure begins. Oral surgery includes a variety of surgical procedures utilizing various instruments. Maintaining an aseptic environment before, during, and after each procedure is important. The dental assistant must learn about commonly used drugs, medical history screening, and the instrument and procedure names, uses, and transfer methods in order to anticipate and respond to the needs of the patient and dentist throughout the preparation, completion, and postoperative phases of surgery. All procedures related to the surgery must be thoroughly and accurately documented in the patient's record.

LEARNING ACTIVITIES AND STUDY AIDS

Review the following study aids and/or complete the activities to ensure that you have achieved the learning objectives for this chapter.

1. Describe the specialty of oral and maxillofacial surgery.

2. List four patient conditions that may compromise a patient's well-being during surgery and the treatment modifications that should be made for these patients.

3. Make a series of flash cards. On one side list a type of surgical instrument. On the other side state its use. Turn these in to your instructor to ensure accuracy, then use these as study tools for exams.

4. Describe the procedures necessary to maintain asepsis.

5. Complete the following table by providing an explanation of why each procedure is performed.

Table 46-1

Procedure	Performed to . . .
Alveolectomy	
Alveoloplasty	
Apicoectomy	
Arthrotomy	
Biopsy	
Cleft lip, palate, or tongue surgery	
Cyst removal	
Drainage of infection	
Exodontia	
Exostosis surgery	
Fracture reduction	
Frenectomy	
Genioplasty	
Gingivectomy	

Gingivoplasty	
Implant surgery	
Orthognathic surgery	
Periodontal flap surgery	
Surgery to remove oral pathology	

6. On the day of surgery, list what the dental assistant should accomplish prior to the patient going into surgery.

7. List pre- and postoperative directions for surgical patients. Feel free to use an additional piece of paper if more room for your information is required.

8. Explain the function of sutures, and list the steps in their removal.

9. Define alveolitis, and describe its treatment.

10. Explain the importance of informed consent and documentation in the oral and maxillofacial surgery practice.

MEDICAL TERMINOLOGY REVIEW

Use a dictionary and/or your textbook to define the following terms.

alveolitis _____

angina pectoris _____

ankyloglossia _____

crepitus _____

diastema _____

xodontia _____

uxate _____

nalady _____

nalignant _____

ericoronitis _____

tosis _____

epticemia _____

tility gloves _____

BBREVIATIONS

BOMS _____

HA _____

DS _____

PM _____

CDC _____

CODA _____

DANB _____

DS _____

MD _____

DA _____

MF _____

V _____

ED _____

MD _____

MJ _____

CRITICAL THINKING

1. What are the general duties/responsibilities of the dental surgical assistant? How can these duties/skills be learned?

2. What is the number one way (action) to decrease or eliminate cross-contamination from patient to patient, staff to patient, and patient to staff? How many times per day should this action be performed and for how long?

3. Why is pharmacology an important learning curve for the surgical assistant to possess? Provide at least one example of why the dental assistant should thoroughly review the patient's medical and dental history before each procedure.

CHAPTER REVIEW TEST

MULTIPLE CHOICE

Circle the letter of the correct answer.

1. All of the following help to reduce legal vulnerability in the dental office EXCEPT:
   a. clear communication
   b. sound business management practices
   c. abbreviated documentation
   d. understandable oral and written instructions
   e. patient's questions answered

2. All dental surgical instruments are classified as _____ instruments and must be _____.

   a. critical; cleaned and sterilized
   b. semicritical; cleaned and disinfected
   c. vulnerable; disposable
   d. fomites; thoroughly washed with soap and hot water, then air dried

3. Define crepitus.

   a. restricted movement when a cleft palate has not been corrected
   b. a blockage in the duct opening of a minor salivary gland
   c. a surgical procedure to remove a nonmalignant epithelial tumor
   d. grating, cracking, or popping sounds when the TMJ is moved

4. The beaks of maxillary forceps are offset, that is, _____ the curvature of the plier-shaped handles, and are given _____ designations.

   a. sharply angled toward; C or L   c. thinner and longer than; X, T, or M
   b. angled away from; S, I, or Z   d. shorter and wider than; L or R

5. Surgical burs are larger than operative burs and are used to:

   a. remove bone   d. a and c
   b. exzpose root tips   e. all of the above
   c. divide teeth

6. Instruments on surgical preset trays or cassettes are arranged:

   a. in order of use
   b. by instrument function
   c. according to size
   d. with handles pointed toward the surgeon or assistant as indicated

7. The goal of surgical asepsis is:

   a. sterility   c. elimination of infection
   b. cleanliness   d. cross-contamination

8. This type of gloves is worn when sterilizing or disinfecting instruments.

   a. latex   c. disposable
   b. vinyl   d. utility

9. Handwashing must be completed:

   a. at the start and end of each day   d. a and c
   b. between patients   e. all of the above
   c. before gloving and after removing gloves

10. This drug is frequently given as an antianxiety premedication.

   a. lidocaine   c. epinephrine
   b. valium   d. mepivacaine

TRUE/FALSE

ndicate whether the statement is true (T) or false (F).

_____ 1. Antiseptics are harsh chemicals applied to inert surfaces.

_____ 2. Pregnant patients should not ordinarily be treated during their first trimester.

_____ 3. Birth control pill effectiveness may be decreased by the use of certain antibiotics.

_____ 4. Diabetic patients should be given late afternoon appointments so their blood glucose will be under better control.

_____ 5. Pain is a subjective "fifth vital sign" that is reported by the patient on a scale of 1 to 10.

_____ 6. In 2007, the AHA increased the number and variety of conditions for which it recommends patients about to undergo dental surgery receive antibiotic premedication.

_____ 7. Patients with cardiac problems should not receive anesthetics containing epinephrine.

_____ 8. Informed consent means consent the patient gives freely when he/she understands the risks, benefits, and alternatives of proceeding with recommended surgery or not.

_____ 9. A frenectomy is plastic surgery of the bone and soft tissue of the chin.

_____ 10. When soft tissue covers part of an erupting or impacted last molar and collects food and debris, the treatment of choice is genioplasty.

FILL IN THE BLANK

Using words from the list below, fill in the blanks to complete the following statements.

bone file	mouth gag	surgical aspirator tip
dressing pliers	retractor	surgical chisel
elevator	root tip pick	surgical curette
forceps		

1. This instrument is a type of tweezers used for grasping and holding: _____.
2. This instrument is used for grasping and removing a tooth: _____.
3. This instrument is used for holding tissue away from the operating field: _____.
4. This instrument is used for raising the tooth from its socket: _____.
5. This instrument is used for loosening and elevating broken root parts: _____.
6. This instrument is used for evacuating blood and other fluids from the mouth: _____
7. This instrument is used to hold the mouth open when the patient is unconscious: _____.
8. This instrument is used to spoon out infectious material, lesions, and debris: _____.
9. This instrument is used to smooth bone after a tooth is extracted: _____.
10. This instrument is used to chip away bone and section impacted teeth: _____.

CHAPTER 47
Pediatric Dentistry

CHAPTER OUTLINE

Review the Chapter Outline. If any content area is unclear, review that area before beginning the workbook exercises.

   A.   The Pediatric Team

   B.   The Pediatric Dental Office

   C.   The Pediatric Patient
       1. Childhood Stages

   D.   Patients with Special Needs
       1. Physical Conditions
       2. Mentally Challenged
       3. Other Mental Disorders

   E.   Diagnosis and Treatment Planning
       1. Behavior Management Techniques

   F.   Preventive Dentistry Procedures
       1. Coronal Polishing
       2. Fluoride Treatments
       3. Placement of Pit and Fissure Sealants
       4. Mouthguard
       5. Interceptive Orthodontics

   G.   Restorative Procedures
       1. Restorative Equipment

   H.   Endodontic Procedures

   I.   Prosthodontic Procedures

   J.   Dental Trauma

   K.   Reporting Child Abuse and Neglect

CHAPTER REVIEW

The following is a summary of the chapter. If any of this material is unclear, review it in the textbook again.

Pediatric dentists treat children from infancy to eighteen years of age, and some compromised adults. Procedures for children are similar to those for adults, except that their small mouth size means special instruments and supplies need to be used and their behavior is less constrained. It is important for the dental assistant to learn and practice behavior management techniques: friendliness, honesty, distraction, assistance with general anesthesia and mild sedation, modeling, the use of gentle restraints, and voice control. Using simple language the child or mentally challenged adult can understand is helpful. Employing the tell-show-do method of explaining procedures that are about to occur will do much to defuse anxiety and engage the child's natural curiosity. Accidental trauma occurs frequently during the childhood years,

primarily from falls, so special techniques have been developed to deal with the injured teeth. Routin(
procedures include placement of restorations, coronal polishing, fluoride treatments, placement of pit an(
fissure sealants, construction of mouthguards, and interceptive orthodontic treatments.

LEARNING ACTIVITIES AND STUDY AIDS

Review the following study aids and/or complete the activities to ensure that you have achieved the learn-
ing objectives for this chapter.

1. List and describe the roles of the pediatric dentistry team members.

2. To understand more about the signs of child abuse and the methods of reporting, go online or to your
   local library and conduct research. On a separate piece of paper, write a one-page report on your
   findings, and cite your resources.

3. Discuss the pediatric patient in relation to changing needs as age increases.

4. Explain the pediatric diagnosis and treatment planning process.

5. List and define the four common pediatric preventive dentistry treatments.

6. Discuss the common types of restorations provided to pediatric patients.

7. Make a series of flash cards. On one side of each card, list a behavior management technique. On the other side, describe the technique. Turn your flash cards into your instructor to receive a grade for your efforts. Use the flash cards as a study tool for upcoming exams.

8. Differentiate restorative, endodontic, and prosthodontic procedures, and state when each type of procedure is commonly used.

9. List and describe the four common types of dental trauma children experience.

10. Discuss the types of behavior management techniques that can be used on a pediatric patient who is visiting the dental office for the first time. Utilize an additional piece of paper if more room for your information is needed.

MEDICAL TERMINOLOGY REVIEW

Use a dictionary and/or your textbook to define the following terms.

alveolus _____

autonomy _____

avulsed _____

coronal _____

decalcification _____

dexterity _____

Down syndrome _____

exfoliate _____

nitrous oxide _____

nonvital _____

open bay _____

papoose board _____

pulpectomy _____

pulpotomy _____

space maintainer _____

t-band _____

traumatic intrusion _____

vital tooth _____

ABBREVIATIONS

IQ _____

CRITICAL THINKING

1. What are some attributes of a pediatric dental assistant? Why are these important when working with younger patients?

2. Why is it important for a dental assistant to know the childhood stages of development when working in a pediatric office?

3. List and discuss as many different types of behavior management as you can, then describe them and discuss their efficacy during treatment.

4. What is the key to preventing decay in the younger patient? Who plays an active role in this prevention aspect?

CHAPTER REVIEW TEST

MULTIPLE CHOICE

Circle the letter of the correct answer.

1. Typically plants are discouraged in a pediatric dental office because of their potential to _____ the child.
   a. poison
   b. activate an allergy of
   c. injure
   d. carry disease to

2. The open bay pediatric dental office design helps to discourage:
   a. anxiety
   b. acting out
   c. parental discipline
   d. isolation

3. Children should be communicated with according to their _____ age.
   a. chronological
   b. mental
   c. emotional
   d. a and c
   e. all of the above

4. Children of this age are extremely curious and want to understand what is happening.

   a. elementary school age
   b. teenagers
   c. preschoolers
   d. toddlers

5. Development of socialization and emergence of peer pressure as an important influence begin during these years:

   a. preschool
   b. adolescent
   c. teenage
   d. elementary school age

6. Children with this level of mental disability are usually able to be treated in the dental office.

   a. mild
   b. moderate
   c. severe
   d. a and possibly b
   e. all of the above

7. Select the following characteristics that are associated with Down syndrome.

   a. peg-shaped teeth
   b. almond-shaped eyes
   c. delayed eruption schedule
   d. a and c
   e. all of the above

8. Who must be present to complete a medical/dental history form for the pediatric patient?

   a. parent
   b. legal guardian
   c. caretaker
   d. a or b
   e. b or c

9. A child's first dental appointment should occur:

   a. between twelve and twenty-four months of age
   b. by three years of age
   c. before the child begins school
   d. when the child experiences a dental problem

10. The key to effective pediatric dentistry is:

   a. prevention
   b. early intervention
   c. restoration as needed
   d. consultation as needed

TRUE/FALSE

Indicate whether the statement is true (T) or false (F).

_____ 1. Children can be instructed to begin flossing for themselves when the permanent teeth begin to erupt.

_____ 2. Children begin to have the dexterity to clean their tooth surfaces effectively at approximately six years of age.

_____ 3. Sealants are placed mainly on the lingual surfaces of anterior teeth because this is where the greatest number of cavities occur.

_____ 4. Interceptive orthodontic procedures are performed primarily to save space and reduce the need for orthodontic care.

_____ 5. Amalgam is often chosen for restoring a child's tooth because it is more esthetic.

_____ 6. The procedure needed for treatment of an injured tooth will depend primarily on the child's age.

_____ 7. Stainless steel crowns are used for children because of their ease of placement.

_____ 8. Although they are occasionally needed, partial and full dentures cannot be constructed to fit a child's small mouth.

_____ 9. Traumatic avulsion occurs primarily in the anterior area of the mouth.

_____ 10. The determining factors for success in replantation of a tooth are the length of elapsed time to replantation, care of the tooth before arrival at the office, and condition of the periodontal ligament on office arrival.

FILL IN THE BLANK

Using words from the list below, fill in the blanks to complete the following statements.

appearance	explain	protrusion of anterior teeth
autonomy	fun	self-interest
can't happen to me	honest	should
dentist	inappropriate dress for the weather	splint

1. Tooth displacement is ordinarily treated with repositioning and a _____.

2. Signs of child neglect can include extensive decay, poor hygiene, and _____.

3. It is preferable for the _____ to report suspected child abuse or neglect.

4. Dental personnel can earn patients' trust by being _____ about treatment procedures and taking the time to _____ how equipment operates.

5. The pediatric dental office should be friendly, welcoming, comfortable, and _____.

6. The major emerging need of a toddler patient is _____.

7. A toddler's parent _____ be in the operatory when the child is being treated.

8. The preadolescent patient is motivated primarily by _____ and _____.

9. The _____ mentality is pervasive throughout adolescence.

10. Thumb sucking can cause _____.

CHAPTER 48

Coronal Polish

CHAPTER OUTLINE

Review the Chapter Outline. If any content area is unclear, review that area before beginning the workbook exercises.

    A. Coronal Polish
        1. Indications for Coronal Polishing
        2. Selective Polishing
        3. Polishing Esthetic Restorations

    B. Dental Stains

    C. Coronal Polishing Materials and Equipment
        1. Abrasives
        2. Prophylaxis Angle and Handpiece

    D. Coronal Polishing Steps
        1. Sequence of Polishing
        2. Flossing after Polishing
        3. Evaluation of Polishing

CHAPTER REVIEW

The following is a summary of the chapter. If any of this material is unclear, review it in the textbook again.

Coronal polishing is the removal of stains and soft deposits from the coronal surfaces of the teeth. It can be completed by dentists, dental hygienists, and in some states, dental assistants. Even though polishing is not usually needed for health reasons, patients are keenly concerned about their smile and want to improve its appearance by having their teeth polished. A dental assistant needs to have knowledge of the coronal polishing procedure and be able to set up, complete, and clean after polishing. It is important for dental assistants to consult the state dental practice act to learn whether they are permitted to polish teeth in their state, and if yes, whether special training and/or credentialing is required.

LEARNING ACTIVITIES AND STUDY AIDS

Review the following study aids and/or complete the activities to ensure that you have achieved the learning objectives for this chapter.

1. In the following table, list the indications and contraindications for coronal polishing.

    Table 48-1

Indications	Contraindications

2. Define selective polishing, and state why it is practiced.

3. List and state the usual source of dental stains.

4. Differentiate soft and hard deposits, and identify which type can be removed by polishing.

5. Differentiate handpieces, angles, cups, and brushes, and describe the use of each.

6. On a separate piece of paper, make a table that includes common abrasives, their abrasive level, and the typical use of each type.

7. List the general principles of polishing technique, and state why each is important.

8. List the steps of a coronal polishing procedure.

9. Explain why correct positioning and speed are so important when using the prophy angle and handpiece.

10. Describe how polishing is evaluated.

MEDICAL TERMINOLOGY REVIEW

Use a dictionary and/or your textbook to define the following terms.

abrasion _____

chlorhexidine _____

clinical crown _____

coronal _____

endogenous stain _____

exogenous stain _____

extrinsic stain _____

fluorosis _____

fulcrum _____

intrinsic stain _____

prophylaxis _____

subgingival _____

supragingival _____

ABBREVIATIONS

None used in this chapter.

CRITICAL THINKING

1. What is a coronal polishing, and why is it performed?

2. Why must a dental assistant be competent in the knowledge of how to either perform a coronal polish or assist with one?

3. What are some contraindications for coronal polishing?

4. What is selective polishing?

CHAPTER REVIEW TEST

MULTIPLE CHOICE

Circle the letter of the correct answer.

1. Why is dental floss used with a gentle sliding motion?

   a. removes more retained abrasive
   b. prevents injury to the gingival tissue
   c. removes remaining bits of stain
   d. prevents lingering malodor in the mouth

2. Select the methods that are used to evaluate the adequacy of a coronal polishing procedure.

   a. mirror
   b. tongue
   c. disclosing solution
   d. a and c
   e. all of the above

3. The mandibular arch is positioned _____ to the floor when the mandibular teeth are polished.

   a. in vertical relationship
   b. perpendicular
   c. parallel
   d. at a right angle

4. Stability of the operating hand during polishing is provided by use of a:

   a. fulcrum
   b. retraction device
   c. polishing cup
   d. handpiece

5. The operator can best reach into the gingival margin to polish the cervical area of the tooth by:

   a. using strong pressure
   b. flaring the polishing cup
   c. revving the polishing engine to more than 20,000 rpm
   d. all of the above

6. Abrasive paste must be kept _____ while it is being used in the mouth.

   a. on very low speed
   b. on very high speed
   c. dry
   d. moist

7. Why are teeth selectively polished?

    a. polishing invariably damages the pulp of the tooth
    b. patients routinely ask for selective polishing
    c. polishing is similar to massaging the teeth
    d. polishing removes a small layer of fluoride-rich outer enamel

8. Teeth should be polished using these types of abrasives.

    a. extra fine
    b. fine
    c. medium

    d. a and b
    e. b and c

9. Green stain is found more often in:

    a. children
    b. adults

    c. men
    d. women

10. Extrinsic stains develop from:

    a. within the tooth
    b. environmental sources

    c. tetracycline antibiotic
    d. using coarse abrasives

TRUE/FALSE

Indicate whether the statement is true (T) or false (F).

_____ 1. It is important to chart the patient's restorations prior to polishing the teeth.

_____ 2. Coarse abrasives are recommended for use on esthetic restorations.

_____ 3. Hard deposits such as calculus can best be removed by polishing them away.

_____ 4. Endogenous stains result from disturbances in tooth development.

_____ 5. Dental stains are primarily an esthetic concern.

_____ 6. Chlorhexidine stain adheres only to tooth structure, not the plaque or soft tissue.

_____ 7. The mildest abrasive paste that is compatible with removing a stain should be selected for polishing the stained tooth.

_____ 8. Reusable prophylaxis angles should be immersed in disinfectant solution following use.

_____ 9. Coronal polishing is known to scratch some types of esthetic restorations but does not scratch metal.

_____ 10. Synthetic rubber polishing cups are preferred because they do not leave stains on the teeth.

FILL IN THE BLANK

Using words from the list below, fill in the blanks to complete the following statements.

black	orange	tetracycline	brown
red	yellow	chlorhexidine	silex
zirconium silicate	green		

1. _____ stain cannot be polished away.

2. _____ stain is thought to be caused by chromogenic bacteria.

3. Brown and _____ stains are associated with poor oral hygiene.

4. _____ stain may overlie decalcification on the tooth surface.

5. _____ stain is caused by the extended use of mouthwash or toothpaste containing the chemical the stain is named for.

6. _____ stain is more often seen in females who have good hygiene and is likely from natural sources.

7. _____ stain is the result of tar combustion during smoking.

8. _____ stain is used to disclose the presence of plaque.

9. _____ is a mild abrasive.

10. _____ is quite abrasive and is used to remove heavy stain.

CHAPTER 49
Dental Sealants

CHAPTER OUTLINE

Review the Chapter Outline. If any content area is unclear, review that area before beginning the workbook exercises.

    A.   Dental Caries and Sealants

    B.   Indications for Sealants

    C.   Contraindications for Sealants

    D.   Types of Sealant Materials

    E.   Storage and Use of Sealants

    F.   Precautions for Dental Personnel and Patients

    G.   Factors in Sealant Retention

CHAPTER REVIEW

The following is a summary of the chapter. If any of this material is unclear, review it in the textbook again.

A dental sealant is a hard resin coating placed on the pits and fissures of a tooth surface to prevent dental decay. When properly applied and cared for, sealants are effective. Sealants isolate the tooth from sugar and bacteria. They also make the tooth surface smoother, and therefore easier to keep clean. Although sealants are usually placed on children's teeth, both children and adults can benefit from sealant placement. Many states permit dental assistants to apply sealants, although the dental assistant must keep in mind that regulations vary from state to state.

LEARNING ACTIVITIES AND STUDY AIDS

Review the following study aids and/or complete the activities to ensure that you have achieved the learning objectives for this chapter.

1. Discuss the relationship between sealants and dental decay.

2. List four reasons for placing enamel sealants.

3. Describe the patient conditions under which sealants should not be placed.

4. List three types of sealant material and an advantage of each type.

5. Differentiate light cured and self-cured sealant materials, and state an advantage of each type.

6. Differentiate filled and unfilled sealants, and describe an advantage of each type.

7. List two materials used for sealants, and indicate which is preferred.

8. Describe the safety measures a dental assistant should take when placing sealants.

9. Explain how sealant failure can occur and the causes.

10. Describe how a dental assistant checks to ensure that a newly placed sealant was properly applied.

MEDICAL TERMINOLOGY REVIEW

Use a dictionary and/or your textbook to define the following terms.

autopolymerized _____

etchant _____

filler _____

light-cured _____

polymerization _____

resin _____

retention _____

sealant _____

self-cured _____

unfilled _____

ABBREVIATIONS

bis-GMA _____

CRITICAL THINKING

1. What is the purpose for placing dental sealants? What are sealants made of?

2. Can sealants be used only on primary teeth? Are sealants more cost-effective than restorations? Which lasts longer, a restoration or a sealant?

3. If a patient has multiple incipient caries, is it possible to place sealants on these teeth? Who makes the final decision for placing sealants?

4. There are two types of sealants; what considerations would be given to use one type over the other?

CHAPTER REVIEW TEST

MULTIPLE CHOICE

Circle the letter of the correct answer.

1. Etchant material:
   a. roughens the outer layers of enamel
   b. smoothes the tooth surface
   c. polishes the deepest parts of the pits and fissures
   d. strengthens the enamel and dentin

2. Sealant retention is improved when these TWO factors are controlled.
   a. heat
   b. moisture
   c. application speed
   d. etching adequacy

3. Which conditions indicate the teeth should be sealed? Select all that apply.
   a. newly erupted molars
   b. pits and fissures of all teeth
   c. teeth that have been caries free for four years
   d. high number of caries on the occlusal surface

4. Patients prefer clear sealants because they are:
   a. easier to apply
   c. more esthetic
   b. retained longer
   d. clearly visible

5. Materials used for sealants include:
   a. amalgam
   b. composite
   c. glass ionomer
   d. a and b
   e. b and c

6. If the dental assistant uses a one-component sealant, what type of material is being used?

   a. heat cured
   b. light cured
   c. chemically cured
   d. amalgam

7. Sealant materials should be stored:

   a. away from light and air
   b. with container caps on
   c. according to the manufacturer's directions
   d. a and c
   e. all of the above

8. The dental team should take the following safety measures when placing a sealant:

   a. patient and dental team should wear protective eyewear
   b. protective eyewear should be a special amber-colored type during light-curing procedures
   c. team members should wear gloves
   d. if a team member's glove is damaged or penetrated by a chemical, that person should deglove, wash hands, and reglove
   e. all of the above

9. The tissue that can be damaged by not wearing the eyewear recommended for light-curing procedures is the:

   a. salivary gland
   b. kidney
   c. cornea
   d. tongue muscle

10. What are the most common causes of sealant failure?

   a. excess material mixing and inadequate etching
   b. inadequate etching and moisture contamination
   c. moisture contamination and insufficient curing time
   d. insufficient curing time and excess material mixing

TRUE/FALSE

Indicate whether the statement is true (T) or false (F).

_____ 1. Sealants are not recommended for adults.

_____ 2. A fluoride treatment may be completed on a newly sealed tooth to ensure the material is thoroughly set.

_____ 3. Phosphoric acid is the active ingredient in etchant material.

_____ 4. Fillers are used to strengthen sealant material.

_____ 5. Filled sealants that are too high will work their way into correct occlusion through normal use.

_____ 6. Polishing paste that contains fluoride may prevent complete bonding of the sealant to the tooth.

_____ 7. A patient with deep occlusal pits and fissures should receive sealants.

_____ 8. One year is the recommended time that a posterior tooth should be caries free for sealant placement to be contraindicated.

_____ 9. Newly erupted molars with normal or excessively deep pit, fissure, and groove anatomy should receive sealants.

_____ 10. A #1 crosscut bur is used to reduce the thickness of a high sealant.

FILL IN THE BLANK

Using words from the list below, fill in the blanks to complete the following statements.

autopolymerized   each   shallow

decay   resin   skin irritation

dental dam   restoration   years

dentist

1. _____ is the main component of the most commonly used sealant materials.

2. Sealant materials that allow only limited working time after mixing the two components are _____.

3. Sealant integrity should be checked at _____ professional dental examination.

4. Sealants that are properly applied and cared for should be retained for _____.

5. A tooth with a small carious lesion requires examination and decision by a _____ before a sealant is applied.

6. A sealant may be used instead of a _____ for treatment of a small carious lesion.

7. Teeth with _____ grooves do not need sealants.

8. Moisture can be controlled during sealant placement by using cotton rolls or _____.

9. The acrylate or resin that is a component of sealant materials can cause _____.

10. A restoration is recommended if _____ progresses under a sealant.

CHAPTER 50
Orthodontics

CHAPTER OUTLINE

Review the Chapter Outline. If any content area is unclear, review that area before beginning the workbook exercises.

A. The Orthodontist

B. The Orthodontic Assistant

C. The Orthodontic Office

D. Understanding Occlusion
   1. Etiology of Malocclusion

E. The Alignment of Teeth and Arches
   1. Benefits of Orthodontic Treatment

F. Orthodontic Records and Treatment Planning
   1. Medical and Dental History
   2. Physical Growth and Evaluation
   3. Diagnostic Records

G. Case Presentations
   1. Financial Arrangements

H. Specialized Instruments

I. Orthodontic Instruments
   1. Fixed Appliances
   2. Orthodontic Bands
   3. Fitting of Molar Bands
   4. Cementation of Bands
   5. Placing Brackets

J. Auxiliary Wire
   1. Arch Wire
   2. Types of Arch Wire
   3. Shape of Arch Wire
   4. Elastomeric Ties
   5. Power Products

K. Headgear

L. Adjustment Visits

M. Oral Hygiene and Dietary Instructions

N. Completed Treatment
   1. Retention
   2. Retention Appliances

O. Treatment Options

CHAPTER REVIEW

The following is a summary of the chapter. If any of this material is unclear, review it in the textbook again.

Orthodontics is concerned with the development, growth, and positioning of the teeth and facial bones. The orthodontic assistant is a skilled professional who completes many functions alone as well as with the dentist. Orthodontic assisting tasks are performed in four basic areas: records, radiography, patent care, and laboratory work. Although the majority of orthodontic patients are children, adults are now seeking orthodontic care in growing numbers. Orthodontics is an elective service but offers extensive benefits in terms of appearance, speech, health of the teeth and periodontium, and self-esteem. Orthodontic assistants expose and process radiographs and photographs, take and pour impressions, assist with or independently complete a wide variety of patient care tasks, and complete many laboratory procedures. Orthodontic assistants may earn the specialty certification Certified Orthodontic Assistant from the Dental Assisting National Board, Inc.

LEARNING ACTIVITIES AND STUDY AIDS

Review the following study aids and/or complete the activities to ensure that you have achieved the learning objectives for this chapter.

1. List and define Angle's classes of malocclusion. Utilize an additional piece of paper if more room is required for your information.

2. List the types of orthodontic records used for treatment planning.

3. Differentiate interceptive and corrective orthodontics, and give an example of each.

4. Describe the steps in a typical orthodontic treatment case, and state the purpose of each.

5. Explain the use and functions of headgear.

6. Differentiate the available types of separators.

7. Explain the effects that each of the habits listed in the following table can have on the development of the jaw.

Table 50-1

Habit affecting jaw development	Effect
Tongue thrust	
Anterior tongue thrust	
Lateral tongue thrust	
Thumb and finger sucking	
Bruxism	
Mouth breathing	

8. Describe the function of arch wire. Differentiate the different types of arch wire, and state why each is used. Feel free to use an additional piece of paper for your answer if needed.

9. Discuss the importance of retainer appliances and follow-up treatment.

10. Describe the align technology that is now available as a treatment option.

MEDICAL TERMINOLOGY REVIEW

Use a dictionary and/or your textbook to define the following terms.

arch wire _____

auxiliary _____

corrective orthodontics _____

dentofacial _____

distoclusion _____

fetal molding _____

interceptive orthodontics _____

ligature _____

mesioclusion _____

retainer _____

ABBREVIATIONS

PVS _____

TMA _____

CRITICAL THINKING

1. What is orthodontics, and what is the role of the dental assistant in this specialty?

2. Why is it important to see patients as young as possible for preventive orthodontic treatment?

3. What are some of the most common reasons patients see an orthodontist?

4. You have a patient who has presented to your office for an evaluation. What are the two most common x-rays you will expose, and what other diagnostic records might you obtain?

CHAPTER REVIEW TEST

MULTIPLE CHOICE

Circle the letter of the correct answer.

1. Dentofacial orthopedics refers to:
   a. movement of teeth to effect proper occlusion
   b. diagnosis of jaw and skull deformities
   c. guidance of facial development
   d. removal or stabilization of primary teeth

2. Neutroclusion is present when the _____ cusp of the _____ first molar fits into the _____ groove of the _____ first molar.
   a. mesiobuccal; maxillary; mesiobuccal; mandibular
   b. mesiolingual; maxillary; mesiolingual; mandibular
   c. distobuccal; mandibular; distobuccal; maxillary
   d. distolingual; mandibular; distolingual; maxillary

3. The incisors are in labioversion, and the maxillary first molar is too mesial in _____ malocclusion.
   a. Class I
   b. Class II, Division I
   c. Class II, Division II
   d. Class III

4. Genetic factors are related to these occlusion problems:
   a. stress and strain on muscle attachments
   b. direct injury to permanent teeth
   c. fetal molding and trauma during birth
   d. supernumerary and congenitally missing teeth

5. Patients with these conditions should receive clearance from their physicians before beginning active orthodontic treatment.
   a. history of rheumatic fever, endocrine problems, prolonged bleeding
   b. diabetes, pregnancy, joint replacement
   c. multiple sclerosis, asthma, varicella (shingles)
   d. autism, detached retina, history of retinal cancer

6. Which of the following is part of the examination process before an orthodontic diagnosis and treatment plan are prepared?
   a. radiographs
   b. photographs
   c. impressions/models
   d. medical/dental history
   e. all of the above

7. Which of the following is used to assess growth by recording the movement of the positions of specified landmarks in relation to each other?
   a. clinical examination
   b. panoramic radiograph
   c. cephalometric tracing
   d. facial photograph

8. Which of the following patient data is protected health information?
   a. any information that can be used to identify the patient
   b. any information assigned by an official agency
   c. information the patient requests be kept confidential
   d. information the dental practice assigns

9. Who owns the original of a patient's dental record?
   a. patient
   b. billing company
   c. insurance company
   d. dentist

10. Which federal agency handles complaints about violations? HIPPA
    a. Department of Elderly Affairs
    b. Indian Health Service
    c. Office of Civil Rights
    d. Health Education Department

TRUE/FALSE

ndicate whether the statement is true (T) or false (F).

_____ 1. Bands to be cemented in place can be adapted either in the patient's mouth or on his/her diagnostic cast.

_____ 2. The timely use of an arch expanded effectively minimizes or eliminates the need for braces when the patient gets older.

_____ 3. Fixed appliances exert more pressure and can achieve more complex movement than removable appliances.

_____ 4. The mechanical forces used to modify or correct facial growth are force, torque, and pressure over time.

_____ 5. A ligature director seats and positions a band around the tooth.

_____ 6. The type of dental care a patient has sought in the past is typically not indicative of the type of orthodontic patient he/she will be.

_____ 7. Orthognathic surgery is completed to prevent jaw abnormalities.

_____ 8. In Class II malocclusion, the mandibular first molar is too distal to the maxillary first molar by the width of a premolar.

_____ 9. Patients with Class I malocclusion have no deficiencies in occlusion, either anteriorly or posteriorly.

_____ 10. Occlusion refers to the relationships between the maxillary and mandibular teeth when the jaws are opened approximately $1 - 1\frac{1}{2}$ mm.

FILL IN THE BLANK

Using words from the list below, fill in the blanks to complete the following statements.

band driver   glass ionomer   orthodontic scaler
bird beak pliers   Hawley retainer   palatal expander
bracket forceps   headgear   separator
distal end-cutting pliers

1. This instrument is used to place orthodontic brackets and remove elastic rings and excess material: _____.

2. This instrument is used to seat and position the band on the tooth: _____.

3. This instrument is used to carry the bracket and place it on the tooth: _____.

4. This type of pliers is used for seating separating springs and bending arch wire: _____.

5. This type of pliers is used to cut and hold the ends of arch wires that protrude slightly from buccal tubes: _____.

6. This common type of appliance is used to retain the tooth position.

7. This type of appliance is used to widen the maxillary arch: _____.

8. This type of appliance is used to transfer neck force to the maxillary first molar in order to distalize it: _____.

9. This type of auxiliary aid is used to provide space between teeth to enable correct placement of the orthodontic bands: _____.

10. _____ cement is frequently used to bond orthodontic bands to teeth because it releases fluoride into the adjacent enamel.

CHAPTER 51
Assisting in Emergency Care

CHAPTER OUTLINE

Review the Chapter Outline. If any content area is unclear, review that area before beginning the workbook exercises.

A. Preventing Medical and Dental Emergencies

B. Emergency Preparedness

C. Responsibilities of Each Team Member

D. Recognizing an Emergency

E. Protocol for Emergency Situations

F. Cardiopulmonary Resuscitation

G. Emergency Equipment and Supplies

H. Oxygen

I. Emergency Responses

J. Shock Recognition and Treatment

K. Drug- and Materials-Sensitivity-Related Emergencies

L. Cardiac Emergencies

M. Respiratory Emergencies

N. Other Emergencies

O. Dental Emergencies

P. Documentation of an Emergency

CHAPTER REVIEW

The following is a summary of the chapter. If any of this material is unclear, review it in the textbook again.

An emergency is a situation or occurrence of a serious nature, developing suddenly and unexpectedly, and demanding immediate action. The dental team must be prepared to offer emergency care in the unfortunate event that an emergency arises. As a dental assistant, prevention and knowing one's responsibility as part of the dental team helps to ensure that the team works effectively together when faced with an emergency. Prevention consists of information, patient medical and dental history, vital signs, and being able to recognize symptoms and signs of an event. The dental team establishes guidelines for emergency practice drills with each member assuming certain responsibilties. Practicing the emergency drills throughout the year helps to better prepare team members for handling an event. It is important for dental assistants to keep up-to-date with cardiopulmonary resuscitation training, defibrillation, obtaining vital signs, and basic life support standards. The dental office emergency supplies should have valid expiration dates and equipment checked monthly for working conditions. The dental assistant is trained in assessing events such as patient syncope, allergic reactions, and anaphylactic shock. Three common cardiovascular emergencies are likely to occur in dental offices: angina pectoris, myocardial infarction, and cardiac arrest.

LEARNING ACTIVITIES AND STUDY AIDS

Review the following study aids and/or complete the activities to ensure that you have achieved the learning objectives for this chapter.

1. Differentiate a symptom and a sign.

2. List the ABCDs of life support.

3. The American Dental Association (ADA) suggests the following items be included in an emergency kit.

Table 51-1

Drug/Product	Usage
A.	preloaded syringes
B.	counteracts the effects of histamine and relieves allergies
C.	injection form for seizures
D.	in injection form that lessens the sensory function to the brain and relieves pain or anxiety
E.	for high blood pressure

F.	sugar packets or frosting, administered sublingually
G.	for chest pain, spray, sublingual tablets, or transdermal patches
H.	inhaler relaxes the bronchi in the event of an asthma attack
I.	ammonia inhalant, a respiratory stimulant used for syncope patients
J.	AED
K.	O_2

4. In the following table, place the appropriate letter of each term or abbreviation in Column A with the appropriate definition in Column B.

Table 51-2

Column A	Column B
A. CPR	_____ insufficient blood flow to the brain resulting from a change in position
B. AED	_____ heart attack
C. syncope	_____ heart disease causing chest pain
D. postural hypotension	_____ a chronic brain disorder characterized by recurrent seizures
E. acute myocardial infraction	_____ emergency medical system
F. respiratory arrest	_____ a stroke
G. angina pectoris	_____ breathing has stopped
H. EMS 911	_____ automated external defibrillator
I. cerebrovascular accident	_____ most common medical emergency, caused by an unbalanced distribution of blood to the brain and the rest of the body
J. epilepsy	_____ cardiopulmonary resuscitation

5. Diabetes has become a more common disease. Conduct research online or in your school or local library. Research the various types of diabetes, causes of each, signs and symptoms, treatments available, and statistics related to this disease in the United States. Prepare a short PowerPoint presentation to present your findings. On a separate piece of paper, cite your resources. Be prepared to present/discuss your information in class.

6. List the symptoms of a postextraction hemorrhage and treatment to stop the bleeding.

7. To learn about the Good Samaritan laws in your state, go online and conduct research. Write a synopsis and explanation of the law. Cite your sources.

8. List the details that are entered into the patient's chart after a dental office emergency.

9. Outline what a dental assistant should do for each of the following conditions that may occur as an emergency in a dental office.

Table 51-3

Condition	Treatment
Syncope (fainting)	
Postural hypotension	
Angina pectoris	
Myocardial infarction	
Stroke	
Hyperventilation	
Asthma	
Allergic reaction	

(*continued*)

(*continued*)

Seizure	
Hyperglycemia	
Hypoglycemia	

10. Explain the best time to schedule an appointment for a diabetic patient.

MEDICAL TERMINOLOGY REVIEW

Use a dictionary and/or your textbook to define the following terms.

allergen _____

alveolitis _____

anaphylactic shock _____

angina pectoris _____

arteriosclerosis _____

asthma _____

asthma attack _____

automated external defibrillator _____

cerebrovascular accident (CVA) _____

congestive heart failure _____

crash cart _____

diabetes mellitus _____

diabetes type I _____

diabetes type II _____

edema _____

epilepsy _____

eugenol _____

gel form _____

grand mal seizure _____

hyperglycemia _____

hyperventilation _____

hypoglycemia _____

myocardial infarction _____

nitroglycerin _____

petit mal seizure _____

postural hypotension _____

symptom _____

syncope _____

ventricular fibrillation _____

ABBREVIATIONS

AED _____

AHA _____

ARC _____

BLS _____

CPR _____

EMS _____

EMT _____

IDDM _____

NIDDM _____

O$_2$ _____

CRITICAL THINKING

1. You are assisting during a routine restorative appointment on a patient replacing a composite on # 8–MIFL. All of a sudden the patient grabs his/her throat and begins wheezing and states that he/she is having trouble breathing. You have already administered a local anesthetic: lidocaine with epinephrine 1:100K. You are the only one in the treatment room; what do you do?

2. What is the best way to prevent a medical emergency in the dental office?

3. According to the American Dental Association, what type of items should be contained in an emergency kit? List the items, and describe their use. Why is this list of emergency items important for the dental assistant to know?

CHAPTER REVIEW TEST

MULTIPLE CHOICE

Circle the letter of the correct answer.

1. A sign of syncope is:
   a. tightness in the chest
   b. increased blood pressure
   c. rapid heart rate
   d. wheezing

2. The pain of _____ can be relieved by the administration of nitroglycerin.
   a. a cerebrovascular accident
   b. an acute myocardial infarction
   c. an asthmatic attack
   d. angina pectoris

3. The abbreviation EMS stands for:
   a. early medical station
   b. emergency medical service
   c. essential medical standards
   d. everything medically standard

4. If a patient becomes extremely anxious about a dental procedure, he/she may:
   a. hyperventilate
   b. hypoventilate
   c. become hyperglycemic
   d. become hypoglycemic

5. A(n) _____ can cause an allergic reaction.
   a. allergen
   b. analgesic
   c. antihistamine
   d. anaphylactic

6. Time is critical when administering CPR because brain damage can occur within _____ minutes after an arrest.
   a. 10 to 15
   b. 5 to 10
   c. 4 to 6
   d. 2 to 5

7. In the step ABCD of CPR, the letter "D" stands for:
   a. deformation
   b. defibrillation
   c. dense breathing
   d. doctor

8. In CPR, the compression-to-ventilation ratio is _____ for all victims of any age, except newborn babies
   a. 15:2
   b. 15:1
   c. 30:2
   d. 30:1

9. If an asthma patient experiences an episode of asthma, the dental assistant should position the patient in the upright position and use his/her _____ to relax the bronchioles.
   a. bronchitis
   b. bronchorestrictor
   c. breather
   d. bronchodilator

10. Another term for a stroke is:
    a. cerebrovascular accident
    b. cerebrovascular incident
    c. cerebrovascular area
    d. cerebrovascular attack

TRUE/FALSE

Indicate whether the statement is true (T) or false (F).

_____ 1. A hemorrhage is when an artery ruptures and the area is filled with blood.

_____ 2. A sign of a cerebrovascular accident is chest pain.

_____ 3. Practice drills for handling office emergencies do not need to be performed routinely.

_____ 4. If an individual is having a heart attack, the greatest risk occurs within the first fifteen minutes of the onset of symptoms.

_____ 5. Cardiac arrest is when circulation and respiration cease and vital organs are deprived of oxygenated blood.

_____ 6. Epilepsy is a chronic brain disorder characterized by recurrent seizures.

_____ 7. An abnormal heart rhythm is called ventricular fibrillation.

_____ 8. Ammonia inhalant is a cardiac stimulant used for angina.

_____ 9. Oxygen is used for all stroke patients.

_____ 10. Oxygen is very flammable.

FILL IN THE BLANK

Using words from the list below, fill in the blanks to complete the following statements

diabetes mellitus	postural hypotension	epilepsy
acute myocardial infarction	petite mal seizure	ammonia
anaphylactic reaction	automated external defibrillator (AED)	Type I
defibrillation	Type II	

1. _____ is a seizure whereby the patient exhibits a blank stare, a twitch, or blinks rapidly.

2. The term "sweet urine" refers to _____.

3. Many dental offices are equipped with an _____, which is an advanced computer that assesses the patient's condition and cardiac rhythms.

4. The term "critical link" in the chain of survival refers to early _____.

5. _____, also known as orthostatic hypotension, is the second-leading cause of syncope in dental offices.

6. _____ causes muscle contractions, which causes more blood flow to the brain.

7. _____ is a severe allergic reaction.

8. When a portion of the myocardium (heart muscle) dies from lack of oxygen caused by narrowing or blockage of the arteries, the patient is experiencing a(n) _____.

9. _____ is a chronic brain disorder characterized by recurrent seizures.

10. Diabetes _____ primarily affects children.

CHAPTER 52

Communication Techniques

CHAPTER OUTLINE

Review the Chapter Outline. If any content area is unclear, review that area before beginning the workbook exercises.

   A. Communication Process

   B. Verbal Communication
      1. Understanding Human Needs

   C. Nonverbal Communication

   D. The Listening Process

   E. Communication with Members of the Dental Team
      1. Channels of Communication
      2. Barriers to Communication

   F. Cultural Diversity

   G. Phone Skills
      1. Answering Machine and Voice Mail
      2. Placing a Patient on Hold
      3. Screening Calls
      4. Taking Messages
      5. Answering Services

   H. Office Equipment

   I. Written Communications
      1. Letters

   J. Dental Office Procedure Manual

CHAPTER REVIEW

The following is a summary of the chapter. If any of this material is unclear, review it in the textbook again.

Good communication skills are the key to building effective relationships with patients, employers, and colleagues. Communication involves both sending and receiving messages, because both sender and receiver must understand the information being conveyed. Messages can be sent consciously or unwittingly. Consequently, a message may convey the information intended to be sent or something else entirely. It is important for the dental assistant to be aware of all of the messages he/she is sending, as well as the interpretation likely to be placed on them by others. It is also important for the dental assistant to listen and observe the behavior of others carefully, so as to accurately receive and interpret the information others are sending.

LEARNING ACTIVITIES AND STUDY AIDS

Review the following study aids and/or complete the activities to ensure that you have achieved the learning objectives for this chapter.

1. Determine how you would respond to the following telephone calls. Then identify the principles that made you choose to respond as you did. Utilize an additional piece of paper as needed to record your information.

    a. You answer the phone by saying, "Good afternoon, Dr. Smithson's office. This is Marie. How may I help you?" The caller responds, "Quiero concertar un cita." How will you respond?

    b. You answer the phone as above, and the caller responds, "This is Mrs. Johnson. Dr. Smithson referred my daughter Mary to an orthodontist, Dr. Sikes. We went for a consultation yesterday, and I don't want to continue going there." How will you respond?

2. Differentiate verbal and nonverbal communication, and describe means of making each more effective.

3. On a separate piece of paper, write a business letter. Make sure the spacing is correct, and the contents are well stated with accurate spelling and grammar. After writing the letter, use a pen to point out each part of the letter such as the letterhead, salutation, and so forth.

4. List the principles of effective telephone etiquette.

5. Discuss how cultural differences can impact communication.

6. Describe means of lessening miscommunication in intercultural communication.

7. Describe Maslow's hierarchy of needs.

8. List and define the different channels of communication in a dental office.

9. Describe the different types of interpersonal conflict.

10. Discuss how appropriate management of conflict can result in improved dental practice functioning.

MEDICAL TERMINOLOGY REVIEW

Use a dictionary and/or your textbook to define the following terms.

cultural diversity _____

downward channel communication _____

horizontal channel communication _____

informal channel communication _____

nonverbal communication _____

objective fears _____

receiver _____

salutation _____

sender _____

subjective fears _____

upward channel communication _____

ABBREVIATIONS

HIPAA _____

CRITICAL THINKING

1. Why is it important for a dental assistant to understand the principles of effective communication? How can this knowledge enhance communication between patients and office staff?

2. How would you describe the placement of veneers for a patient? Remember to include what they are, why they are a good choice for this patient, and the benefits of veneers over other restorations.

3. There are two types of fears that patients may come into your office with; describe these fears, and how it is best to deal with these "fearful" patients.

4. Your patient has just come into your office and is trembling, crying, and short of breath—although he/she is there only for a routine prophylaxis. How would you deal with this patient and try to calm him/her down?

CHAPTER REVIEW TEST

MULTIPLE CHOICE

Circle the letter of the correct answer.

1. Describe communication.
   a. two-way sharing of information
   b. may be written or spoken
   c. may be verbal or nonverbal
   d. a and c
   e. all of the above

2. Patients evaluate their experience in the dental office on the basis of how they are treated:
   a. on the telephone
   b. during interactions with front office personnel
   c. personally in the treatment room
   d. a and c
   e. all of the above

3. The essential component of an effective message is that the:
   a. receiver understands the message
   b. sender transmits the message clearly
   c. appropriate channel is selected for message transmission
   d. message is conveyed personally

4. The essential prerequisite to effective patient communication is to:
   a. provide the message in writing as well as through spoken words
   b. convey the meaning of the message precisely
   c. think before speaking
   d. defuse the patient's anxiety and fear

5. Discovering what motivates a patient to accept treatment is key to effective communication of:

    a. procedures that will be performed
    b. fees for treatment received
    c. positive outcomes
    d. treatment options

6. To meet the needs of a patient who is dental phobic, the dental team must take extra steps to provide a _____ atmosphere.

    a. positive   d. a and c
    b. sincere   e. all of the above
    c. respectful

7. If the dental team is running behind schedule, waiting patients should be:

    a. informed and given a choice to reschedule or wait
    b. rescheduled for the following week at the same time
    c. asked to return tomorrow at the same time
    d. completed before the day is over

8. When a patient is angry, it is the job of the dental team to:

    a. inform the dentist
    b. learn what the problem is
    c. tell the patient the office policies and procedures
    d. avoid rescheduling that patient

9. The key to effective communication among members of a dental team is:

    a. placing the dentist's needs first   c. teamwork
    b. efficiency   d. working with similar personalities

10. Which of the following is a barrier to effective communication among the dental team?

    a. monitoring and exploiting the grapevine as appropriate
    b. cross-training team members
    c. lack of frequent personal interaction
    d. lack of clarity regarding roles and responsibilities

TRUE/FALSE

Indicate whether the statement is true (T) or false (F).

_____ 1. All conflict in the dental office should be avoided if possible.

_____ 2. The dental assistant should be open to discussion of a patient's culture if the patient so chooses.

_____ 3. A nonjudgmental attitude is important to the demonstration of acceptance and respect of a culture different than one's own.

_____ 4. Although beliefs about health and illness are important within a culture, they rarely influence a specific patient's behavior.

_____ 5. In some cultures, patients may prefer not to know about their diagnoses and treatments because they fear the words themselves may inflict harm.

_____ 6. When answering the phone in a professional office, it is important to speak more rapidly than usual so as not to waste expensive time.

_____ 7. The phone should be answered within three rings.

_____ 8. A caller may be placed on hold for up to two minutes.

_____ 9. With specific exceptions, a patient asking to speak with the dentist is politely informed that the dentist is with a patient and asked if the phone answerer may take a message.

_____ 10. Receiving or placing personal calls during working hours is acceptable so long as the calls are not too long.

FILL IN THE BLANK

Using words from the list below, fill in the blanks to complete the following statements.

acceptable	entire office team	personal
health information	active	everyone
positive	as soon as	open
proofread	belonging	passive
safety	discomfort	

1. Messages should be retrieved from an answering or message service _____ the office is _____.

2. Under HIPAA, _____ is responsible for protecting the patient's privacy.

3. It is _____ for the dental assistant to choose and customize a letter template and style from a word processing program.

4. In letter writing, the use of _____ verbs is preferable to the use of _____ verbs.

5. Use _____ words and tones in professional writing.

6. Before being sent, a letter should always be _____ to ensure complete accuracy in form and content.

7. _____ should not be sent via e-mail.

8. The office manual should be developed by the _____.

9. The word *pain* is rarely used in a dental office; this more effective word is used instead: _____.

10. Creation of a warm, supportive environment in the dental office helps to meet the patients' needs for _____ and _____.

CHAPTER 53
Practice Management Procedures

CHAPTER OUTLINE

Review the Chapter Outline. If any content area is unclear, review that area before beginning the workbook exercises.

    A. Operating Procedure Manuals
        1. Procedure Formats

    B. Computer Applications in the Dental Office
        1. Software and Hardware
        2. Computer Safety
        3. The Future of Computers in the Dental Office

    C. Record Keeping
        1. Clinical Records
        2. Guidelines to Record Keeping

    D. Filing and Storing of Patient Records
        1. Storing Files
        2. Rules for Filing
        3. Methods for Filing

    E. Appointment Scheduling
        1. The Appointment Book
        2. Using the Appointment Book
        3. Scheduling Systems

    F. Preventive Recall Programs

    G. Inventory Management
        1. Equipment
        2. Supplies
        3. Inventory Systems

    H. Equipment Repairs

CHAPTER REVIEW

The following is a summary of the chapter. If any of this material is unclear, review it in the textbook again.

Effective practice management procedures are required if a dental practice is to run smoothly, efficiently, and profitably. Such procedures include the development and use of an operating manual, records filing, management and storage, appointment scheduling, operation of a patient recall program, management of the equipment and supplies inventory, and maintenance and repair of the equipment used in the practice. Smooth, efficient operation is promoted by the standardization of policies and procedures and use of an office manual. Additionally, the routine use of systematic procedures to accomplish tasks encourages their completion at a high level of quality. There are different systems from which to choose, but the key is to choose and practice the best systems for the practice under consideration.

LEARNING ACTIVITES AND STUDY AIDS

Review the following study aids and/or complete the activities to ensure that you have achieved the learning objectives for this chapter.

1. Mrs. Caren Bolek has just finished her current series of appointments and has been asked to return for a recall appointment in four months. It is now February. During what month should she return? When should a recall reminder be sent to her? With whom should her next appointment be made?

2. Go online and search for the *easy*dental computer practice management system. Make a list of the functions that can be completed using this program. Then go online and search for the Dentrix and Eaglesoft practice management systems. Explain the functions that can be completed by these systems. Note your resources for your information.

3. List and define four types of appointment scheduling techniques.

4. Discuss the advantages and disadvantages of different types of preventive recall programs.

5. Explain why good record keeping is important.

6. Describe the available types of filing systems.

7. List the principles of alphabetical filing.

8. Differentiate tag and bar code inventory management systems, and state the advantages of each.

9. On a separate piece of paper, place each of the following names in correct order for alphabetical filing. Begin with the name nearest the beginning of the alphabet and end with the name nearest the end.

Table 53-1

Julie M. Jackson	Janet K. Johnson (Mrs. Andrew)	Phillip W. Jackson
Siobhan McNabb	Sally Wheaton	James J. Johnson, III
James J. Johnson, IV	The Rev. Andrew Johnson	Sarah Wilson
Judith Anne MacGillicuddy		

10. List measures that may be taken to protect the dental assistant during computer use.

1. Because your computer program is down today, have Emélia complete the new patient registration form so you can enter the data in your computer later. Be sure you have her sign it. (For the purpose of this learning activity, you are Emélia). Use the information on Emélia as provided to complete the Patient Registration Form.

PATIENT REGISTRATION FORM
(Please Print)

Date _____

Patient's
Name _____ DOB _____/_____/_____
      First   Middle   Last   Month   Day   Year

Address _____ Phone (_____) _____ - _____
      Street   City   State   Zip   Area

Alternate Phone _____ SS # _____ - _____ - _____ Occupation _____

Method of Payment (circle):   Cash   Check   Credit Card   Insurance Copayment

Primary Insurance Company _____ Policy/Group # _____

Medicare # _____ Medicaid # _____

Person
Responsible
for Payment _____ Relationship _____
      First   Middle   Last

Address _____ Phone (_____) _____ - _____
      Street   City   State   Zip   Area

Employer _____ Department _____

Address _____ Phone (_____) _____ - _____
      Street   City   State   Zip   Area

Emergency
Contact _____ Phone (_____) _____ - _____
                                    Area

Address _____ Phone (_____) _____ - _____
      Street   City   State   Zip   Area

How were you referred to this office? _____
_____

Statement of Financial Responsibility: I, _____, do hereby agree to pay all charges incurred by the above listed patient. I further understand that these charges are my responsibility, regardless of insurance coverage.

Responsible Person's Signature: _____

Emélia Garcia lives at 2872 Hope Street in Ashaway, RI. She has recently moved here with her mother, Hermana Rodriguez, and does not know the zip code for this address. Their telephone number is 401.123.7654. Emélia is working as a secretary, and Hermana is working as a loom operator at Richmond Lace, 22 Main Street, Richmond. Emélia is bilingual, with Spanish as her first language and English her second. Hermana speaks only Spanish. Richmond Lace provides dental insurance through Delta Dental of Massachusetts, and you have made a copy of Emélia's insurance card for Dr. Smithson's records. Neither Emélia nor Hermana has any other dental insurance coverage, and the appointment today will be Emélia's first use of her new insurance. Dr. Smithson prefers that records be filed alphabetically but does assign patient numbers because so many names are similar. You assign Emélia patient number 47298, and note on your records that she was born April 12, 1972. Her Social Security number is 262-83-9788. Emélia's insurance is Delta Dental. Her numbers are: Group number 77842, Subscriber number 174169932849.

Once the form is filled out, go online to the United States Postal Service site and find the correct zip code for Ashaway, RI. Then provide it on the form.

12. Using the following schedule, matrix off the following times:

        Office hours: 9:30–5:00

        Lunch hour: 12:00–1:30

The doctor likes to leave at least two half-hour slots open for emergencies.

        Ed Trombley—M composite #7, first appointment, 1 hour

        Jerry Richard—DO amalgam #28, 11:00 appointment, 45 minutes

        Janet Orlando—Deliver PFM crown, 11:45 appointment, 15 minutes

        Lena Mezza—Simple extraction #16, 1:30 appointment, 1 hour

        Emélia Garcia—Class II restoration, 3:00 appointment, $1\frac{1}{2}$ hours

Monday, June 8, 20xx
9:00 a.m.
9:15 a.m.
9:30 a.m.
9:45 a.m.
10:00 a.m.
10:15 a.m.
10:30 a.m.
10:45 a.m.
11:00 a.m.
11:15 a.m.
11:30 a.m.
11:45 a.m.
12:00 p.m.
12:15 p.m.
12:30 p.m.
12:45 p.m.
1:00 p.m.

1:15 p.m.	
1:30 p.m.	
1:45 p.m.	
2:00 p.m.	
2:15 p.m.	
2:30 p.m.	
2:45 p.m.	
3:00 p.m.	
3:15 p.m.	
3:30 p.m.	
3:45 p.m.	
4:00 p.m.	
4:15 p.m.	
4:30 p.m.	
4:45 p.m.	
5:00 p.m.	
5:15 p.m.	
5:30 p.m.	

MEDICAL TERMINOLOGY REVIEW

Use a dictionary and/or your textbook to define the following terms.

calibration _____

credit slip _____

double-booking _____

ergonomics _____

lead time _____

modified wave scheduling _____

operating procedure manual _____

reorder point _____

shelf life _____

wave scheduling _____

ABBREVIATIONS

CPU _____

CRITICAL THINKING

1. What is an operating procedure manual? Why is it important to the dental office?

2. Why are ergonomics important when using the computer? Describe what ergonomics are, and provide some ideas of how to correctly posture oneself when using the computer.

3. Why is office practice management such an important operation within the dental office? What are some business practices specific to the dental office?

CHAPTER REVIEW TEST

MULTIPLE CHOICE

Circle the letter of the correct answer.

1. Policies are:
   a. guides for action to be taken
   b. systematic statements of uniform means of working
   c. written directions for completing some function or task
   d. collections of methods that must be followed

2. The overall purpose of a procedures manual is:
   a. easy dissemination of technical knowledge
   b. coordination of policies with procedures
   c. quality management and control
   d. compliance with OSHA and HIPAA mandates

3. The advantage of an electronic procedures manual is:
   a. everything is in one place but can be carried to where it is needed
   b. convenience of information access and replacement
   c. HIPAA inspectors can see that all necessary procedures have been followed
   d. all team members can look at it simultaneously

4. Select TWO characteristics of office hardware that indicate it needs to be updated.
   a. storage capacity of unit is diminished
   b. unit can no longer support the necessary software
   c. retrieval of records from the unit is difficult
   d. inputting records into the unit takes time

5. The primary function of a computer in a dental office is:
   a. saving the office manager time
   b. saving the space taken up by files
   c. data standardization
   d. data management

6. Backup of computer data should be completed:
   a. daily
   b. weekly
   c. monthly
   d. as convenient

7. The patient's dental chart contains all of the following EXCEPT:
   a. radiographs
   b. examination records
   c. financial information
   d. prescriptions

8. Legally, the _____ owns the patient's chart and the _____ owns the information it contains.
   a. patient; dentist
   b. dentist; patient
   c. dentist; dentist
   d. patient; patient

9. Which of the following is NOT an appropriate guideline for dental practice record keeping?
   a. Date every entry.
   b. Sign all entries.
   c. Maintain the confidentiality of health information.
   d. Use red ink for emergency entries.

10. Patient files should be kept for:
    a. one year past their last appointment
    b. three years
    c. seven years
    d. indefinitely

TRUE/FALSE

Indicate whether the statement is true (T) or false (F).

_____ 1. No clinical charts or financial records should be visible on the desk or in the operatory for other patients to view.

_____ 2. Although specific health information may not be placed on the outside of a patient's chart, a color coding system may be used.

_____ 3. Out guides are rarely used anymore because they require excessive time to fill out and place.

_____ 4. Papers, such as lab or x-ray reports, should be formally released before being filed.

_____ 5. Paper files should be arranged so the newest entries are on top.

_____ 6. Numeric filing systems are best suited for use in small, one-dentist practices.

_____ 7. When filing, nothing comes before something.

_____ 8. When filing, hyphenated names are considered separately and filed under the first letter of the second name.

_____ 9. A married woman's chart is filed under her husband's first and last names.

_____ 10. Confidentiality is most easily maintained in an alphabetical filing system.

FILL IN THE BLANK

Using words from the list below, fill in the blanks to complete the following statements.

operating manuals	software	time buffer
alphabetical	the patient	ergonomics
capital purchases	"paperless"	filing
numeric		

1. _____ are generally notebooks or three-ring binders that contain written directions for completing some function or task.

2. The _____ is the part of the computer system that manages the data and is not visible.

3. _____ are the body mechanics that are considered in using equipment and tools by a human.

4. Many offices are already considered "_____" with electronic charting, appointments, billing, and radiology.

5. Consent forms for releasing files must be signed by _____.

6. _____ is the act of preserving and protecting the files, including arranging them so that they can be retrieved quickly.

7. _____ filing is the oldest, most common system for any information that is ordered.

8. _____ filing systems are recommended for extremely large practices with over 5,000 charts.

9. One strategy that is recommended to help keep the office flowing smoothly is to leave two open appointment slots available each day. This is known as a _____.

10. _____ are normally those items that cost at least $500 and include things like furniture.

CHAPTER 54
Financial Management

CHAPTER OUTLINE

Review the Chapter Outline. If any content area is unclear, review that area before beginning the workbook exercises.

A. Accounting
   1. Percentages
   2. Decimals
B. Preventive Account Management
   1. Collecting Financial Data and Information
   2. Fees and Financial Arrangements
C. Accounts Receivable
   1. Types of Accounts Receivable
   2. Managing Accounts Receivable
D. Collections
   1. Collection Letters
   2. Collection Calls
E. Accounts Payable Management
   1. Types of Expenses
   2. Budgeting
F. Writing Checks
G. Payroll
   1. Employee Pay Record

CHAPTER REVIEW

The following is a summary of the chapter. If any of this material is unclear, review it in the textbook again.

A dental practice is a business as well as a health service agency. A business must be run efficiently and profitably if it is to support its owners and employees. The dental assistant who manages the finances, variously termed a front desk assistant, office manager, practice manager, or administrative assistant, has an important role to play in ensuring the practice is efficient and profitable. Basic accounting and bookkeeping knowledge and skill are required to be successful in this position, as are the ability to discuss financial arrangements with patients, collect monies owed to the practice, pay bills accurately and on time, and work with insurance companies, suppliers, financial service agencies, accountants, and other employees. It is imperative that the financial assistant pay attention to detail. The desk is the hub of a dental practice. A practice that is well run financially is a pleasure to work in.

LEARNING ACTIVITIES AND STUDY AIDS

Review the following study aids and/or complete the activities to ensure that you have achieved the learning objectives for this chapter.

1. In conformance with Dr. Smithson's policies, because Emélia is a new patient, she was booked with the dental hygienist for a cleaning and examination. When she called for her appointment, she stated her reason for wanting to see the dentist was because it was "time for a checkup." Again in conformance with Dr. Smithson's policies, the hygienist will also take whatever radiographs are indicated once he sees Emélia's medical/dental history and the conditions in her mouth. During the appointment the hygienist did the cleaning and examination and took four posterior bitewings. During the examination he found an MO cavity on tooth #31. Emélia takes good care of her teeth and was dismayed to find she has a cavity. The fees charged were $62.00 for the x-rays, $76.00 for the cleaning, and $34.00 for the examination. Richmond Lace's plan with Delta Dental covers all three services, once per year for the bitewings and twice per year for the cleaning and examination. None of the services require preauthorization. Emélia's deductible is $150.00. Determine how much Delta Dental will pay, and how much Emélia must pay.

2. Explain the procedure and rationale for conducting a credit check.

3. You have just received a statement from the bank detailing this month's transactions. The balance at the end of last month was $15,256.35. Deposits were $11,234.40. Checks that were written totaled $1201.42. There is one outstanding check for $3,201.00. There were no service fees. What should the balance be in your checkbook? Your checkbook lists the balance as $21,188.33. What is the most likely explanation for the error? What should be done to reconcile the two balances?

4. On a separate piece of paper, write a pay letter to Mr. Kenneth Colson of 1936 A Street, Bradford, RI 02808. Assume today is October 3, 2009. He has owed Dr. Smithson $431.00 since May 2008 and although he agreed to pay $25.00 per month in November, he has not yet paid anything on the bill. Use block style and be firm but positive. Remember to use correct capitalization, punctuation, spelling, and grammar.

5. Discuss procedures for collection of past due accounts.

6. Describe the process of aging accounts.

7. The office is planning to buy a new laser printer. The cost is $564.82 plus tax of 7%. What will the total cost of the printer be? Once it has been purchased, will you record the bill as an account receivable or account payable? Must the old printer be recycled?

8. Dr. Smithson hired a new dental assistant yesterday, and she has arrived for her appointment with you to complete the necessary paperwork. What form will you need to have her complete in order to make the appropriate tax deductions from her paycheck? What is done with this form?

9. The new assistant is Maria Montecalvo. She lives at 91 Main Street, Wakefield, RI 02879. Her Social Security number is 862-40-0012. She will be paid $20.00/hour for a 40-hour workweek. She is a single mother with two children, all of whom she claims as dependents. Help Maria complete the following W-4 form.

Figure 54-1

Form W-4 (2008)

Purpose. Complete Form W-4 so that your employer can withhold the correct federal income tax from your pay. Consider completing a new Form W-4 each year and when your personal or financial situation changes.

Exemption from withholding. If you are exempt, complete **only** lines 1, 2, 3, 4, and 7 and sign the form to validate it. Your exemption for 2008 expires February 16, 2009. See Pub. 505, Tax Withholding and Estimated Tax.

Note. You cannot claim exemption from withholding if (a) your income exceeds $900 and includes more than $300 of unearned income (for example, interest and dividends) and (b) another person can claim you as a dependent on their tax return.

Basic instructions. If you are not exempt, complete the **Personal Allowances Worksheet** below. The worksheets on page 2 adjust your withholding allowances based on itemized deductions, certain credits,

adjustments to income, or two-earner/multiple job situations. Complete all worksheets that apply. However, you may claim fewer (or zero) allowances.

Head of household. Generally, you may claim head of household filing status on your tax return only if you are unmarried and pay more than 50% of the costs of keeping up a home for yourself and your dependent(s) or other qualifying individuals. See Pub. 501, Exemptions, Standard Deduction, and Filing Information, for information.

Tax credits. You can take projected tax credits into account in figuring your allowable number of withholding allowances. Credits for child or dependent care expenses and the child tax credit may be claimed using the **Personal Allowances Worksheet** below. See Pub. 919, How Do I Adjust My Tax Withholding, for information on converting your other credits into withholding allowances.

Nonwage income. If you have a large amount of nonwage income, such as interest or dividends, consider making estimated tax

payments using Form 1040-ES, Estimated Tax for Individuals. Otherwise, you may owe additional tax. If you have pension or annuity income, see Pub. 919 to find out if you should adjust your withholding on Form W-4 or W-4P.

Two earners or multiple jobs. If you have a working spouse or more than one job, figure the total number of allowances you are entitled to claim on all jobs using worksheets from only one Form W-4. Your withholding usually will be most accurate when all allowances are claimed on the Form W-4 for the highest paying job and zero allowances are claimed on the others. See Pub. 919 for details.

Nonresident alien. If you are a nonresident alien, see the Instructions for Form 8233 before completing this Form W-4.

Check your withholding. After your Form W-4 takes effect, use Pub. 919 to see how the dollar amount you are having withheld compares to your projected total tax for 2008. See Pub. 919, especially if your earnings exceed $130,000 (Single) or $180,000 (Married).

Personal Allowances Worksheet (Keep for your records.)

A Enter "1" for **yourself** if no one else can claim you as a dependent . . . . **A** _____

B Enter "1" if:
- You are single and have only one job; or
- You are married, have only one job, and your spouse does not work; or
- Your wages from a second job or your spouse's wages (or the total of both) are $1,500 or less.

. . **B** _____

C Enter "1" for your **spouse.** But, you may choose to enter "-0-" if you are married and have either a working spouse or more than one job. (Entering "-0-" may help you avoid having too little tax withheld.) . . . . **C** _____

D Enter number of **dependents** (other than your spouse or yourself) you will claim on your tax return . . . . . . **D** _____

E Enter "1" if you will file as **head of household** on your tax return (see conditions under **Head of household** above) . **E** _____

F Enter "1" if you have at least $1,500 of **child or dependent care expenses** for which you plan to claim a credit . . **F** _____

(**Note.** Do **not** include child support payments. See Pub. 503, Child and Dependent Care Expenses, for details.)

G **Child Tax Credit** (including additional child tax credit). See Pub. 972, Child Tax Credit, for more information.
- If your total income will be less than $58,000 ($86,000 if married), enter "2" for each eligible child.
- If your total income will be between $58,000 and $84,000 ($86,000 and $119,000 if married), enter "1" for each eligible child plus "1" **additional** if you have 4 or more eligible children. . . . . **G** _____

H Add lines A through G and enter total here. (**Note.** This may be different from the number of exemptions you claim on your tax return.) ▶ **H** _____

For accuracy, complete all worksheets that apply.
- If you plan to **itemize or claim adjustments to income** and want to reduce your withholding, see the **Deductions and Adjustments Worksheet** on page 2.
- If you have **more than one job** or are **married and you and your spouse both work** and the combined earnings from all jobs exceed $40,000 ($25,000 if married), see the **Two-Earners/Multiple Jobs Worksheet** on page 2 to avoid having too little tax withheld.
- If **neither** of the above situations applies, **stop here** and enter the number from line H on line 5 of Form W-4 below.

- **Cut here and give Form W-4 to your employer. Keep the top part for your records.** - - - - - - - - - - - - - - - - -

Form **W-4**	**Employee's Withholding Allowance Certificate**	OMB No. 1545-0074
Department of the Treasury Internal Revenue Service	▶ **Whether you are entitled to claim a certain number of allowances or exemption from withholding is subject to review by the IRS. Your employer may be required to send a copy of this form to the IRS.**	2008

1 Type or print your first name and middle initial.	Last name	**2** Your social security number

Home address (number and street or rural route)

3 ☐ Single ☐ Married ☐ Married, but withhold at higher Single rate.
Note. If married, but legally separated, or spouse is a nonresident alien, check the "Single" box.

City or town, state, and ZIP code

4 If your last name differs from that shown on your social security card, check here. You must call 1-800-772-1213 for a replacement card. ▶ ☐

5 Total number of allowances you are claiming (from line **H** above **or** from the applicable worksheet on page 2) | **5** |

6 Additional amount, if any, you want withheld from each paycheck . . . . | **6** $ |

7 I claim exemption from withholding for 2008, and I certify that I meet **both** of the following conditions for exemption.
- Last year I had a right to a refund of **all** federal income tax withheld because I had **no** tax liability **and**
- This year I expect a refund of **all** federal income tax withheld because I expect to have **no** tax liability.

If you meet both conditions, write "Exempt" here . . . . ▶ | **7** |

Under penalties of perjury, I declare that I have examined this certificate and to the best of my knowledge and belief, it is true, correct, and complete.

Employee's signature
(Form is not valid unless you sign it.) ▶ _____ Date ▶ _____

8 Employer's name and address (Employer: Complete lines 8 and 10 only if sending to the IRS.) | **9** Office code (optional) | **10** Employer identification number (EIN) |

For Privacy Act and Paperwork Reduction Act Notice, see page 2. Cat. No. 10220Q Form **W-4** (2008)

Deductions and Adjustments Worksheet

Note. Use this worksheet *only* if you plan to itemize deductions, claim certain credits, or claim adjustments to income on your 2008 tax return.

1   Enter an estimate of your 2008 itemized deductions. These include qualifying home mortgage interest, charitable contributions, state and local taxes, medical expenses in excess of 7.5% of your income, and miscellaneous deductions. (For 2008, you may have to reduce your itemized deductions if your income is over $159,950 ($79,975 if married filing separately). See *Worksheet 2* in Pub. 919 for details.)   . .   **1** $ _____

2   Enter: $\left\{\begin{array}{l}\text{\$10,900 if married filing jointly or qualifying widow(er)}\\\text{\$ 8,000 if head of household}\\\text{\$ 5,450 if single or married filing separately}\end{array}\right\}$ . . . .   **2** $ _____

3   **Subtract** line 2 from line 1. If zero or less, enter "-0-"   . . . .   **3** $ _____

4   Enter an estimate of your 2008 adjustments to income, including alimony, deductible IRA contributions, and student loan interest   **4** $ _____

5   **Add** lines 3 and 4 and enter the total. (Include any amount for credits from *Worksheet 8* in Pub. 919)   **5** $ _____

6   Enter an estimate of your 2008 nonwage income (such as dividends or interest)   . . . .   **6** $ _____

7   **Subtract** line 6 from line 5. If zero or less, enter "-0-"   . . . .   **7** $ _____

8   **Divide** the amount on line 7 by $3,500 and enter the result here. Drop any fraction   . . . . .   **8**   _____

9   Enter the number from the **Personal Allowances Worksheet,** line H, page 1   . . . .   **9**   _____

10 **Add** lines 8 and 9 and enter the total here. If you plan to use the **Two-Earners/Multiple Jobs Worksheet,** also enter this total on line 1 below. Otherwise, **stop here** and enter this total on Form W-4, line 5, page 1   **10**   _____

Two-Earners/Multiple Jobs Worksheet (See *Two earners or multiple jobs* on page 1.)

Note. Use this worksheet *only* if the instructions under line H on page 1 direct you here.

1   Enter the number from line H, page 1 (or from line 10 above if you used the **Deductions and Adjustments Worksheet**)   **1**   _____

2   Find the number in **Table 1** below that applies to the **LOWEST** paying job and enter it here. **However,** if you are married filing jointly and wages from the highest paying job are $50,000 or less, do not enter more than "3."   . . . .   **2**   _____

3   If line 1 is **more than or equal to** line 2, subtract line 2 from line 1. Enter the result here (if zero, enter "-0-") and on Form W-4, line 5, page 1. **Do not** use the rest of this worksheet   . . . .   **3**   _____

Note. If line 1 is *less than* line 2, enter "-0-" on Form W-4, line 5, page 1. Complete lines 4–9 below to calculate the additional withholding amount necessary to avoid a year-end tax bill.

4   Enter the number from line 2 of this worksheet   . . . .   **4**   _____

5   Enter the number from line 1 of this worksheet   . . . .   **5**   _____

6   **Subtract** line 5 from line 4   . . . .   **6**   _____

7   Find the amount in **Table 2** below that applies to the **HIGHEST** paying job and enter it here   . . . .   **7** $ _____

8   **Multiply** line 7 by line 6 and enter the result here. This is the additional annual withholding needed   . .   **8** $ _____

9   Divide line 8 by the number of pay periods remaining in 2008. For example, divide by 26 if you are paid every two weeks and you complete this form in December 2007. Enter the result here and on Form W-4, line 6, page 1. This is the additional amount to be withheld from each paycheck   . . . .   **9** $ _____

Table 1				Table 2			
Married Filing Jointly		**All Others**		**Married Filing Jointly**		**All Others**	
If wages from **LOWEST** paying job are—	Enter on line 2 above	If wages from **LOWEST** paying job are—	Enter on line 2 above	If wages from **HIGHEST** paying job are—	Enter on line 7 above	If wages from **HIGHEST** paying job are—	Enter on line 7 above
$0 - $4,500	0	$0 - $6,500	0	$0 - $65,000	$530	$0 - $35,000	$530
4,501 - 10,000	1	6,501 - 12,000	1	65,001 - 120,000	880	35,001 - 80,000	880
10,001 - 18,000	2	12,001 - 20,000	2	120,001 - 180,000	980	80,001 - 150,000	980
18,001 - 22,000	3	20,001 - 27,000	3	180,001 - 310,000	1,160	150,001 - 340,000	1,160
22,001 - 27,000	4	27,001 - 35,000	4	310,001 and over	1,230	340,001 and over	1,230
27,001 - 33,000	5	35,001 - 50,000	5				
33,001 - 40,000	6	50,001 - 65,000	6				
40,001 - 50,000	7	65,001 - 80,000	7				
50,001 - 55,000	8	80,001 - 95,000	8				
55,001 - 60,000	9	95,001 - 120,000	9				
60,001 - 65,000	10	120,001 and over	10				
65,001 - 75,000	11						
75,001 - 100,000	12						
100,001 - 110,000	13						
110,001 - 120,000	14						
120,001 and over	15						

10. Describe standard taxes withheld from employee paychecks.

11. The young man who delivers the neighborhood newspaper has just arrived at the office to collect his weekly fee. Although the office is closed on Sundays and Mondays, the paper is delivered seven days per week and costs $1.25 on weekdays and Saturdays, $2.75 on Sunday. Complete a petty cash voucher, using today's date, and pay the young man for the current week. The person who also initials the voucher with you as an acceptable expense is Derek Johnson, the hygienist. This will be the fourth petty cash voucher filled out this week, and Dr. Smithson's accountant categorizes the charges for the newspaper as a Publications cost.

Amount _____   No. _____

RECEIPT OF PETTY CASH

_____, 20____

For _____

Charge to _____

Approved by   Received by

_____   _____

12. Before you leave today, you must make a deposit slip to take to the bank on your way home. You received the following checks:

From	Check Number	Amount
Angela Johnson	212	125.00
David Baynes	8593	75.00
Maria Rodriguez	27	242.00
Beth Moore	318	34.00
Megan Ward	7601	790.00
John Lusitano	354	50.00
Angel Ricardo	5586	100.00

You also received $20.00 cash from Mary Grande.
Complete the following deposit slip.

FIRST COMMERCIAL

Deposit Ticket

DATE_____
DEPOSITS MAY NOT BE AVAILABLE FOR IMMEDIATE WITHDRAWAL

CASH　　　　　　◆ __ __ __ __ __ __ __ __

CHECKS

_____　　　　◆ __ __ __ __ __ __ __ __

_____　　　　◆ __ __ __ __ __ __ __ __

_____　　　　◆ __ __ __ __ __ __ __ __

_____　　　　◆ __ __ __ __ __ __ __ __

_____　　　　◆ __ __ __ __ __ __ __ __

_____　　　　◆ __ __ __ __ __ __ __ __

_____　　　　◆ __ __ __ __ __ __ __ __

TOTAL　　　　　◆ __ __ __ __ __ __ __ __

$ __ __ __ __ __ __ __.__ __

I:000216913: 02 20011893"· 8724

MEDICAL TERMINOLOGY REVIEW

Use a dictionary and/or your textbook to define the following terms.

accounts payable _____

accounts receivable _____

aging account _____

bonded _____

deposit slip _____

expenditures _____

fixed expenses _____

gross salary _____

net salary _____

overhead _____

pegboard system _____

variable expenses _____

walk-out statement _____

ABBREVIATIONS

FEIN _____

FICA _____

FUTA _____

IRS _____

CRITICAL THINKING

1. At the end of every business day the front office personnel or dental assistant must match the daily posting of payments with cash or other payments in the cash drawer. Why is this function so important to the dental office that it must be done on a daily basis?

2. If you must send a patient account for collection, what guidelines must be followed? What might you do prior to sending an account to collection?

3. Why is it important for a dental office to accurately and promptly bill patients for services? Why does a dental assistant need to be concerned with these front office duties?

CHAPTER REVIEW TEST

MULTIPLE CHOICE

Circle the letter of the correct answer.

1. Accounting involves the _____ of monies received and paid.
   a. classifying
   b. recording
   c. verifying
   d. a and c
   e. all of the above

2. 20% of $1050.00 =
   a. $20.10
   b. $21.00
   c. $210.00
   d. none of the above

3. A patient's financial information is obtained:
   a. through the patient registration form
   b. prior to his initial appointment
   c. at the close of her initial appointment
   d. a and b
   e. a and c

4. Which of the following is true?
   a. preventive account management is that portion of financial management that consists of assessing patients' ability to pay contracted fees
   b. patient permission is required before reports are requested from credit reporting agencies
   c. inclusion of usual, customary, and reasonable fees into the office accounting system is necessary to comply with dental law
   d. payment or financial arrangements should be made as soon as services have been rendered

5. A monthly account of business transactions is a:
   a. billing statement
   b. walk-out statement
   c. credit slip
   d. financial reconciliation

6. Financial discussions should always be conducted in a _____ place and remain _____.

    a. private; at the oral level
    b. private; confidential
    c. business office; unresolved until written
    d. business office; as understood by the patient

7. An employee may be bonded to protect the office against:

    a. a dentist's illness
    b. being sued
    c. employee theft
    d. a patient's failure to pay

8. This financial record is used to document every patient and every financial transaction.

    a. charge slip
    b. daily journal
    c. billing statement
    d. cash receipt

9. When the patient pays using this method, the practice pays a processing fee.

    a. credit card
    b. check
    c. insurance benefit
    d. cash

10. A bank deposit should be made:

    a. daily
    b. weekly
    c. monthly
    d. as convenient

TRUE/FALSE

Indicate whether the statement is true (T) or false (F).

_____ 1. A check should be stamped with a restrictive endorsement as soon as it is received and recorded.

_____ 2. Audit reports track daily transactions and verify that all transactions were posted correctly.

_____ 3. Accounts receivable reports track the monies the dental practice owes to suppliers.

_____ 4. An account aging report is completed to track accounts that are overdue by 30, 60, or 90 days.

_____ 5. A certified check must be countersigned in the presence of the person accepting the check as payment.

_____ 6. For courtesy's sake, a telephoned reminder that an account is past due always precedes a written reminder.

_____ 7. When making a collection call, it is important to first confirm that the receiver of the call is the responsible party for the bill in question.

_____ 8. Because a petty cash fund is used to pay minor expenses, it is not necessary to maintain strict accounting of monies paid from it.

_____ 9. All unpaid bills should be placed in an accounts payable folder that is organized by expense category and the date the bill is due.

_____ 10. Outstanding checks are those that have not been returned by the bank at the time the check register is being reconciled with the bank statement.

FILL IN THE BLANK

Using words from the list below, fill in the blanks to complete the following statements.

ten	fair	receipt
computerized	fee	W-2
confidential	four	W-4
confirmation letter	gross salary	

1. It is required by law that payroll records be kept for _____ years.

2. A _____ form is completed for each new employee to determine what amount of his/her salary should be withheld for income tax purposes.

3. _____ is the amount an employee earns before deductions have been taken out.

4. A _____ is given to each employee each year, generally no later than January 31, to be filed with his/her federal and state income tax returns.

5. The type of accounting system that provides the greatest time saving for the financial assistant, the greatest accuracy in calculations, and the greatest versatility in compiling helpful reports is a _____ system.

6. The Fair Debt Collection Practices Act was passed to ensure debtors receive _____, _____ treatment.

7. The disadvantage of using an agency for collecting overdue accounts is the _____ that must be paid.

8. When a debtor agrees in a collection call to pay an amount or on a schedule that is agreeable to the dental practice, this oral agreement must be followed with a _____.

9. A patient who pays in cash must always be given a _____.

10. Checks and automatic payments should be sent _____ days prior to their due date to ensure adequate processing time.

CHAPTER 55
Dental Insurance

CHAPTER OUTLINE

Review the Chapter Outline. If any content area is unclear, review that area before beginning the workbook exercises.

A. Dental Insurance Terminology
B. Dental Insurance Plans
   1. Dental HMOs and DMOs
   2. Dental Preferred Provider Organizations
   3. Dental Indemnity Plans
   4. Exclusive Provider Organizations
   5. Alternative Plans
   6. Determining Eligibility
   7. Determining Benefits
   8. Clarifying Primary and Secondary Carriers
   9. Coordination of Benefits
   10. Understanding Limitations and Frequencies
C. Dental Procedure Codes
   1. CDT Categories (Current Dental Terminology)
D. Processing Claims
   1. Electronic Claims Submission
   2. Filling out the ADA Claim Form
   3. Clean Claims
   4. Filling out the Patient Registration Form
   5. HIPAA and Electronic Transactions
E. Management of Claims

CHAPTER REVIEW

The following is a summary of the chapter. If any of this material is unclear, review it in the textbook again.

The majority of dental fees are now paid at least partially by an insurance carrier. Specific forms and rules apply to the generation and submission of insurance claim forms. A dental assistant must be familiar with the specialized vocabulary of dental insurance: its types, their provisions, the relationships between different insurance plans, and the forms and procedures used to process claims. Computerization and standardization of claims generation and processing has made the process easier and more efficient. Attention to detail will enable the dental assistant to file and process claims quickly, an important tool in maintaining patient goodwill, practice profitability, and good relationships with the insurance carriers.

LEARNING ACTIVITIES AND STUDY AIDS

Review the following study aids and/or complete the activities to ensure that you have achieved the learning objectives for this chapter.

1. State the means by which dental insurance may be obtained.

2. Complete the following table by providing a description of each type of insurance plan.

Table 55-1

Type of insurance plan	Description
Dental HMO	
DMO	
PPO	
Indemnity plan	
EPO	
DR	

3. In the following table, provide the definition for each term.

Table 55-2

Term	Definition
Subscriber	
Deductible	
Managed care	
Closed panel	
Copay	
Indemnity	
Eligibility	
Waiting period	
Benefit	
Dual coverage	
Primary carrier	
Procedure code	
Claim form	
Carrier	

4. Identify the procedure code ranges for diagnostic, preventive, and restorative services.

5. Explain processing, tracking, and management of dental insurance claims.

6. Discuss the importance of educating patients regarding the provisions of their dental insurance plans.

7. Describe the provisions of the HIPAA Act of 1996.

8. Discuss how claims are allocated between primary and secondary carriers.

9. Describe a subscriber number.

10. List the two tooth numbering systems that are acceptable for use on an ADA insurance claim form.

11. Complete the following claim form to send to Delta Dental for collection of the money owed to Dr. Smithson for treating Emélia García. (The fees charged were $62.00 for the x-rays, $76.00 for the cleaning, and $34.00 for the examination.) Use the same patient information as provided in Chapter 53 for Emélia.

Dental Claim Form

HEADER INFORMATION

1. Type of Transaction (Mark all applicable boxes)

☐ Statement of Actual Services ☐ Request for Predetermination/Preauthorization

2. Predetermination/Preauthorization Number

△ DELTA DENTAL   P.O. Box 9695   **Customer Service**
Boston, MA 02114   800-872-0500

INSURANCE COMPANY/DENTAL BENEFIT PLAN INFORMATION

3. Company/Plan Name, Address, City, State, Zip Code

POLICYHOLDER/SUBSCRIBER INFORMATION (For Insurance Company Named in #3)

12. Policyholder/Subscriber Name (Last, First, Middle Initial, Suffix) Address, City, State, Zip Code

13. Date of Birth (MM/DD/CCYY)	14. Gender ☐ M ☐ F	15. Policyholder/Subscriber ID (SSN or ID#)
16. Plan/Group Number	17. Employer Name	

OTHER COVERAGE

4. Other Dental or Medical Coverage? ☐ No (Skip 5-11) ☐ Yes (Complete 5-11)

5. Name of Policyholder/Subscriber in #4 (Last, First, Middle Initial, Suffix)

6. Date of Birth (MM/DD/CCYY)	7. Gender ☐ M ☐ F	8. Policyholder/Subscriber ID (SSN or ID#)
9. Plan/Group Number	10. Patient's Relationship to Person Named in #5 ☐ Self ☐ Spouse ☐ Dependent ☐ Other	

11. Other Insurance Company/Dental Benefit Plan Name, Address, City, State. Zip Code

PATIENT INFORMATION

18. Relationship to Policyholder/Subscriber Named in #12 Above
☐ Self ☐ Spouse ☐ Dependent ☐ Other

19. Student Status ☐ FTS ☐ PTS

20. Name (Last, First, Middle Initial, Suffix), Address, City, State, Zip Code

21. Date of Birth (MM/DD/CCYY)	22. Gender ☐ M ☐ F	23. Patient ID/Account # (Assigned by Dentist)

RECORD OF SERVICES PROVIDED

	24. Procedure Date (MM/DD/CCYY)	25. Area of Oral Cavity	26. Tooth System	27. Tooth Number(s) or Letter(s)	28. Tooth Surface	29. Procedure Code	30. Description	31. Fee
1								
2								
3								
4								
5								
6								
7								
8								
9								
10								
11							32. Other Fee(s)	
12								
13							33. Total Fee	

34. Remarks

AUTHORIZATIONS

35. I have been informed of the treatment plan and associated fees. I agree to be responsible for all charges for dental services and materials not paid by my dental benefit plan, unless prohibited by law, or the treating dentist or dental practice has a contractual agreement with my plan prohibiting all or a portion of such charges. To the extent permitted by law, I consent to your use and disclosure of my protected health information to carry out payment of activities in connection with this claim.

X _____
Patient/Guardian signature   Date

36. I hereby authorize and direct payment of the dental benefits otherwise payable to me, directly to the below named dentist or dental entity.

X _____
Subscriber signature   Date

ANCILLARY CLAIM/TREATMENT INFORMATION

37. Place of Treatment
☐ Provider's Office ☐ Hospital ☐ ECF ☐ Other

38. Number of Enclosures (00-99)
Radiograph(s) ☐ Oral Image(s) ☐ Model(s) ☐

39. Is Treatment for Orthodontics?
☐ No (Skip 40-41) ☐ Yes (Compete 40-41)

40. Date Appliance Placed (MM/DD/CCYY)

41. Months of Treatment Remaining

42. Replacement of Prosthesis? ☐ No ☐ Yes (Complete 43)

43. Date Prior Placement (MM/DD/CCYY)

44. Treatment Resulting from
☐ Occupational illness/injury ☐ Auto accident ☐ Other accident

45. Date of Accident (MM/DD/CCYY)

46. Auto Accident State

BILLING DENTIST OR DENTAL ENTITY (Leave blank if dentist or dental entity is not submitting claim on behalf of the patient or insured/subscriber)

47. Name, Address, City, State, Zip Code

48. NPI	49. License Number	50. SSN or TIN
51. Phone Number ( ) -	51A. Additional Provider ID	

TREATING DENTIST AND TREATMENT LOCATION INFORMATION

52. I hereby certify that the procedures as indicated by date are in progress (for procedures that require multiple visits) or have been completed.

X _____
Signed (Treating Dentist)   Date

53. NPI	54. License Number
55. Address, City, State, Zip Code	56. Provider Specialty Code
57. Phone Number ( ) -	58. Additional Provider ID

To reorder call Grossman Marketing Group at 1-800-368-1368

12. When completing the claim form, what reference do you need to consult to determine the current dental procedure numbers and names so that you can complete the Record of Services Provided? If the office does not have a copy, where can you purchase this information?

MEDICAL TERMINOLOGY REVIEW

Use a dictionary and/or your textbook to define the following terms.

allowable charges _____

benefit _____

copay _____

deductible _____

exclusive provider organization _____

explanation of benefits _____

individual deductible _____

managed care _____

national provider identifier _____

preferred provider organization _____

upcoding _____

waiting period _____

ABBREVIATIONS

ADA _____

CDT _____

CHAMPUS _____

COBRA _____

DMO _____

DR _____

EOB _____

EPO _____

FMX _____

HHS _____

HIPAA _____

HMO _____

LEAT _____

NPI _____

PPO _____

CRITICAL THINKING

1. What is the difference between a managed care dental insurance plan and a PPO? How can knowing this help a dental assistant provide assistance to patients?

2. Why is it important to determine that the patient is eligible for receiving benefits under an insurance plan before providing treatment?

3. What is the difference between having a primary and secondary insurance carrier? Why does the business manger and the dental assistant need to know about these types of coverage?

CHAPTER REVIEW TEST

MULTIPLE CHOICE

Circle the letter of the correct answer.

1. All of the following are purposes of dental insurance plans EXCEPT:
   a. encourage patients to seek preventive care
   b. provide reimbursement to the insured for the cost of dental care
   c. reduce dental patient fears
   d. control health insurance costs

2. The dental insurance subscriber is:
   a. the employer who offers the benefit
   b. the individual who holds the insurance policy
   c. any person covered under the plan
   d. any person who is currently eligible for benefits

3. The amount of money the patient must pay before the insurance plan will start to pay is the:
   a. deductible
   b. maximum allowable charge
   c. eligibility period
   d. copay

4. Dentists who choose to become a member of a PPO agree to accept:
   a. the PPO payment as payment in full
   b. all patients sent by the insurance company
   c. discounted fees
   d. payment on the basis of number of patients served

5. If a subscriber is laid off from, loses, or leaves his/her job, he/she is eligible to continue coverage under the provisions set forth by:
   a. DMO
   b. HMO
   c. PPO
   d. COBRA

6. The dental assistant must verify _____ that patients with Medicaid dental insurance remain eligible for benefits.
   a. at each appointment
   b. monthly
   c. quarterly
   d. semiannually

7. If LEAT is a provision of the patient's insurance plan, the plan may:
   a. agree to pay for a less expensive alternative than the preferred procedure
   b. refuse to pay for a procedure that is actually present on its schedule of allowances
   c. propose a schedule of maximum allowable charges
   d. all of the above

8. The primary carrier for a subscriber with dual coverage is the plan held by the:
   a. spouse with the earlier birthday
   b. larger employer
   c. earliest date of purchase
   d. subscriber

9. Through the coordination of benefits rule, total payments to a subscriber with dual coverage may not exceed:
   a. 100% of charges
   b. 150% of charges
   c. 200% of charges
   d. there is no maximum; 100% of benefits may be collected from both carriers

10. Who is ultimately responsible for any fees not covered by the insurance company?
    a. dentist
    b. primary carrier
    c. secondary carrier
    d. patient/subscriber

TRUE/FALSE

Indicate whether the statement is true (T) or false (F).

_____ 1. It is the dentist and staff members' responsibility to explain to the patient why treatment is in his/her best interest regardless of any limitations of his/her insurance plan.

_____ 2. Dental procedure codes are based on the category of service being performed.

_____ 3. Dental procedure codes may be used from a CDT book published for any of the past three years.

_____ 4. Electronic claims are submitted to the appropriate insurance carrier, which then forwards them to a clearinghouse for verification before they can be paid.

_____ 5. An electronic claim form may be rejected if the number of procedures reported exceeds the number of lines on the form.

_____ 6. A claim is filed with the primary and secondary carriers at the same time, so their respective staffs can calculate the relative amounts each carrier will pay.

_____ 7. The provider specialty code indicates the procedure for which reimbursement is being claimed.

_____ 8. A clean claim is one that has been processed and paid, and for which all follow-up paper work has been completed.

_____ 9. The patient's signature is kept on file so this can be noted when a claim is submitted electronically.

_____ 10. HIPAA requires any dentist who submits health information in an electronic form to use a standard format and ADA procedure codes.

FILL IN THE BLANK

Using words from the list below, fill in the blanks to complete the following statements.

17	dependents	predetermination
authorized	employer	tax identification number
D0100-D0999	individual	upcoding
D4000-D4999		

1. Claim status tracking may reveal the claim has received _____, has been paid, or needs revision and resubmission.

2. _____ billing for services not provided, and performing unsuitable or unnecessary services, are examples of dental insurance fraud.

3. Dental offices have _____ policies and procedures for handling insurance claims in the office.

4. A common provision of insurance plans is to cover the subscriber's _____ only up to a certain age.

5. Preventive services such as cleaning, fluoride treatments, sealants, and nutrition or tobacco counseling are indicated using ADA procedure codes in the _____ range.

6. Periodontics services, such as surgical and nonsurgical services, are indicated using ADA procedure codes in the _____ range.

7. The group number of an insurance plan identifies the _____.

8. Using the universal tooth numbering system, a mandibular left third molar to be removed would be designated as tooth # _____.

9. When the patient gives permission for disclosure of protected health information to an insurance carrier, the patient has _____ the disclosure.

10. When a claim form requests the dentist's TIN, it is asking for his/her _____.

CHAPTER 56

Marketing Your Skills

CHAPTER OUTLINE

Review the Chapter Outline. If any content area is unclear, review that area before beginning the workbook exercises.

A. Professional Career Goal Opportunities
   1. Career Opportunities
B. Locating Employment Opportunities
C. The Résumé and Cover Letter
   1. The Résumé
   2. The Cover Letter
D. The Interview and Follow-up
E. Employment Negotiations
   1. Salary and Benefits
   2. Letter of Agreement or Employee Contract
F. Rights as an Employee
   1. Americans with Disabilities Act
   2. Family and Medical Leave Act
G. Advancing One's Career
   1. The Importance of Attitude and Healthy Living

CHAPTER REVIEW

The following is a summary of the chapter. If any of this material is unclear, review it in the textbook again.

The big day is here; you are finishing your training program and are ready to seek a position where you can use your many new skills. How do you go about it? First, clarify your goals. Do you want to work in a private office; public health facility; hospital dental clinic; dental or dental assisting school; as a salesperson, consultant, or insurance reviewer; in research; or in forensics? Use multiple sources of information to locate available jobs: classified advertisements in the newspaper, school placement offices, Internet sources, employment/temporary agencies, professional organization contacts, and networking. Create a résumé and cover letter that showcase your skills. Prepare well for your employment interviews, dress professionally, and follow up in a professional manner. Negotiate a suitable contract and once hired, continue to improve and expand your skills.

LEARNING ACTIVITIES AND STUDY AIDS

Review the following study aids and/or complete the activities to ensure that you have achieved the learning objectives for this chapter.

1. Identify nine different areas of dental assisting employment.

2. Suggest six different means of learning about available dental assisting positions.

3. On a separate piece of paper, create your résumé . Type and proofread it prior to submitting to your instructor for a grade. Ensure that all required information is provided.

4. Discuss how to be prepared for a job interview. Write out a list of fifteen questions that you might ask a perspective employer.

5. On a separate piece of paper, create a cover letter to go with your résumé. Prior to submitting to your instructor, be sure and proof read your work to ensure accuracy in format and grammar.

6. Describe the provisions of the Americans with Disabilities Act.

7. Explain the provisions of the Family and Medical Leave Act.

8. Define salary, and list the types of benefits that may be included in the salary package of a particular organization.

9. Discuss how a dental assistant may improve and expand his/her job skills.

10. On a separate piece of paper, write a thank-you letter that you might send after an interview. Check for accuracy prior to submitting to your instructor for a grade.

MEDICAL TERMINOLOGY REVIEW

Use a dictionary and/or your textbook to define the following terms.

Americans with Disabilities Act _____

cover letter _____

demeanor _____

Family and Medical Leave Act _____

Federal Equal Opportunity and Employment Act _____

forensic _____

résumé _____

solo practice _____

ABBREVIATIONS

ADA _____

ADAA _____

CDA _____

CEU _____

CPR _____

DANB _____

FMLA _____

OSAP _____

OSHA _____

PTO _____

CRITICAL THINKING

1. Why is it important to evaluate one's goals before searching for a career in dental assisting?

2. What are some questions that you can ask yourself before looking for a job to help evaluate your career goals?

3. What types of opportunities are available for employment as a dental assistant? Provide reasons for why you would or would not want to work in each one of these settings.

4. What are some resources that a dental assistant might use to find a job? Why would the settings selected vary depending on the individual?

5. What makes a résumé effective?

CHAPTER REVIEW TEST

MULTIPLE CHOICE

Circle the letter of the correct answer.

1. When goals are defined, they should be:
   a. measurable
   b. specific
   c. based on the dental assistant's aims
   d. a and c
   e. all of the above

2. The number of dental assisting jobs is expected to _____ through the year 2012.
   a. increase
   b. decrease
   c. remain static
   d. a prediction cannot be made at this time

3. The section of the newspaper in which employers advertise available dental assisting jobs is the _____ section.
   a. lifestyle
   b. economic
   c. classified
   d. health

4. A written résumé should be on _____ paper and have absolutely correct spelling, grammar, punctuation, and capitalization.
   a. gently striped
   b. white or light gray
   c. eye-catching color
   d. yellow or light green

5. Select the e-mail address that would be appropriate to include on a résumé.
   a. ashleysexkitten@hotmail.com
   b. callmebaby@msn.com
   c. tangolady@earthlink.net
   d. mncosta@cox.net

6. When preparing a résumé, educational institutions attended and positions held should be listed:
   a. most recent first
   b. earliest date first
   c. only if they are relevant to the position sought
   d. with explanation for any gap periods

7. It is ideal if a résumé can be:
   a. at least five pages in length
   b. at least three pages long
   c. no more than two pages long
   d. kept to one page

8. The TWO items that make an initial statement about the dental assistant to a potential employer prior to the interview are the:
   a. recommendation letters
   b. résumé
   c. cover letter
   d. assistant's manner of dress

9. A dental assistant should research the organization to which he/she is applying for a job because:
   a. employers are impressed when an applicant knows about their company
   b. it is important to know the salary, benefits, and hours of the position before seeking it
   c. the assistant can determine if the company's philosophy fits her own
   d. a and c
   e. all of the above

0. The best approach to take if asked about your weaknesses during a job interview is to:
   a. turn your weakness into an advantage
   b. indicate that you have never been told you have any
   c. humorously turn the inquiry away
   d. any of the above

TRUE/FALSE

Indicate whether the statement is true (T) or false (F).

_____ 1. Personal questions are illegal in the interview process.

_____ 2. A job applicant should never discuss salary and benefits on the initial job interview.

_____ 3. It is acceptable to wear scrubs to an interview unless the position being sought is front desk assistant.

_____ 4. Once a job interview is complete, the interviewee should thank the interviewer for his/her time and shake his/her hand.

_____ 5. A handwritten thank-you note should be mailed to the interviewer approximately one week after the interview took place.

_____ 6. It is acceptable to chew gum during an interview, provided the chewing is discreet.

_____ 7. Cell phones should be turned off during an interview.

_____ 8. Salary includes the hourly wage plus benefits of a position.

_____ 9. The Fair Labor Standards Act requires that employees be paid sick time.

_____ 10. Probation, also termed provisional employment, is usually for a period of 90 days.

FILL IN THE BLANK

Using words from the list below, fill in the blanks to complete the following statements.

twelve	clinical	one
fifteen	compassionate	taxes
fifty	dentalworkers.com	word of mouth
business	disability	

1. The Federal Equal Opportunity and Employment Act prohibits discrimination on the basis of race, color, religion, sex, national origin, age, marital status, political affiliation, or _____.

2. The Americans with Disabilities Act applies to workplaces with _____ or more employees.

3. The Family and Medical Leave Act applies to workplaces with _____ or more employees.

4. National DANB certification in dental assisting requires the certificant to complete _____ CEUs of education annually.

5. Membership in the American Dental Assistants Association Fellowship program is awarded to dental assistants who complete documented additional education in _____ or _____ dental assisting.

6. A solo dental practice has _____ dental practitioner(s).

7. The Web site _____ is extremely helpful to dental assistants seeking to learn about available jobs.

8. A dental assistant should be prompt, motivated, enthusiastic, and _____.

9. Public health dental facilities are ordinarily funded through _____.

10. Networking is meeting people and gaining job information through _____.

Procedure 12-1

Disinfecting a Treatment Room

Objective: Demonstrate how to properly disinfect a treatment room.

Equipment and Supplies Needed: PPE (utility gloves, eyewear, mask), intermediate-level disinfectant, and paper towels or 4 × 4 gauze.

Notes to the Student:

Skills Assessment Requirements

Read and familiarize yourself with the procedure; complete the minimum practice requirements. Document information when appropriate to demonstrate proper charting techniques. Complete each procedure within a reasonable amount of time, with a minimum of 85% accuracy.

POINT VALUE ◆ = 5 points ∗ = 10 points		PRACTICE TRIAL	GRADED TRIAL # 1	GRADED TRIAL # 2	NOTES:
1. ◆	Put on PPE.				
2. ∗	Prepare disinfectant according to manufacturer's instructions.				
3. ◆	Spray towels with disinfectant and wipe surfaces (precleaning).				
4. ∗	Spray disinfectant on clean paper towel or gauze. Allow disinfectant to contact surface for the recommended amount of time.				
5. ∗	If surface is still wet after contact time, wipe dry with clean towel.				

(continued)

POINT VALUE ♦ = 5 points * = 10 points		PRACTICE TRIAL	GRADED TRIAL # 1	GRADED TRIAL # 2	NOTES:
6. *	When using disinfectant wipes, follow the manu-facturer's instructions, don appropriate PPE and wipe surface, discard towelette, wipe surface with new towelette, allow to dry.				

Document:

Document information for proper charting of this procedure.

Grading

Points earned	_____		
Points possible	_____	50	50
Percent grade (Points earned/Points possible)	_____		
Pass:	_____	❑ YES ❑ NO ❑ N/A	❑ YES ❑ NO ❑ N/A

Instructor Sign-Off

Instructor: _____ Date: _____

Procedure 12-2
Placing and Removing Surface Barriers

Objective: Demonstrate how to properly place and remove surface barriers.

Equipment and Supplies Needed: antimicrobial soap, utility gloves, and plastic surface barriers.

Notes to the Student:

Skills Assessment Requirements

Read and familiarize yourself with the procedure; complete the minimum practice requirements. Document information when appropriate to demonstrate proper charting techniques. Complete each procedure within a reasonable amount of time, with a minimum of 85% accuracy.

POINT VALUE ♦ = 5 points ✳ = 10 points	PRACTICE TRIAL	GRADED TRIAL # 1	GRADED TRIAL # 2	NOTES:
1. ♦ Wash and dry hands using proper hand hygiene techniques.				
2. ♦ Select appropriate surface barriers for clean surface.				
3. ✳ Place barrier securely on dental chair or other surface so it does not fall off. If barrier comes off, then the surface will require disinfecting.				
4. ✳ Wear utility gloves to remove contaminated barriers; discard barrier in contaminated or general waste container.				
5. ✳ Remove, wash, disinfect, and dry utility gloves. Then wash hands.				
6. ✳ Apply fresh surface barriers for the next patient.				

(continued)

Document:

Document information for proper charting of this procedure.

Grading

Points earned	_____		
Points possible	_____	50	50
Percent grade (Points earned/Points possible)	_____		
Pass:	_____	❏ YES ❏ NO ❏ N/A	❏ YES ❏ NO ❏ N/A

Instructor Sign-Off

Instructor: _____ Date: _____

Procedure 12-3

CDC Recommendations for Hand Antisepsis Washing

Objective: Demonstrate how to properly wash hands and apply antisepsis CDC procedures.

Supplies Needed: alcohol-based hand rub, anti-microbial liquid soap, and hand/nail scrub brush, paper towel.

Notes to the Student:

Skills Assessment Requirements

Read and familiarize yourself with the procedure; complete the minimum practice requirements. Document information when appropriate to demonstrate proper charting techniques. Complete each procedure within a reasonable amount of time, with a minimum of 85% accuracy.

	POINT VALUE ◆ = 5 points ✳ = 10 points	PRACTICE TRIAL	GRADED TRIAL # 1	GRADED TRIAL # 2	NOTES:
A.	**Procedure Steps for Alcohol-Based Hand Rubs**				
1. ◆	Apply hand rub in palm of hand.				
2. ◆	Rub hands together.				
3. ✳	Be sure all surfaces of hands and fingers are covered with the rub. Rub until dry on the hands and fingers.				
B.	**Procedure Steps for Hand Hygiene**				
1. ✳	Wet hands first.				
2. ✳	Apply soap to hands.				
3. ✳	Use brush to scrub fingernails on each hand.				
4. ✳	Rub hands together vigorously for 15 seconds.				

(continued)

POINT VALUE ♦ = 5 points ✳ = 10 points		PRACTICE TRIAL	GRADED TRIAL # 1	GRADED TRIAL # 2	NOTES:
5. ✳	Cover all surfaces of hands and fingers with soap, washing from top to bottom of each finger and thumb.				
6. ✳	Rinse hands with cool water.				
7. ✳	Dry hands with clean, disposable paper towel.				
8. ✳	Use paper towel when touching the faucet to turn off the water. Dispose of paper towel in general waste.				

Document:

Document information for proper charting of this procedure.

Grading

Points earned	_____		
Points possible	_____	100	100
Percent grade (Points earned/Points possible)	_____		
Pass:	_____	❑ YES ❑ NO ❑ N/A	❑ YES ❑ NO ❑ N/A

Instructor Sign-Off

Instructor: _____ Date: _____

Procedure 12–4
Infection Control in the Darkroom

Objective: Demonstrate how to maintain proper control in the darkroom.

Supplies Needed: paper towel, gloves, plastic bag or paper cup, and lead foil container.

Notes to the Student:

Skills Assessment Requirements

Read and familiarize yourself with the procedure; complete the minimum practice requirements. Document information when appropriate to demonstrate proper charting techniques. Complete each procedure within a reasonable amount of time, with a minimum of 85% accuracy.

POINT VALUE ◆ = 5 points ✳ = 10 points		PRACTICE TRIAL	GRADED TRIAL # 1	GRADED TRIAL # 2	NOTES:
1. ◆	Place paper towel and cup next to processor in the darkroom.				
2. ◆	Wash hands and put on new gloves.				
3. ✳	Ensure safety light is turned on before touching the contaminated film.				
4. ✳	Open the film packets and allow film to drop on paper towel.				
5. ✳	Allow lead foil to drop in lead foil container.				
6. ◆	Place empty film packets in cup, remove gloves, and discard both.				
7. ◆	Place films in the processor with bare hands, being careful to touch the edges only.				

(continued)

Document:

Document information for proper charting of this procedure.

Grading

Points earned	_____		
Points possible	_____	50	50
Percent grade (Points earned/Points possible)	_____		
Pass:	_____	❏ YES ❏ NO ❏ N/A	❏ YES ❏ NO ❏ N/A

Instructor Sign-Off

Instructor: _____ Date: _____

Procedure 12–5
Infection Control with a Daylight Loader

Objective: Demonstrate how to properly follow infection control guidelines when using a daylight loader.

Supplies Needed: paper towels, two pairs of gloves, disposable cup or plastic bag, and lead foil container.

Notes to the Student:

Skills Assessment Requirements

Read and familiarize yourself with the procedure; complete the minimum practice requirements. Document information when appropriate to demonstrate proper charting techniques. Complete each procedure within a reasonable amount of time, with a minimum of 85% accuracy.

POINT VALUE ◆ = 5 points ✳ = 10 points		PRACTICE TRIAL	GRADED TRIAL # 1	GRADED TRIAL # 2	NOTES:
1. ✳	After exposing film and placing contaminated film in cup, remove gloves and wash and dry hands.				
2. ✳	Place a barrier (paper towel or plastic barrier) inside, on the bottom of the daylight loader.				
3. ✳	Place the cup with contaminated film, a clean pair of gloves, an empty cup, and the lead foil container in the daylight loader.				
4. ✳	Place clean hands into the sleeves of the loader, then put on clean gloves.				
5. ✳✳	Open film packets and drop film into empty cup, drop lead foil in container, and then place contaminated film packets back into contaminated cup.				

(continued)

POINT VALUE ♦ = 5 points ✳ = 10 points		PRACTICE TRIAL	GRADED TRIAL # 1	GRADED TRIAL # 2	NOTES:
6. ✳	After the film packets are opened, remove gloves by turning them inside out.				
7. ✳	Insert film into processor with bare hands.				
8. ✳	When the film has been loaded, remove hands from loader.				
9. ✳	Don clean gloves, open top of the loader, and remove and discard contaminated items.				

Document:

Document information for proper charting of this procedure.

Grading

Points earned	_____		
Points possible	_____	100	100
Percent grade (Points earned/Points possible)	_____		
Pass:	_____	❏ YES ❏ NO ❏ N/A	❏ YES ❏ NO ❏ N/A

Instructor Sign-Off

Instructor: _____ Date: _____

Procedure 15-1
Applying a Topical Fluoride

Objective: Demonstrate how to administer a topical fluoride treatment.

Equipment and Supplies Needed: basic setup: mirror, explorer, cotton pliers, saliva ejector, high-volume evacuator tip (HVE), air/water syringe tip, 2 × 2 gauze squares, topical fluoride solution, proper size fluoride trays, and watch with a second hand.

Notes to the Student:

Skills Assessment Requirements

Read and familiarize yourself with the procedure; complete the minimum practice requirements. Document information when appropriate to demonstrate proper charting techniques. Complete each procedure within a reasonable amount of time, with a minimum of 85% accuracy.

POINT VALUE ◆ = 5 points ✱ = 10 points		PRACTICE TRIAL	GRADED TRIAL # 1	GRADED TRIAL # 2	NOTES:
1. ✱	Seat the patient upright in the dental chair and adjust the headrest. Place the patient napkin around the neck. Explain the procedure to the patient and instruct the patient to not swallow the fluoride.				
2. ✱	Ensure the disposable fluoride trays will cover all teeth but not extend too far distal.				
3. ✱	Fill both trays about one-third full with topical fluoride. Show the patient how to use the saliva ejector.				
4. ✱	Dry the teeth with 2 × 2 gauze squares or by blowing air with the air/water syringe.				
5. ✱	Insert the loaded fluoride trays carefully. Place one on the lower arch and the other on the upper arch. Move the trays around to disperse the fluoride.				

(continued)

POINT VALUE ♦ = 5 points * = 10 points		PRACTICE TRIAL	GRADED TRIAL # 1	GRADED TRIAL # 2	NOTES:
6. *	Place the saliva ejector between the arches and have the patient gently close.				
7. *	Look at the second hand on your watch to ensure the fluoride treatment is in place for the entire specified time. Most fluoride treatments require one full minute.				
8. *	Remove the trays and quickly use the HVE to completely remove all fluoride from the teeth. Tell the patient not to swallow.				
9. *	When dismissing the patient, tell her that she may spit into the sink, but instruct her not to rinse or drink anything for at least 30 minutes to allow the fluoride to work.				
10. *	Be sure to enter the fluoride treatment procedure and patient instructions in the patient's dental record.				

Document:

Document information for proper charting of this procedure.

Grading

Points earned	_____		
Points possible	_____	100	100
Percent grade (Points earned/Points possible)	_____		
Pass:	_____	❑ YES ❑ NO ❑ N/A	❑ YES ❑ NO ❑ N/A

Instructor Sign-Off

Instructor: _____ Date: _____

Procedure 17-1
Processing Contaminated Instruments

Objective: Demonstrate how to properly process contaminated instruments.

Equipment and Supplies Needed: PPE (utility gloves, mask, protective eyewear and clothing), contaminated instruments, holding solution, ultrasonic cleaner, instrument sterilization wrap, and sterilizer.

Notes to the Student:

Skills Assessment Requirements

Read and familiarize yourself with the procedure; complete the minimum practice requirements. Document information when appropriate to demonstrate proper charting techniques. Complete each procedure within a reasonable amount of time, with a minimum of 85% accuracy.

POINT VALUE ♦ = 5 points ✳ = 10 points		PRACTICE TRIAL	GRADED TRIAL #1	GRADED TRIAL #2	NOTES:
1. ✳	After patient dismissal, discard all contaminated disposables in dental operatory.				
2. ✳	Wearing PPE, including utility gloves, transport instruments to processing area. Use container to transport loose instruments.				
3. ✳	Submerge instruments in a holding/precleaning solution. (This step can be skipped if the assistant has time to place the instruments in the ultrasonic cleaner immediately.)				
4. ✳	After disinfecting dental treatment room, return to processing area and rinse holding solution off of instruments.				

(continued)

POINT VALUE ♦ = 5 points ✳ = 10 points		PRACTICE TRIAL	GRADED TRIAL # 1	GRADED TRIAL # 2	NOTES:
5. ✳	Place instruments in ultrasonic cleaner. Do not hand scrub instruments. (Instrument cassettes can also be placed in a washer/disinfector.)				
6. ✳	Determine which instruments will be heat processed and which will be processed in the chemical liquid sterilant.				
7. ✳	Dry and lubricate handpieces and hinged instruments to prevent corrosion.				
8. ✳	Wrap and prepare instruments according to the type of sterilization process used.				
9. ✳	Load into sterilizer.				
10. ✳	Store sterile instrument packages in a storage place away from contaminated instruments.				

Document:

Document information for proper charting of this procedure.

Grading

Points earned	_____		
Points possible	_____	100	100
Percent grade (Points earned/Points possible)	_____		
Pass:	_____	❏ YES ❏ NO ❏ N/A	❏ YES ❏ NO ❏ N/A

Instructor Sign-Off

Instructor: _____ Date: _____

Procedure 17-2
Operating the Ultrasonic Cleaner

Objective: Demonstrate how to properly operate the ultrasonic cleaner.

Equipment and Supplies Needed: PPE (utility gloves, mask, protective eyewear and clothing), ultrasonic cleaner, ultrasonic solution.

Notes to the Student:

Skills Assessment Requirements

Read and familiarize yourself with the procedure; complete the minimum practice requirements. Document information when appropriate to demonstrate proper charting techniques. Complete each procedure within a reasonable amount of time, with a minimum of 85% accuracy.

POINT VALUE ♦ = 5 points ✳ = 10 points		PRACTICE TRIAL	GRADED TRIAL # 1	GRADED TRIAL # 2	NOTES:
1. ♦	Don PPE, including utility gloves, mask, and protective eyewear and clothing.				
2. ✳	Remove instruments from holding solution. Remove lid from ultrasonic cleaner.				
3. ♦	Ensure cleaner is filled with water and the appropriate ultrasonic solution. (Check manufacturer's instructions.)				
4. ✳✳	Place loose instruments or instrument cassettes in ultrasonic basket; gently submerge into cleaner, carefully avoiding excess splash.				
5. ✳✳	Replace lid and turn on cycle to desired time (typically between 6 and 12 minutes).				

(*continued*)

POINT VALUE ♦ = 5 points ✳ = 10 points		PRACTICE TRIAL	GRADED TRIAL # 1	GRADED TRIAL # 2	NOTES:
6. ✳✳	When the cleaning cycle is complete, remove basket and rinse with tap water.				
7. ✳✳	Tip basket onto a clean towel, remove instruments, and replace basket and lid on ultrasonic cleaner.				

Document:

Document information for proper charting of this procedure.

Grading

Points earned	_____		
Points possible	_____	100	100
Percent grade (Points earned/Points possible)	_____		
Pass:	_____	❏ YES ❏ NO ❏ N/A	❏ YES ❏ NO ❏ N/A

Instructor Sign-Off

Instructor: _____ Date: _____

Procedure 17-3
Testing the Ultrasonic Cleaner

Objective: Demonstrate how to properly test the ultrasonic cleaner.

Equipment and Supplies Needed: ultrasonic cleaner, fresh ultrasonic solution, and foil.

Notes to the Student:

Skills Assessment Requirements

Read and familiarize yourself with the procedure; complete the minimum practice requirements. Document information when appropriate to demonstrate proper charting techniques. Complete each procedure within a reasonable amount of time, with a minimum of 85% accuracy.

POINT VALUE ◆ = 5 points ✳ = 10 points		PRACTICE TRIAL	GRADED TRIAL # 1	GRADED TRIAL # 2	NOTES:
1. ✳	Use regular household aluminum foil; cut a piece to fit the width of the cleaner.				
2. ✳	Prepare fresh cleaner solution and fill the ultrasonic tank according to manufacturer's directions.				
3. ✳	Insert the foil vertically into the ultrasonic tank.				
4. ✳✳	Hold the foil steady. Turn the machine on for 20 to 30 seconds.				

Document:

Document information for proper charting of this procedure.

(continued)

Grading

Points earned	_____		
Points possible	_____	50	50
Percent grade (Points earned/Points possible)	_____		
Pass:	_____	❑ YES ❑ NO ❑ N/A	❑ YES ❑ NO ❑ N/A

Instructor Sign-Off

Instructor: _____ Date: _____

Procedure 17-4
Performing Biological Monitoring

Objective: Demonstrate how to properly perform biologic monitoring.

Equipment and Supplies Needed: PPE (exam gloves, mask, protective eyewear and clothing), biological indicator (spore test), sterilizer bag/wrap, autoclave, and sterilization monitoring log.

Notes to the Student:

Skills Assessment Requirements

Read and familiarize yourself with the procedure; complete the minimum practice requirements. Document information when appropriate to demonstrate proper charting techniques. Complete each procedure within a reasonable amount of time, with a minimum of 85% accuracy.

POINT VALUE ♦ = 5 points ✳ = 10 points		PRACTICE TRIAL	GRADED TRIAL # 1	GRADED TRIAL # 2	NOTES:
1. ✳	Don appropriate PPE.				
2. ✳	Put the biological indicator in a sterilizing bag.				
3. ✳	Place in the center of the instrument load; place instrument packs in the sterilizer.				
4. ✳	Process through a normal cycle.				
5. ✳	Remove PPE; wash and dry hands.				
6. ✳✳	Record date of test, type of sterilizer, temperature, time, and the name of the person doing the test.				

(continued)

POINT VALUE ♦ = 5 points ✳ = 10 points		PRACTICE TRIAL	GRADED TRIAL # 1	GRADED TRIAL # 2	NOTES:
7. ✳	When cycle is complete, remove processed biological indicator.				
8. ✳	Mail processed indicator and control to the monitoring service.				
9. ✳	Document results on log when received.				

Document:

Document information for proper charting of this procedure.

Grading

Points earned	_____		
Points possible	_____		
Percent grade (Points earned/Points possible)	_____	100	100
Pass:	_____	❏ YES ❏ NO ❏ N/A	❏ YES ❏ NO ❏ N/A

Instructor Sign-Off

Instructor: _____ Date: _____

Procedure 17-5
Operating the Autoclave

Objective: Demonstrate how to properly operate the autoclave.

Equipment and Supplies Needed: PPE (gloves, utility gloves, mask, protective eyewear and clothing), autoclave, contaminated instruments, instrument lubricant, instrument packaging, distilled water, and internal indicators.

Notes to the Student:

Skills Assessment Requirements

Read and familiarize yourself with the procedure; complete the minimum practice requirements. Document information when appropriate to demonstrate proper charting techniques. Complete each procedure within a reasonable amount of time, with a minimum of 85% accuracy.

POINT VALUE ♦ = 5 points * = 10 points		PRACTICE TRIAL	GRADED TRIAL # 1	GRADED TRIAL # 2	NOTES:
1. ♦	Don appropriate PPE (mask, eye protection, and utility gloves).				
2. ♦	Lubricate instruments as needed.				
3. *	Insert internal indicator in each package; seal package and label.				
4. ♦	Remove contaminated utility gloves. Don clean exam gloves to touch the sterilizer controls.				
5. ♦	Use distilled water to fill the chamber or tank up to "fill line." (Check manufacturer's instructions).				

(continued)

POINT VALUE ♦ = 5 points ✳ = 10 points		PRACTICE TRIAL	GRADED TRIAL # 1	GRADED TRIAL # 2	NOTES:
6. ✳	Check pressure gauge to ensure it is at zero. Never open door if pressure gauge is not at zero.				
7. ✳	Load autoclave with larger packages on the bottom. Don't overfill; ensure there is space between the packages so the steam can circulate.				
8. ✳	Turn control valve to "fill." The chamber will fill with water.				
9. ♦	Close and secure door.				
10. ✳	Turn control valve to "Steam/ Sterilize."				
11. ✳	Pressure and temperature must be reached prior to setting the timer. (Remove PPE.)				
12. ♦	After the cycle, vent the steam.				
13. ♦	Allow instruments to dry and cool before removing from chamber.				
14. ♦	Store cooled sterilized instruments.				

Document:

Document information for proper charting of this procedure.

Grading

Points earned	_____		
Points possible	_____	100	100
Percent grade (Points earned/Points possible)	_____		
Pass:	_____	❑ YES ❑ NO ❑ N/A	❑ YES ❑ NO ❑ N/A

Instructor Sign-Off

Instructor: _____ Date: _____

Procedure 17-6

Operating the Chemical Vapor Sterilizer

Objective: Demonstrate how to properly operate the chemical vapor sterilizer.

Equipment and Supplies Needed: PPE (gloves, utility gloves, mask, protective eyewear and clothing), contaminated instruments, internal indicators, sterilization bag/wrap, chemical sterilizer, and chemical.

Notes to the Student:

Skills Assessment Requirements

Read and familiarize yourself with the procedure; complete the minimum practice requirements. Document information when appropriate to demonstrate proper charting techniques. Complete each procedure within a reasonable amount of time, with a minimum of 85% accuracy.

POINT VALUE ♦ = 5 points ✳ = 10 points		PRACTICE TRIAL	GRADED TRIAL # 1	GRADED TRIAL # 2	NOTES:
1. ✳	Don appropriate PPE (mask, eye protection, and utility gloves).				
2. ✳	Ensure instruments are free of debris and dry prior to packaging them.				
3. ✳	Insert process indicator in package.				
4. ✳	Remove contaminated utility gloves. Don clean exam gloves to touch sterilizer controls.				
5. ✳	Ensure chemical is placed in the sterilizer. (Check manufacturer's instructions).				
6. ✳	Load chamber with instrument packs.				

(continued)

POINT VALUE ♦ = 5 points ✳ = 10 points		PRACTICE TRIAL	GRADED TRIAL # 1	GRADED TRIAL # 2	NOTES:
7. ✳	Set appropriate time, temperature, and pressure. (Remove PPE.)				
8. ✳	Vent sterilizer.				
9. ✳	Remove instruments when cool.				
10. ✳	Store cooled sterilized instruments.				

Document:

Document information for proper charting of this procedure.

Grading

Points earned	_____		
Points possible	_____		
Percent grade (Points earned/Points possible)	_____	100	100
Pass:	_____	❑ YES ❑ NO ❑ N/A	❑ YES ❑ NO ❑ N/A

Instructor Sign-Off

Instructor: _____ Date: _____

Procedure 17-7
Sterilizing Handpieces

Objective: Demonstrate how to properly sterilize handpieces.

Equipment and Supplies Needed: PPE (gloves, utility gloves, mask, protective eyewear and clothing), moist gauze, handpiece lubricant, dental unit, sterilization bag, internal indicator, and autoclave.

Notes to the Student:

Skills Assessment Requirements

Read and familiarize yourself with the procedure; complete the minimum practice requirements. Document information when appropriate to demonstrate proper charting techniques. Complete each procedure within a reasonable amount of time, with a minimum of 85% accuracy.

POINT VALUE ♦ = 5 points ✳ = 10 points	PRACTICE TRIAL	GRADED TRIAL # 1	GRADED TRIAL # 2	NOTES:
1. ✳ ✳ Keep the handpiece attached with bur after treatment. Don appropriate PPE (mask, eye protection, and utility gloves) and run for 20 to 30 seconds to flush air/water lines.				
2. ✳ Wipe off debris with moist gauze.				
3. ✳ Clean/lubricate internal parts of handpiece. (Use manufacturer's instructions for lubrication.)				
4. ✳ ✳ Reattach handpiece to unit; run lubricant through.				
5. ✳ ✳ Insert handpiece and internal indicator in sterilizing bag. Remove contaminated utility gloves and don clean exam gloves before touching the sterilizer controls.				

(continued)

POINT VALUE ♦ = 5 points ✳ = 10 points		PRACTICE TRIAL	GRADED TRIAL #1	GRADED TRIAL #2	NOTES:
6. ✳	Place in autoclave or Chemiclave for the required time, temperature, and pressure.				
7. ✳	Prior to using, ensure the handpiece is cool. Open the end of the bag and lubricate if recommended by manufacturer. The handpiece is now ready to use on the next patient.				

Document:

Document information for proper charting of this procedure.

Grading

Points earned	_____		
Points possible			
Percent grade (Points earned/Points possible)	_____	100	100
Pass:	_____	❑ YES ❑ NO ❑ N/A	❑ YES ❑ NO ❑ N/A

Instructor Sign-Off

Instructor: _____ Date: _____

Procedure 20-1
Opening the Dental Office

Objective: Demonstrate how to open the dental office.

Notes to the Student:

Skills Assessment Requirements

Read and familiarize yourself with the procedure; complete the minimum practice requirements. Document information when appropriate to demonstrate proper charting techniques. Complete each procedure within a reasonable amount of time, with a minimum of 85% accuracy.

POINT VALUE ♦ = 5 points ✳ = 10 points		PRACTICE TRIAL	GRADED TRIAL # 1	GRADED TRIAL #2	NOTES:
1. ♦	Arrive early enough to complete tasks needed to create an on-time and smooth flow for the daily patient schedule.				
2. ♦	Turn on all master switches to lights, radiology and dental units, clinical computers, central air compressors, vacuum system, and regulator for nitrous oxide sedation system.				
3. ✳	Flush water through waterlines for a minimum of two to four minutes.				
4. ✳	Open valves on the nitrous oxide and oxygen tanks.				
5. ✳	Turn on the x-ray film processor. Change water and replenish tanks to appropriate levels with processing solutions, as necessary.				

(continued)

POINT VALUE ♦ = 5 points ✳ = 10 points		PRACTICE TRIAL	GRADED TRIAL # 1	GRADED TRIAL # 2	NOTES:
6. ✳	Check the reception room for neatness, organize magazines and books, straighten chairs, turn on lights, and unlock and open patient doors.				
7. ♦	Print and post copies of schedules in designated areas throughout office.				
8. ♦	Check answering machine for messages.				
9. ✳	Review patient schedule and ensure that all patient records and x-ray/laboratory results are available for patients on the day's schedule.				
10. ✳	Dress in appropriate OSHA-required attire for the clinical treatment rooms. Perform a 60-second thorough hand washing.				
11. ♦	Turn on and complete sterilization from prior day. Check sterilizer's fluid levels, complete any overnight and/or cold sterile procedures, and change disinfectant solutions as needed.				
12. ♦	Prepare rooms for daily patients: • Check and restock supplies. • Place barriers. • Fill water reservoir/bottles. • Prepare tray and instruments for first patients.				
13. ♦	Prepare operatory completely before seating patient.				
14. ♦	Greet and seat patient on time for first appointment.				

Document:

Document information for proper charting of this procedure.

Grading

Points earned	_____		
Points possible	_____	100	100
Percent grade (Points earned/Points possible)	_____		
Pass:	_____	❏ YES ❏ NO ❏ N/A	❏ YES ❏ NO ❏ N/A

Instructor Sign-Off

Instructor: _____ Date: _____

Procedure 20-2
Closing the Dental Office

Objective: Demonstrate how to close the dental office.

Notes to the Student:

Skills Assessment Requirements

Read and familiarize yourself with the procedure; complete the minimum practice requirements. Document information when appropriate to demonstrate proper charting techniques. Complete each procedure within a reasonable amount of time, with a minimum of 85% accuracy.

POINT VALUE ◆ = 5 points ＊ = 10 points		PRACTICE TRIAL	GRADED TRIAL # 1	GRADED TRIAL # 2	NOTES:
1. ◆	Wear appropriate personal protective equipment (PPE) for exposure control.				
2. ＊	Complete operatory room cleanup and preparation. This may include: • Performing an extensive cleaning of the dental chair and dental unit • Flushing air/water syringes and handpieces • Running evacuation cleaner through vacuum lines • Cleaning traps and filters • Maintaining water reservoirs/bottle • Wiping down with disinfectants all surfaces in the operatory room.				
3. ＊	Sterilize all instruments and setup trays for the next day. Empty ultrasonic solutions and be sure all overnight or cold sterilization instruments are fully submerged into solutions.				

(continued)

POINT VALUE ♦ = 5 points ✳ = 10 points		PRACTICE TRIAL	GRADED TRIAL # 1	GRADED TRIAL # 2	NOTES:
4. ♦	Empty waste cans and replace fresh plastic liners.				
5. ✳	Make sure all laboratory cases have been sent to the lab and next day cases have been checked in and received from the lab.				
6. ✳	Complete processing, mount and file patient x-rays, turn off water supply to processor, and turn off/shut down according to manufacturer's instructions.				
7. ✳	Wipe down with disinfectant solutions all surfaces and turn off darkroom lights, including safe light.				
8. ✳	Turn off all master switches to equipment in the operatories, each radiology and dental unit, central sterilization, lights, computers, any small equipment that may have been used during the day, and regulator for nitrous oxide sedation system.				
9. ✳	Close valves on the nitrous oxide and oxygen tanks.				
10. ✳	Remove and dispose of PPE in appropriate container prior to leaving treatment area according to OSHA requirements.				
11. ✳	Straighten reception area, lock patient doors, turn off any machinery and clean staff lounge, back up computers, turn off business equipment and computers, turn on answering machine, and ensure all charts have been pulled for the next day.				

Document:

Document information for proper charting of this procedure.

Grading

Points earned	_____		
Points possible	_____	100	100
Percent grade (Points earned/Points possible)	_____		
Pass:	_____	❑ YES ❑ NO ❑ N/A	❑ YES ❑ NO ❑ N/A

Instructor Sign-Off

Instructor: _____ Date: _____

Procedure 21-1
Preparing the Patient for the Extraoral and Intraoral Dental Examinations

Objective: Demonstrate how to properly set up and prepare for performing the extraoral and intraoral examinations.

Equipment and Supplies Needed: basic setup (mirror, explorer, cotton pliers), periodontal probe, articulating paper and holder, 2 × 2 gauze squares, patient record, black ink pen, dental chart, and red/blue pencil or a computer that is ready to receive input.

Notes to the Student:

Skills Assessment Requirements

Read and familiarize yourself with the procedure; complete the minimum practice requirements. Document information when appropriate to demonstrate proper charting techniques. Complete each procedure within a reasonable amount of time, with a minimum of 85% accuracy.

POINT VALUE ♦ = 5 points ✳ = 10 points		PRACTICE TRIAL	GRADED TRIAL # 1	GRADED TRIAL # 2	NOTES:
1. ✳✳	While escorting the patient to the treatment room, observe his general appearance, gait, speech, and eyes for anything unusual.				
2. ✳✳	Seat the patient comfortably in the dental chair; adjust the headrest and light. Place the patient napkin around the patient's neck. Ensure the patient has eye protection.				
3. ✳✳	Explain to the patient that the dentist is going to perform a complete dental exam, which includes gently feeling the face and neck with the hands and fingers and then performing an examination of the mouth.				

(*continued*)

POINT VALUE ♦ = 5 points ✳ = 10 points		PRACTICE TRIAL	GRADED TRIAL # 1	GRADED TRIAL # 2	NOTES:
4. ✳ ✳	Organize the dental record and chart on a flat surface, or set up the computer and prepare to document the examination as the dentist dictates his or her findings.				
5. ✳ ✳	Tell the dentist that the patient is ready and prepare to record the findings of the exam.				

Document:

Document information for proper charting of this procedure.

Grading

Points earned	_____		
Points possible			
	_____		
Percent grade (Points earned/Points possible)	_____	100	100
Pass:	_____	❏ YES ❏ NO ❏ N/A	❏ YES ❏ NO ❏ N/A

Instructor Sign-Off

Instructor:_____ Date: _____

Procedure 23-1
Taking Temperature Orally

Objective: Demonstrate how to properly take an oral temperature.

Equipment and Supplies Needed: digital thermometer, probe covers, waste container, pen and chart.

Notes to the Student:

Skills Assessment Requirements

Read and familiarize yourself with the procedure; complete the minimum practice requirements. Document information when appropriate to demonstrate proper charting techniques. Complete each procedure within a reasonable amount of time, with a minimum of 85% accuracy.

POINT VALUE ♦ = 5 points * = 10 points		PRACTICE TRIAL	GRADED TRIAL # 1	GRADED TRIAL # 2	NOTES:
1. ♦	Wash your hands.				
2. *	Seat the patient and explain what you are about to do.				
3. ♦	Place the thermometer in the probe cover and throw out the extra paper.				
4. ♦	Turn the thermometer on.				
5. ♦	With the patient seated, have the patient open his mouth and lift his tongue.				
6. *	Place the thermometer under the tongue and have the patient close his mouth gently without biting down.				
7. *	Leave the probe in place until it beeps, signaling the registration of the temperature.				

(continued)

POINT VALUE ◆ = 5 points ✳ = 10 points		PRACTICE TRIAL	GRADED TRIAL #1	GRADED TRIAL #2	NOTES:
8. ✳	Remove the probe from the patient's mouth.				
9. ✳	Read the results from the thermometer.				
10. ✳	Remove the probe cover and throw it in the trash.				
11. ✳	Record the results in the patient's chart.				
12. ◆	Put the thermometer in its proper storage place.				
13. ◆	Wash your hands.				

Document:

Document information for proper charting of this procedure.

Grading

Points earned	_____		
Points possible			
Percent grade (Points earned/Points possible)	_____	100	100
Pass:	_____	❏ YES ❏ NO ❏ N/A	❏ YES ❏ NO ❏ N/A

Instructor Sign-Off

Instructor: _____ Date: _____

Procedure 23-2
Measuring Blood Pressure

Objective: Demonstrate how to properly take blood pressure.

Equipment and Supplies Needed: stethoscope, sphygmomanometer, disinfectant and gauze, pen and chart.

Notes to the Student:

Skills Assessment Requirements

Read and familiarize yourself with the procedure; complete the minimum practice requirements. Document information when appropriate to demonstrate proper charting techniques. Complete each procedure within a reasonable amount of time, with a minimum of 85% accuracy.

POINT VALUE ♦ = 5 points ✳ = 10 points		PRACTICE TRIAL	GRADED TRIAL # 1	GRADED TRIAL # 2	NOTES:
1. ♦	Wash your hands.				
2. ♦	Disinfect the earpieces of the stethoscope. Place both the stethoscope and working sphygmomanometer on the counter in the treatment room.				
3. ♦	Seat the patient upright.				
4. ♦	Explain in general terms what you will be doing.				
5. ♦	Have the patient remove any long-sleeved shirt, sweater, or coat so the bend of the elbow is exposed. Locate the brachial artery (inside the elbow crease closest to the body).				
6. ♦	Center the cuff according to the artery arrow found on the cuff. Position the cuff about one to two inches above the bend of the elbow. Close the inflator valve with the thumbscrew. Do not tighten too hard.				

(continued)

POINT VALUE ♦ = 5 points ✳ = 10 points		PRACTICE TRIAL	GRADED TRIAL # 1	GRADED TRIAL # 2	NOTES:
7. ♦	Find the brachial pulse with your first finger.				
8. ✳	Pump the cuff until you cannot feel the pulse any more, and then pump the cuff another 20 to 30 mm Hg. This number will usually be between 160 and 180 mm Hg for a normal reading.				
9. ♦	Put the stethoscope in your ears, pointing the earpieces forward.				
10. ✳	Place the diaphragm of the stethoscope over the brachial artery and hold it in place with a thumb. Make sure the arm stays positioned at a straight angle.				
11. ✳	Deflate the cuff slowly, at a rate of about 2 to 4 mm Hg per second by opening the thumbscrew slightly.				
12. ♦	Listen. The first sound and its corresponding number represent the measurement of the systolic number.				
13. ♦	Continue deflation of the cuff, listening to the pulse. The last sound marks the number of the diastolic reading. Continue deflating for another 10 millimeters to ensure that the last sound has been heard.				
14. ♦	Open the thumbscrew all the way and let the air out of the bladder rapidly.				
15. ♦	Remove the cuff from the patient's arm.				
16. ♦	Disinfect the earpieces of the stethoscope.				
17. ♦	Wash hands and record the procedure and the measurement on the patient's chart.				

Document:

Document information for proper charting of this procedure.

Grading

Points earned	_____		
Points possible	_____		
Percent grade (Points earned/Points possible)	_____	100	100
Pass:	_____	❑ YES ❑ NO ❑ N/A	❑ YES ❑ NO ❑ N/A

Instructor Sign-Off

Instructor: _____ Date: _____

Procedure 23-3
Taking Pulse and Respirations

Objective: Demonstrate how to properly take pulse and respirations.

Supplies Needed: stopwatch, pen, and chart.

Notes to the Student:

Skills Assessment Requirements

Read and familiarize yourself with the procedure; complete the minimum practice requirements. Document information when appropriate to demonstrate proper charting techniques. Complete each procedure within a reasonable amount of time, with a minimum of 85% accuracy.

POINT VALUE ♦ = 5 points ✳ = 10 points		PRACTICE TRIAL	GRADED TRIAL #1	GRADED TRIAL #2	NOTES:
1. ✳	Wash your hands.				
2. ✳	Seat the patient and explain what you are about to do, but do not mention that you will be counting the respirations. (A patient who knows she is being watched may change her breathing subconsciously.)				
3. ✳	Ask the patient for her wrist.				
4. ✳	Try to lay the wrist on the arm of the chair or a table nearby.				
5. ✳	Locate the radial pulse by running your finger down the thumb to the first bony protrusion on the inner aspect of the wrist. Pull your fingers to the inside until they fall into the first divot. The pulse should be felt there.				

(continued)

POINT VALUE ♦ = 5 points ∗ = 10 points		PRACTICE TRIAL	GRADED TRIAL # 1	GRADED TRIAL # 2	NOTES:
6. ♦	Use the stopwatch to start counting the pulse.				
7. ∗	Count for 30 seconds and remember the number.				
8. ∗	Count the respirations for the next 30 seconds and remember the number.				
9. ∗	Multiply the numbers by two and record the readings in the chart.				
10. ∗	Record any irregularity in pulse and/or breathing.				
11. ♦	Wash your hands.				

Document:

Document information for proper charting of this procedure.

Grading

Points earned	_____		
Points possible	_____		
Percent grade (Points earned/Points possible)	_____	100	100
Pass:	_____	❏ YES ❏ NO ❏ N/A	❏ YES ❏ NO ❏ N/A

Instructor Sign-Off

Instructor: _____ Date: _____

Procedure 26-1
Placing the High-Volume Evacuator Tips

Objective: Demonstrate how to place the high-volume evacuator tips, including maxillary right posterior, maxillary left posterior, mandibular right posterior, mandibular left posterior, maxillary anterior facial, maxillary anterior lingual, mandibular facial, and mandibular anterior lingual tip placements.

Equipment and Supplies Needed: high volume evacuator (HVE), cotton rolls, air/water syringe, basic setup, and dental handpiece.

Notes to the Student:

Skills Assessment Requirements

Read and familiarize yourself with the procedure; complete the minimum practice requirements. Document information when appropriate to demonstrate proper charting techniques. Complete each procedure within a reasonable amount of time, with a minimum of 85% accuracy.

POINT VALUE ♦ = 5 points ∗ = 10 points		PRACTICE TRIAL	GRADED TRIAL # 1	GRADED TRIAL # 2	NOTES:
A.	**Procedure Steps for HVE Maxillary Right Posterior Tip Placement**				
1. ∗	Place the HVE tip in the holder by pushing the end of the tip into the HVE hose.				
2. ∗	Position the tip near the lingual surface, just distal to the tooth being worked on.				
3. ♦	The bevel of the tip should be parallel to the lingual surface of the teeth.				
B.	**Procedure Steps for HVE Maxillary Left Posterior Tip Placement**				
1. ∗	Place the HVE tip in the holder by pushing the end of the tip into the HVE hose.				

(continued)

	POINT VALUE ♦ = 5 points ✳ = 10 points	PRACTICE TRIAL	GRADED TRIAL # 1	GRADED TRIAL # 2	NOTES:
2. ♦	Position the tip of the evacuator parallel to the buccal surface of the teeth.				
3. ♦	To maintain patient comfort, the tip can rest on a cotton roll.				
4. ♦	The tip may need to be utilized to retract the cheek away from the working area.				
C.	**Procedure Steps for HVE Mandibular Right Posterior Tip Placement**				
1. ✳	Place the HVE tip in the holder by pushing the end of the tip into the HVE hose.				
2. ✳	Position the tip across the mandibular left teeth between the lingual surface of the teeth and the tongue.				
3. ✳	The tip should be parallel to the lingual surface of the teeth.				
4. ♦	A cotton roll may be utilized to assist in retracting the tongue away from the operator's field of vision.				
D.	**Procedure Steps for HVE Mandibular Left Posterior Tip Placement**				
1. ✳	Place the HVE tip in the holder by pushing the end of the tip into the HVE hose.				
2. ✳	The tip of the beveled portion of the HVE tip should be positioned parallel to the buccal surface of the teeth.				
3. ✳	The tip may need to be utilized to retract the cheek away from the working area.				
E.	**Procedure Steps for HVE Maxillary Anterior Facial Tip Placement**				
1. ✳	Place the HVE tip in the holder by pushing the end of the tip into the HVE hose.				

POINT VALUE ♦ = 5 points ✳ = 10 points		PRACTICE TRIAL	GRADED TRIAL # 1	GRADED TRIAL #2	NOTES:
2. ✳	Place the tip parallel to the facial of the anterior teeth when the operator is preparing a tooth from the lingual surface of the tooth.				
F.	**Procedure Steps for HVE Maxillary Anterior Lingual Tip Placement**				
1. ✳	Place the HVE tip in the holder by pushing the end of the tip into the HVE hose.				
2. ✳	The evacuator tip is placed on the lingual surface of the anterior teeth when the operator is preparing a tooth from the facial surface of the tooth.				
G.	**Procedure Steps for HVE Mandibular Facial Tip Placement**				
1. ✳	Place the HVE tip in the holder by pushing the end of the tip into the HVE hose.				
2. ✳	The evacuator tip is positioned on a cotton roll near the facial surface of the mandibular teeth when the operator is preparing a tooth from the lingual side of the tooth.				
3. ✳	The beveled portion of the tip should retract the lower lip and should be parallel to the facial surface.				
H.	**Procedure Steps for HVE Mandibular Anterior Lingual Tip Placement**				
1. ✳	Place the HVE tip in the holder by pushing the end of the tip into the HVE hose.				
2. ♦	The evacuator tip is positioned with the bevel parallel to the lingual surface of the teeth when the operator is preparing a tooth from the facial surfaces.				

(continued)

Document:

Enter the appropriate information in the chart below.

Grading

Points earned	_____		
Points possible	_____	200	200
Percent grade (Points earned/Points possible)	_____		
Pass:	_____	❑ YES ❑ NO ❑ N/A	❑ YES ❑ NO ❑ N/A

Instructor Sign-Off

Instructor: _____ Date: _____

Procedure 26-2
Performing a Limited Mouth Rinse

Objective: Demonstrate how to perform a limited mouth rinse.

Equipment Needed: saliva ejector and air/water syringe.

Notes to the Student:

Skills Assessment Requirements

Read and familiarize yourself with the procedure; complete the minimum practice requirements. Document information when appropriate to demonstrate proper charting techniques. Complete each procedure within a reasonable amount of time, with a minimum of 85% accuracy.

POINT VALUE ♦ = 5 points ∗ = 10 points		PRACTICE TRIAL	GRADED TRIAL # 1	GRADED TRIAL # 2	NOTES:
1. ∗ ∗ ♦	The limited mouth rinse is generally performed by one operator utilizing the saliva ejector and the air/water syringe simultaneously.				
2. ∗ ∗ ♦	Turn on the suction and position the tip toward the site for a limited area rinse. The tip of the saliva ejector can be used to retract the cheeks when rinsing on each side of the oral cavity.				
3. ∗ ∗ ♦	Spray the combination of air and water (aerated spray) onto the site to be rinsed. The aerated spray provides enough force to thoroughly clean the area.				
4. ∗ ∗ ♦	Suction all fluid and debris from the area, being sure to remove all fluids.				

(continued)

Document:

Enter the appropriate information in the chart below.

Grading

Points earned	_____		
Points possible	_____	100	100
Percent grade (Points earned/Points possible)	_____		
Pass:	_____	❑ YES ❑ NO ❑ N/A	❑ YES ❑ NO ❑ N/A

Instructor Sign-Off

Instructor: _____ Date: _____

Procedure 26-3
Performing a Complete Mouth Rinse

Objective: Demonstrate how to perform a complete mouth rinse.

Equipment Needed: air/water syringe, and saliva ejector or HVE.

Notes to the Student:

Skills Assessment Requirements

Read and familiarize yourself with the procedure; complete the minimum practice requirements. Document information when appropriate to demonstrate proper charting techniques. Complete each procedure within a reasonable amount of time, with a minimum of 85% accuracy.

POINT VALUE ♦ = 5 points ✳ = 10 points	PRACTICE TRIAL	GRADED TRIAL # 1	GRADED TRIAL # 2	NOTES:
1. ✳✳ When performing a two-person complete mouth rinse procedure, the dentist will operate the air/water syringe and the assistant will operate the HVE. When performing a one-person complete mouth rinse procedure, the operator will hold the air/water syringe in one hand and the saliva ejector in the other.				
2. ✳✳ The operator should have the patient turn his or her head toward the operator to allow for the water to pool on one side making it easier for removal.				
3. ✳✳ Turn on the HVE and position it carefully in the vestibule so that it does not come into contact with any soft tissue.				

(continued)

POINT VALUE ♦ = 5 points ✳ = 10 points		PRACTICE TRIAL	GRADED TRIAL # 1	GRADED TRIAL # 2	NOTES:
4. ✳✳	With the HVE in position, direct the air/water syringe from the patient's maxillary right across to the side closest to the operator, spraying all surfaces.				
5. ✳✳	Continue down to the mandibular arch, following the same sequence. This pattern of rinsing forces the debris to the posterior region of the mouth where the suction tip is positioned for easier removal of fluid and debris.				

Document:

Enter the appropriate information in the chart below.

Grading

Points earned	_____		
Points possible	_____	100	100
Percent grade (Points earned/Points possible)	_____		
Pass:	_____	❑ YES ❑ NO ❑ N/A	❑ YES ❑ NO ❑ N/A

Instructor Sign-Off

Instructor: _____ Date: _____

Procedure 26-4
Placing a Dental Dam

Objective: Demonstrate how to place a dental dam.

Equipment and Supplies Needed: dental dam stamp or template, dental dam material, dental dam frame, clamp with ligature, dental dam punch, dental dam forceps, dental dam lubricant, and dental floss.

Notes to the Student:

Skills Assessment Requirements

Read and familiarize yourself with the procedure; complete the minimum practice requirements. Document information when appropriate to demonstrate proper charting techniques. Complete each procedure within a reasonable amount of time, with a minimum of 85% accuracy.

POINT VALUE ♦ = 5 points ✳ = 10 points		PRACTICE TRIAL	GRADED TRIAL # 1	GRADED TRIAL # 2	NOTES:
1. ♦	Following the administration of the local anesthetic, explain the procedure to the patient.				
2. ♦	Determine which teeth are to be isolated. Examine the patient's oral cavity to determine the anchor tooth, shape of the arch, tooth alignment, missing teeth, and the presence of crowns and bridges.				
3. ✳	Stamp the rubber dam material with the rubber dam stamp or mark the desired position if using the dental dam template.				

(continued)

POINT VALUE ♦ = 5 points ✳ = 10 points		PRACTICE TRIAL	GRADED TRIAL # 1	GRADED TRIAL # 2	NOTES:
4. ✳	Use the dental dam punch to punch the holes in the rubber dam. Punch the holes according to the size of the tooth to be restored with the key punch hole being the largest to accommodate the anchor tooth and the clamp.				
5. ✳	Select the clamp or several clamps to try on the tooth. Clamp design (winged or wingless) and the mesiodistal and faciolingual width of the CEJ should be considered.				
6. ✳	After choosing the appropriate clamp for the desired tooth, place the floss or waxed tape ligature on the bow of the desired dental dam clamp.				
7. ✳	Place the clamp on the beaks of the dental dam forceps and lock the forceps into the open position by spreading the jaws of the forceps open.				
8. ✳	Position the clamp securely on the anchor tooth (one tooth just distal to the tooth being treated). To open the jaws of the clamp, gently squeeze the forceps handle to release the locking bar.				
9. ✳	Fit the lingual jaws of the clamp on the lingual side of the tooth first. Next, spread the clamp open slightly to fit the buccal jaws of the clamp over the height of contour and fit the buccal jaws onto the buccal side of the tooth. Release the pressure on the clamp but do not release the clamp from the forceps.				

POINT VALUE ♦ = 5 points ✳ = 10 points		PRACTICE TRIAL	GRADED TRIAL #1	GRADED TRIAL #2	NOTES:
10. ✳	Check the status of the clamp on the anchor tooth. The jaw points should be placed securely at the CEJ and should not be pinching any gingival tissues. If adjustments are needed, move the wrist to the left and right and by putting more pressure on the distal or mesial of the clamp.				
11. ♦	Apply the rubber dam lubricant to the underside of the dental dam material.				
12. ✳	Place the dental dam over the clamp bow by grasping the dam material and placing the index fingers on each side of the key hole punch. Spread the hole wide enough to slip over the clamp. Stretch the hole over the anchor tooth and one side of the clamp, then expose the other clamp jaw so that the entire clamp and anchor tooth are exposed.				
13. ✳	Pull the dental floss ligature through the dam and drape to the side of the patient's face.				
14. ♦	Place the dental dam napkin around the patient's mouth and underneath the dental dam material.				
15. ♦	Stretch the rubber dam material around the projections of the dental dam frame. The frame can be placed either under or over the dental dam material depending on the choice of frame and operator preference.				
16. ♦	Continue to expose the remaining teeth through each punched hole.				

(continued)

POINT VALUE ♦ = 5 points ✳ = 10 points		PRACTICE TRIAL	GRADED TRIAL #1	GRADED TRIAL #2	NOTES:
17. ♦	Using dental floss, work the dental dam gently between the contacts and below the proximal contacts of each tooth to be isolated.				
18. ♦	Invert or tuck the dam material until all edges of the dam are sealed.				
19. ✳	To increase patient comfort, place a saliva ejector under the frame, dam material, and the patient's tongue.				

Document:

Enter the appropriate information in the chart below.

Grading

Points earned	_____		
Points possible	_____	150	150
Percent grade (Points earned/Points possible)	_____		
Pass:	_____	❏ YES ❏ NO ❏ N/A	❏ YES ❏ NO ❏ N/A

Instructor Sign-Off

Instructor: _____ Date: _____

Procedure 26-5
Removing the Dental Dam

Objective: Demonstrate how to remove a dental dam.

Equipment and Supplies Needed: In addition to the materials already present for the procedure of placing the dental dam (Procedure 26-4), crown and bridge scissors are required for removal.

Notes to the Student:

Skills Assessment Requirements

Read and familiarize yourself with the procedure; complete the minimum practice requirements. Document information when appropriate to demonstrate proper charting techniques. Complete each procedure within a reasonable amount of time, with a minimum of 85% accuracy.

POINT VALUE ♦ = 5 points ✳ = 10 points		PRACTICE TRIAL	GRADED TRIAL # 1	GRADED TRIAL # 2	NOTES:
1. ✳	Explain the procedure to the patient and instruct the patient not to bite down once the dam is removed.				
2. ✳	Stretch the material facially so that you are stretching the material away from the isolated teeth.				
3. ✳ ✳	Working from posterior to anterior, cut each septum (the area of the dam in between each tooth) with the crown and bridge scissors. To protect the patient, slip the index or middle finger underneath the dam material.				

(continued)

POINT VALUE ♦ = 5 points ✳ = 10 points		PRACTICE TRIAL	GRADED TRIAL # 1	GRADED TRIAL # 2	NOTES:
4. ✳ ✳	Using the dental dam forceps, position the beaks in the holes of the clamp, and open the clamp by squeezing the handle to remove the clamp. Usually, the clamp can be lifted straight off the tooth, but if this is not possible, rotate the clamp facially so the jaws clear the lingual and then rotate the clamp lingually to clear the buccal.				
5. ✳	Remove the dam, the frame, and the dental dam napkin from the patient's face.				
6. ✳ ✳	Carefully inspect the material to ensure that all pieces are intact. Lay the dental dam material flat and examine to make certain that all the interseptal material is present. If there are any pieces missing, floss interproximally. This should dislodge any missing segment of the dam material.				
7. ✳	Massage the gingival area around the anchor tooth to increase circulation of the area.				

Document:

Enter the appropriate information in the chart below.

Grading

Points earned	_____		
Points possible	_____	100	100
Percent grade (Points earned/Points possible)	_____		
Pass:	_____	❑ YES ❑ NO ❑ N/A	❑ YES ❑ NO ❑ N/A

Instructor Sign-Off

Instructor: _____ Date: _____

Procedure 26-6
Placing a Quick Dam

Objective: Demonstrate how to place a quick dam.

Equipment and Supplies Needed: quick dam, quick dam template, dental dam punch, dental dam clamps, dental dam forceps, dental floss, and tucking instrument.

Notes to the Student:

Skills Assessment Requirements

Read and familiarize yourself with the procedure; complete the minimum practice requirements. Document information when appropriate to demonstrate proper charting techniques. Complete each procedure within a reasonable amount of time, with a minimum of 85% accuracy.

POINT VALUE ♦ = 5 points ✳ = 10 points		PRACTICE TRIAL	GRADED TRIAL # 1	GRADED TRIAL # 2	NOTES:
1. ♦	Examine the patient's dentition to determine the punch pattern. Make note of any misaligned or missing teeth.				
2. ✳	Use the quick dam template to mark each tooth to be punched and allow for any deviations. Place mark in desired position.				
3. ♦	Punch the marked teeth according to the corresponding hole size for each tooth.				
4. ✳	Without a clamp, fold the ends of the quick dam toward each other and press the sides together.				
5. ✳	Insert the quick dam into the patient's mouth and release the sides. The quick dam fits into the patient's vestibule.				

(continued)

POINT VALUE ♦ = 5 points ✳ = 10 points		PRACTICE TRIAL	GRADED TRIAL # 1	GRADED TRIAL # 2	NOTES:
6. ✳	Slide the dam over the teeth to be isolated. Use dental floss to tuck the dental dam, and secure the dam with floss ligatures on the distal of the last isolated teeth.				
7. ✳	Select a clamp and attach a ligature to the bow of the clamp.				
8. ✳	Secure the clamp in the hole punched for the tooth to be clamped.				
9. ✳	Apply the clamp forceps, and place the clamp over the tooth.				
10. ✳	Once the clamp is securely on the tooth, remove the clamp forceps.				
11. ✳	Place the dam over the teeth to be isolated and tuck the dam.				

Document:

Enter the appropriate information in the chart below.

Grading

Points earned	_____		
Points possible	_____	100	100
Percent grade (Points earned/Points possible)	_____		
Pass:	_____	❑ YES ❑ NO ❑ N/A	❑ YES ❑ NO ❑ N/A

Instructor Sign-Off

Instructor: _____ Date: _____

PROCEDURE 28-1
Applying Topical Anesthetic

Objective: Demonstrate how to properly apply topical anesthetic.

Equipment and Supplies Needed: basic set up, air/water syringe, air evacuator, 2 × 2 sterile gauze squares, topical anesthetic gel ointment, and cotton tip applicator.

Notes to the Student:

Skills Assessment Requirements

Read and familiarize yourself with the procedure; complete the minimum practice requirements. Document information when appropriate to demonstrate proper charting techniques. Complete each procedure within a reasonable amount of time, with a minimum of 85% accuracy.

POINT VALUE ♦ = 5 points ✳ = 10 points		PRACTICE TRIAL	GRADED TRIAL # 1	GRADED TRIAL # 2	NOTES:
1. ♦	Read patient's history.				
2. ♦	Explain the procedure to the patient to avoid any confusion.				
3. ♦	Wait for the dentist to do an oral examination and give you permission to apply topical anesthetic.				
4. ✳	Locate the site of local anesthesia as indicated by the dentist.				
5. ♦	Dry the area with a 2 × 2 cotton gauze. (*Note:* The site should always be dry so that the topical anesthetic is 100% effective.)				
6. ✳	Place a small amount of topical anesthetic on the cotton applicator tip, then place on a 2 × 2 cotton gauze. (*Note:* Never reuse applicator tips.)				

(continued)

POINT VALUE ♦ = 5 points ✳ = 10 points		PRACTICE TRIAL	GRADED TRIAL # 1	GRADED TRIAL # 2	NOTES:
7. ✳	Place the cotton applicator tip with anesthetic at the site of injection.				
8. ✳	If multiple injections will be needed, then apply the topical application to all injection sites.				
9. ✳	Keep the material on the site for three to five minutes.				
10. ♦	Observe and ask patients about the sensation at the site of application.				
11. ✳	Remove any extra material with the air/water syringe and dispose of the cotton applicator.				
12. ✳	Use the evacuation system to suction residual topical anesthetic material.				
13. ♦	Inform the dentist and be prepared to assist in local anesthesia administration.				

Document:

Document information for proper charting of this procedure.

Grading

Points earned	_____		
Points possible	_____		
Percent grade (Points earned/Points possible)	_____	100	100
Pass:	_____	❑ YES ❑ NO ❑ N/A	❑ YES ❑ NO ❑ N/A

Instructor Sign-Off

Instructor: _____ Date: _____

Procedure 28-2
Assembling the Local Anesthetic Syringe

Objective: Demonstrate how to properly assemble the local anesthetic syringe.

Equipment and Supplies Needed: gloves, sterile anesthetic syringe, sterile disposable needles, sterile anesthetic cartridge, 2 × 2 sterile gauze sponge.

Notes to the Student:

Skills Assessment Requirements

Read and familiarize yourself with the procedure; complete the minimum practice requirements. Document information when appropriate to demonstrate proper charting techniques. Complete each procedure within a reasonable amount of time, with a minimum of 85% accuracy.

POINT VALUE ♦ = 5 points ✳ = 10 points		PRACTICE TRIAL	GRADED TRIAL # 1	GRADED TRIAL # 2	NOTES:
A.	**Setting Up the Tray**				
1. ♦	Wash hands and don gloves before preparing the anesthetic syringe.				
2. ✳	Prepare the type of anesthesia based on the dentist's choice. The dentist will determine the type of anesthetic solution needed according to the patient's health history.				
3. ♦	Arrange all supplies on a tray at chairside away from the patient's view.				
B.	**Threading the Needle**				
1. ♦	Select the right size of needle based on infiltration or block anesthesia.				
2. ♦	Remove the plastic cap of the needle from the hub end.				

(continued)

POINT VALUE ♦ = 5 points ✳ = 10 points		PRACTICE TRIAL	GRADED TRIAL # 1	GRADED TRIAL # 2	NOTES:
3. ✳	Screw the needle on the needle end of the syringe, taking care that the end of the needle going inside the syringe does not bend. If the needle bends, retrieve another needle and begin again.				
4. ✳	Make sure the needle is tightly attached to the syringe.				
C.	**Loading the Anesthetic Cartridge into the Syringe**				
1. ✳	Hold the syringe in one hand and use the thumb ring to pull back the plunger.				
2. ✳	Use the other hand to place the cartridge into the syringe with the stopper end toward the plunger.				
3. ✳	Allow the harpoon to engage the stopper by releasing the plunger.				
4. ✳	Make sure that the harpoon is engaged in the stopper by pulling back the thumb ring. (*Note:* This action should be done gently to avoid breaking of the glass cartridge.)				
D.	**Getting the Local Anesthetic Tray**				
1. ♦	Place the loaded syringe on the tray out of the patient's sight.				
2. ♦	Inform the dentist that the setup is ready.				

Document:

Document information for proper charting of this procedure.

Grading

Points earned	_____		
Points possible		100	100
Percent grade (Points earned/Points possible)	_____		
Pass:	_____	❑ YES ❑ NO ❑ N/A	❑ YES ❑ NO ❑ N/A

Instructor Sign-Off

Instructor: _____ Date: _____

PROCEDURE 28-3

Assisting in the Administration of Local Anesthesia

Objective: Demonstrate how to properly assist in applying local anesthetic.

Equipment and Supplies Needed: basic setup, gloves, air/water syringe, evacuator, topical anesthetic ointment, 2 × 2 sterile gauze squares, cotton rolls, cotton applicator tips, assembled local anesthetic syringe (see Procedure 28-2), needle recapper, and a sharps disposal container.

Notes to the Student:

Skills Assessment Requirements

Read and familiarize yourself with the procedure; complete the minimum practice requirements. Document information when appropriate to demonstrate proper charting techniques. Complete each procedure within a reasonable amount of time, with a minimum of 85% accuracy.

POINT VALUE ♦ = 5 points ✳ = 10 points		PRACTICE TRIAL	GRADED TRIAL # 1	GRADED TRIAL # 2	NOTES:
1. ♦	Read patient's history chart.				
2. ♦	Wash hands and don gloves.				
3. ✳	Apply the topical anesthetic to the particular injection site as indicated by the dentist, following the guidelines.				
4. ✳	Dry the area and free it from any saliva.				
5. ♦	Put cotton rolls for isolation of the injection site.				
6. ♦	Loosen the needle guard and transfer the loaded syringe with the thumb ring over the operator's thumb.				
7. ♦	Always transfer the syringe under the patient's chin, so the patient does not see it.				

(continued)

POINT VALUE ♦ = 5 points ∗ = 10 points		PRACTICE TRIAL	GRADED TRIAL #1	GRADED TRIAL #2	NOTES:
8. ♦	Do not release the syringe from your hand until you make sure that the dentist has a firm grip on the thumb ring.				
9. ∗	As the dentist is giving the injection, monitor the patient for any adverse reactions, making sure you portray a calm and relaxed sense of being.				
10. ∗	After the injection is completed, replace the needle guard by using a one-handed scoop technique or recapping device.				
11. ♦	Rinse the patient's mouth with the air/water syringe, and suction with the saliva injector or high-volume evacuator.				
12. ♦	Remove the used needle with the guard in place and dispose of the needle in the sharps container.				
13. ♦	Dispose of the used cartridge in a medical waste receptacle.				
14. ♦	Prepare the anesthetic syringe for sterilization.				
15. ♦	Continue monitoring the patient's reaction throughout the procedure.				
16. ♦	After the surgical procedure is complete, provide patient with postoperative instructions including not to chew on the site for several hours to avoid accidental biting on the cheek or lip.				

Document:

Document information for proper charting of this procedure.

Grading

Points earned	_____		
Points possible	_____	100	100
Percent grade (Points earned/Points possible)	_____		
Pass:	_____	❑ YES ❑ NO ❑ N/A	❑ YES ❑ NO ❑ N/A

Instructor Sign-Off

Instructor: _____ Date: _____

PROCEDURE 28-4
Assisting in the Administration and Monitoring of Nitrous Oxide/Oxygen Sedation

Objective: Demonstrate how to properly assist in the administration and monitoring of nitrous oxide/oxygen sedation.

Equipment and Supplies Needed: gloves, N_2O/O_2 inhalation system tanks, inhalation masks with scavenging system (adult and child sizes), blood pressure cuff, pulse rate tester, and body temperature testing strip.

Notes to the Student:

Skills Assessment Requirements

Read and familiarize yourself with the procedure; complete the minimum practice requirements. Document information when appropriate to demonstrate proper charting techniques. Complete each procedure within a reasonable amount of time, with a minimum of 85% accuracy.

POINT VALUE ♦ = 5 points ✳ = 10 points		PRACTICE TRIAL	GRADED TRIAL #1	GRADED TRIAL #2	NOTES:
A.	**Preparing the Equipment and Patient**				
1. ♦	Read patient's history.				
2. ♦	Wash hands and don gloves.				
3. ♦	Wait for the dentist's permission.				
4. ♦	Select the size of mask for patient after dentist's consent.				
5. ♦	Check all parts of the equipment for any leakage and smooth flow.				
6. ✳	Seat patient, update medical history, and take all vital signs.				

(continued)

POINT VALUE ♦ = 5 points ∗ = 10 points		PRACTICE TRIAL	GRADED TRIAL # 1	GRADED TRIAL # 2	NOTES:
7. ♦	Explain to the patient the use of nitrous oxide and what to expect. Answer all patient questions in easy and clear English.				
8. ♦	Have the patient sign an informed consent form.				
9. ♦	Place the patient in the supine position.				
10. ♦	Instruct the patient not to talk while inhaling the anesthetic agents because leaks and inadequate anesthesia may result.				
11. ∗	Place the mask on the patient and adjust accordingly. Tighten the tubing so it is comfortable on the patient.				
12. ♦	If mask feels uncomfortable to the patient, place a 2 × 2 gauze square under the edge of the mask.				
B.	**Assisting with Administration of Nitrous Oxide Inhalation**				
1. ∗	When the dentist instructs, adjust the flow meter for the oxygen (O_2) only and release the control knob of the green cylinder with O_2. The patient is given 100% oxygen for one minute.				
2. ∗	When the dentist instructs, adjust the N_2O flow in increments of 0.5 to 1 L/min, while reducing the O_2 by the same increments.				
3. ♦	Repeat this process at one-minute intervals until you reach the patient's baseline reading. (*Note:* The patient will start feeling relaxed and slightly sedated.)				
4. ∗	Record the patient's baseline level, while monitoring the patient's reaction throughout the procedure and also recording all vital signs.				

		PRACTICE TRIAL	GRADED TRIAL # 1	GRADED TRIAL # 2	NOTES:
POINT VALUE ♦ = 5 points * = 10 points					
C.	**Assisting with Oxygenation**				
1. ♦	Toward the end of the procedure, N_2O is reduced in the same increments as it was increased. The goal is to have 100% oxygen at the end of the procedure.				
2. ♦	Let the patient breath 100% oxygen for a minimum of five minutes in order to avoid diffusion hypoxia (the feeling of light-headedness).				
3. *	After completion of oxygenation, remove the mask from the patient's nose and place the patient upright slowly because a sudden change of position may cause postural hypotension (fainting).				
4. ♦	Record the patient's baseline level of N_2O and O_2 and also note the patient's response to the analgesia. (*Note:* This recording acts as a reference for future care and is an important legal document.)				
D.	**Dismissing the Patient**				
1. ♦	Check the vital signs and do not let the patient leave until all vital signs are within normal range. (*Note:* If possible, the patient should be escorted by a family member.)				
2. *	To confirm if the patient is fully conscious, the Trieger test can be performed.				
3. ♦	Record all postanesthesia observations and vital signs in the patient's file.				

Document:

Document information for proper charting of this procedure.

(continued)

Grading

Points earned	_____		
Points possible	_____	150	150
Percent grade (Points earned/Points possible)	_____		
Pass:	_____	❑ YES ❑ NO ❑ N/A	❑ YES ❑ NO ❑ N/A

Instructor Sign-Off

Instructor: _____ Date: _____

PROCEDURE 30-1

Processing Dental Film Manually and Performing Infection Control Measures

Objective: Demonstrate how to properly process dental film manually while maintaining infection control.

Equipment and Supplies Needed: gloves, barriers, exposed radiograph, safelight, master tank, thermometer, timer, stirring paddles, x-ray rack, developer and fixer solutions, and pen or pencil.

Notes to the Student:

Skills Assessment Requirements

Read and familiarize yourself with the procedure; complete the minimum practice requirements. Document information when appropriate to demonstrate proper charting techniques. Complete each procedure within a reasonable amount of time, with a minimum of 85% accuracy.

POINT VALUE ♦ = 5 points ✳ = 10 points		PRACTICE TRIAL	GRADED TRIAL # 1	GRADED TRIAL # 2	NOTES:
A.	**Preparation for Film Processing**				
1. ♦	Check developer and fixer solution levels; replenish if low.				
2. ♦	Stir developer and fixer tanks with appropriate paddles.				
3. ♦	Establish chemical and water bath temperatures and ensure that the water bath is circulating.				
4. ♦	Clean counter around the master tank to ensure no chemical solution drops remain. Wash hands.				
5. ♦	Establish that x-ray racks are clean and in working order and label with patient's name and date.				

(continued)

	POINT VALUE ♦ = 5 points ✳ = 10 points	PRACTICE TRIAL	GRADED TRIAL # 1	GRADED TRIAL # 2	NOTES:
6. ♦	Place barriers on darkroom counter with exposed films (still in the disposable container).				
7. ♦	Turn off overhead light and turn on safelight.				
8. ♦	Don gloves.				
B.	**Procedure Steps for Manual Film Processing**				
1. ♦	Carefully remove wrapper from film, not touching the film but allowing it to fall on the clean barrier. (Check state guidelines for proper lead foil disposal in your area.)				
2. ♦	Dispose of contaminated wrapper in the appropriate waste receptacle.				
3. ♦	Remove gloves. Wash and dry hands, being careful not get water droplets on film.				
4. ♦	Carefully attach the film to the rack and check that it is secure. Place film on the rack from the bottom up, alternating sides of the rack.				
5. ♦	Check the temperature of the developing solution to determine the length of time for developing the films.				
6. ♦	Place rack in the developing tank and gently agitate to remove any bubbles and then replace the lid on the tank.				
7. ♦	Set timer for appropriate time (normal developing time is 4½ minutes at 68°F), but always investigate and follow manufacturer's directions.				
8. ♦	Remove from developer after the appropriate time and rinse in the water bath. Gently agitate for 20 seconds.				

POINT VALUE ♦ = 5 points ✳ = 10 points		PRACTICE TRIAL	GRADED TRIAL # 1	GRADED TRIAL # 2	NOTES:
9. ♦	Place into the fixing solution, then replace the lid on the tank and set the timer. The time required to fix the films is double the developing time, but always investigate and follow manufacturer's directions.				
10. ♦	Remove from fixer after the appropriate time and place in the water bath for approximately 20 minutes to do a final wash of the films.				
11. ♦	Remove film from water bath and place film in the film dryer if available or allow to air dry.				
12. ♦	Remove barriers and clean work areas to prepare for the next film processing.				

Document:

Document information for proper charting of this procedure.

Grading

Points earned	_____		
Points possible	_____	100	100
Percent grade (Points earned/Points possible)	_____		
Pass:	_____	❑ YES ❑ NO ❑ N/A	❑ YES ❑ NO ❑ N/A

Instructor Sign-Off

Instructor: _____ Date: _____

PROCEDURE 30-2

Processing Dental Film Automatically and Performing Infection Control Measures

Objective: Demonstrate how to properly process dental film automatically and maintain infection control.

Equipment and Supplies Needed: automatic processor with daylight loader, two disposable containers, exposed radiographs, paper towel, disinfectant, and gloves.

Notes to the Student:

Skills Assessment Requirements

Read and familiarize yourself with the procedure; complete the minimum practice requirements. Document information when appropriate to demonstrate proper charting techniques. Complete each procedure within a reasonable amount of time, with a minimum of 85% accuracy.

	POINT VALUE ♦ = 5 points ✳ = 10 points	PRACTICE TRIAL	GRADED TRIAL # 1	GRADED TRIAL # 2	NOTES:
A.	**Preparing for Film Processing**				
1. ✳	The automatic processor should be turned on at the start of the workday so the chemicals reach recommended temperatures.				
2. ✳	Wash and dry hands.				
3. ✳	Open the top of the daylight loader and place a paper towel on the bottom that will serve as a barrier. Place the disposable containers on the paper towel. One is for the lead foil and the other contains the exposed films but will be used to discard contaminated gloves, paper towel, and film wrapping after the films are loaded into the processor.				

(continued)

POINT VALUE ♦ = 5 points ✳ = 10 points		PRACTICE TRIAL	GRADED TRIAL # 1	GRADED TRIAL # 2	NOTES:
B.	**Procedure Steps for Automatic Film Processing**				
1. ✳	Don gloves and put hands into the sleeves of the daylight loader.				
2. ✳	Unwrap film and feed the film into the machine. When processing multiple films, load them slowly to avoid film overlaps during processing. Alternate slots in the processor.				
3. ✳	Place lead foils in one of the disposable containers and place the film wrappers on the paper towel. (Check state guidelines for proper lead foil disposal in your area.)				
4. ✳	Continue with steps 2 and 3 until all films have been fed into the processor. Then remove gloves, placing them in the center of the paper towel with the film wrappers.				
5. ✳	Using only the corners of the paper towel, wrap the paper towel over the gloves and film wrappers and carefully place them in the empty container where the exposed films were.				
6. ✳	The disposable containers are removed using the lid on the top of the daylight loader. The trash is discarded and the lead foils are taken to the recycling area.				
7. ✳	Disinfect the daylight loader to prevent cross-contamination.				

Document:

Document information for proper charting of this procedure.

Grading

Points earned	_____		
Points possible	_____	100	100
Percent grade (Points earned/Points possible)	_____		
Pass:	_____	❑ YES ❑ NO ❑ N/A	❑ YES ❑ NO ❑ N/A

Instructor Sign-Off

Instructor: _____ Date: _____

PROCEDURE 31-1
Preparing the Patient for Intraoral Radiographs

Objective: Demonstrate how to properly prepare a patient for intraoral radiographs.

Equipment and Supplies Needed: lead apron and thyroid collar, cup or container, and paper towel.

Notes to the Student:

Skills Assessment Requirements

Read and familiarize yourself with the procedure; complete the minimum practice requirements. Document information when appropriate to demonstrate proper charting techniques. Complete each procedure within a reasonable amount of time, with a minimum of 85% accuracy.

POINT VALUE ♦ = 5 points ✳ = 10 points		PRACTICE TRIAL	GRADED TRIAL # 1	GRADED TRIAL # 2	NOTES:
1. ✳✳	Explain the procedure to the patient prior to beginning and ask if he has any questions.				
2. ✳✳	Seat the patient and adjust the chair in an upright position that is at a comfortable working height for the dental assistant.				
3. ✳✳	Adjust the headrest to support and position the patient's head so that the occlusal plane of the maxillary arch is parallel to the floor and the midsagittal plane is perpendicular to the floor.				
4. ✳✳	Have the patient remove all dentures, partials, retainers, eyeglasses, and lip, nose, or oral piercing objects. Place them on a paper towel or in a container.				
5. ✳✳	Place the lead apron with thyroid collar over the patient.				

(continued)

Document:

Document information for proper charting of this procedure.

Grading

Points earned	_____		
Points possible	_____	100	100
Percent grade (Points earned/Points possible)	_____		
Pass:	_____	❏ YES ❏ NO ❏ N/A	❏ YES ❏ NO ❏ N/A

Instructor Sign-Off

Instructor: _____ Date: _____

PROCEDURE 31-2
Assembling the XCP Paralleling Device

Objective: Demonstrate how to properly assembly the XCP paralleling device.

Equipment and Supplies Needed: Rinn XCP device—anterior and posterior, bitewing instruments, and paper towel.

Notes to the Student:

Skills Assessment Requirements

Read and familiarize yourself with the procedure; complete the minimum practice requirements. Document information when appropriate to demonstrate proper charting techniques. Complete each procedure within a reasonable amount of time, with a minimum of 85% accuracy.

POINT VALUE ◆ = 5 points ✳ = 10 points		PRACTICE TRIAL	GRADED TRIAL # 1	GRADED TRIAL # 2	NOTES:
1. ✳	Wash and dry hands. Lay out paper towels on a disinfected countertop.				
2. ✳	Gather the sterilized XCP instrument components for the anterior device: the anterior indicator rod, the blue vertical bite block, and the blue locator ring.				
3. ✳	Insert the two short metal extensions on the anterior indicator rod into the side of the blue bite block.				
4. ✳	Insert the blue locator ring onto the indicator rod so that the blue bite block is centered within the ring.				
5. ✳✳	Gather the components for the posterior XCP device: the posterior indicator rod, the yellow horizontal bite block, and the yellow locator ring.				

(continued)

POINT VALUE ♦ = 5 points ✳ = 10 points		PRACTICE TRIAL	GRADED TRIAL # 1	GRADED TRIAL # 2	NOTES:
6. ✳	Insert the two short metal extensions on the posterior indicator rod into the side of the yellow bite block.				
7. ✳	Insert the red locator ring onto the indicator rod so that the yellow bite block is centered within the ring.				
8. ✳✳	Gather the components for the bitewing XCP device: the bitewing indicator rod, the red bite block, and the red locator ring.				

Document:

Document information for proper charting of this procedure.

Grading

Points earned	_____		
Points possible	_____	100	100
Percent grade (Points earned/Points possible)	_____		
Pass:	_____	❏ YES ❏ NO ❏ N/A	❏ YES ❏ NO ❏ N/A

Instructor Sign-Off

Instructor: _____ Date: _____

PROCEDURE 31-3

Taking Full Mouth Radiographs Using the Paralleling Technique

Objective: Demonstrate how to properly take a full mouth set of radiographs using the paralleling technique.

Equipment and Supplies Needed: Rinn XCP device—anterior, posterior, and periapical film, lead apron with thyroid color, cup or container, cotton rolls, 2 × 2 sterile gauze squares, paper towel, and gloves

Notes to the Student:

Skills Assessment Requirements

Read and familiarize yourself with the procedure; complete the minimum practice requirements. Document information when appropriate to demonstrate proper charting techniques. Complete each procedure within a reasonable amount of time, with a minimum of 85% accuracy.

POINT VALUE ♦ = 5 points ✳ = 10 points		PRACTICE TRIAL	GRADED TRIAL # 1	GRADED TRIAL # 2	NOTES:
1. ♦	Seat the patient comfortably in the chair, explain the procedure, and ask if she has any questions. Drape the lead apron on the patient and assure the patient that the procedure will be completed as quickly as possible. Adjust the control panel settings.				
2. ♦	Adjust the chair in an upright position to a comfortable working height for the dental assistant. Adjust the headrest to support and position the patient's head so that the occlusal plane of the maxillary arch is parallel to the floor and the midsagittal plane is perpendicular to the floor.				
3. ♦	Wash and dry hands. Don gloves. Prepare the film-holding devices.				

(continued)

POINT VALUE ◆ = 5 points ✳ = 10 points		PRACTICE TRIAL	GRADED TRIAL # 1	GRADED TRIAL # 2	NOTES:
4. ◆	Ask the patient to remove any oral prostheses, eyeglasses, earrings, and oral piercings.				
5. ◆	Look inside the mouth to assess the size and shape of the oral cavity and to identify landmarks such as tori that may cause the patient to be uncomfortable during the radiographic procedure.				
6. ✳	Begin the full mouth radiograph series in the anterior by inserting a film vertically into the backing plate of the blue bite block by bending it slightly backwards. Make sure that the smooth (white) side of the film packet is facing the locator ring.				
7. ◆	Place the anterior edge of the bite block on the incisal surface of the maxillary anterior teeth to be radiographed by inserting it at an upward angle for patient comfort. Instruct the patient to close the teeth together slowly but firmly. Slide the locator ring down the indicator rod to near the patient's face, align the PID parallel with the ring, and expose the film. Instruct the patient not to move each time you are ready to expose a radiograph.				
8. ◆	Remove the film and film-holding device carefully from the patient's mouth. Repeat until all prescribed maxillary anterior films have been exposed. Place each exposed film into the cup or container.				

POINT VALUE ♦ = 5 points ✳ = 10 points		PRACTICE TRIAL	GRADED TRIAL #1	GRADED TRIAL #2	NOTES:
9. ✳	Place the anterior edge of the bite block on the incisal surface of the mandibular anterior teeth to be radiographed by inserting it at a downward angle for patient comfort. Instruct the patient to close the teeth together slowly but firmly. Slide the locator ring down the rod to near the patient's face, align the PID parallel with the ring, and expose the film. Remove the film and film-holding device carefully from the patient's mouth. Repeat until all prescribed mandibular anterior films have been exposed.				
10. ♦	Insert a film horizontally into the backing plate of the bite block by bending it slightly backwards. Make sure that the smooth side of the film packet is facing the locator ring.				
11. ♦	Place the bite block on the occlusal surfaces of the posterior teeth to be radiographed by inserting it into the mouth at an upward angle for maxillary teeth and at a downward angle for mandibular teeth. Gently pull the cheek around the indicator rod where necessary so that the XCP device is inside the mouth and not pulling on the cheek area.				
12. ♦	Instruct the patient to close the teeth together slowly but firmly. Slide the locator ring down the rod to near the patient's face, align the PID parallel with the ring, and expose the film. Remove the film and film-holding device carefully from the patient's mouth. Repeat until all prescribed posterior films have been exposed.				

(continued)

POINT VALUE ♦ = 5 points ✳ = 10 points		PRACTICE TRIAL	GRADED TRIAL # 1	GRADED TRIAL # 2	NOTES:
13. ♦	Insert a film into one side of the bracket plate of the bitewing, then slightly flex the film, insert the opposite edge into the other side of the bracket, and center the film. Make sure that the smooth side of the film packet is facing the locator ring.				
14. ♦	Gently place the bite block on the occlusal surfaces of the premolars aligning the anterior border of the film packet with the distal portion of the mandibular cuspid.				
15. ♦	Instruct the patient to close firmly to retain the position of the film. Slide the aiming ring down the indicator rod close to the skin surface and align the PID on the ring. Expose the radiograph and then carefully remove the film and XCP device.				
16. ♦	Repeat for the molar bitewing aligning the anterior border of the film packet with the distal portion of the second premolar.				
17. ♦	Repeat the premolar and molar bitewing radiographs on the opposite side of the patient's mouth.				
18. ♦	When all prescribed radiographs have been completed, remove gloves, wash and dry hands, remove the lead apron from the patient, and release the patient. Transport the films to the processing area. Record the radiographs in the patient's record.				

Document:

Document information for proper charting of this procedure.

Grading

Points earned	_____		
Points possible	_____	100	100
Percent grade (Points earned/Points possible)	_____		
Pass:	_____	❑ YES ❑ NO ❑ N/A	❑ YES ❑ NO ❑ N/A

Instructor Sign-Off

Instructor: _____ Date: _____

PROCEDURE 31-4
Mounting Intraoral Radiographs

Objective: Demonstrate how to properly mount intraoral radiographs.

Supplies Needed: processed radiographs, x-ray mount, pen or pencil, patient chart, x-ray view box, and white paper.

Notes to the Student:

Skills Assessment Requirements

Read and familiarize yourself with the procedure; complete the minimum practice requirements. Document information when appropriate to demonstrate proper charting techniques. Complete each procedure within a reasonable amount of time, with a minimum of 85% accuracy.

POINT VALUE ♦ = 5 points ✳ = 10 points		PRACTICE TRIAL	GRADED TRIAL # 1	GRADED TRIAL # 2	NOTES:
1. ✳	Gather all necessary supplies. Wash and thoroughly dry hands. Select the appropriate size mount and label it with the patient's name and date of exposure.				
2. ✳	On the piece of white paper, identify maxillary and mandibular anterior, maxillary and mandibular posterior, and bitewing views. Group them together with the embossed dot facing up. Handle films by the edges only, never on the front or back.				

(continued)

POINT VALUE ♦ = 5 points ✳ = 10 points		PRACTICE TRIAL	GRADED TRIAL # 1	GRADED TRIAL # 2	NOTES:
3. ✳	Once the films are arranged properly place them into the mount in their correct location. Slide each radiograph completely into the appropriate window on the mount. Mount the bitewing radiographs first. Use them to identify restorations and missing teeth which will assist in mounting the other radiographs.				
4. ✳	Use anatomical landmarks as clues to mount the remaining periapical radiographs.				
5. ✳	After mounting the films, either put them in the patient's chart, or on the view box for the dentist to view.				

Document:

Document information for proper charting of this procedure.

Grading

Points earned	_____		
Points possible	_____	50	50
Percent grade (Points earned/Points possible)	_____		
Pass:	_____	❏ YES ❏ NO ❏ N/A	❏ YES ❏ NO ❏ N/A

Instructor Sign-Off

Instructor: _____ Date: _____

Procedure 33-1
Mixing, Placing, and Carving of Dental Amalgam

Objective: Demonstrate how to properly mix, place, and carve an amalgam restoration.

Equipment and Supplies Needed: amalgam capsule, amalgam well, activator, amalgam carrier, pluggers/condensers, carving and finishing instruments, occlusal paper, and floss.

Notes to the Student:

Skills Assessment Requirements

Read and familiarize yourself with the procedure; complete the minimum practice requirements. Document information when appropriate to demonstrate proper charting techniques. Complete each procedure within a reasonable amount of time, with a minimum of 85% accuracy.

POINT VALUE ♦ = 5 points ✳ = 10 points		PRACTICE TRIAL	GRADED TRIAL #1	GRADED TRIAL #2	NOTES:
1. ♦	Activate the amalgam capsule with the activator.				
2. ✳	Place the capsule into the triturator, close the lid, check for the appropriate settings, and begin trituration.				
3. ♦	Remove the capsule from the triturator, open the capsule, and spill the amalgam into the amalgam well.				
4. ✳	Fill the amalgam carrier by pressing the end of the carrier into the soft amalgam so as to pack the carrier to the top with amalgam. (The dentist may request the small end or the large end of the carrier first.)				

(continued)

POINT VALUE ♦ = 5 points ∗ = 10 points		PRACTICE TRIAL	GRADED TRIAL # 1	GRADED TRIAL # 2	NOTES:
5. ∗	Transfer the carrier to the dentist with the filled end on the carrier toward the preparation to be filled.				
6. ∗	Continue the handoff of the amalgam carrier to and from the assistant to the dentist until the preparation is overfilled.				

Document:

Document information for proper charting of this procedure.

Grading

Points earned	_____		
Points possible	_____	50	50
Percent grade (Points earned/Points possible)	_____		
Pass:	_____	❑ YES ❑ NO ❑ N/A	❑ YES ❑ NO ❑ N/A

Instructor Sign-Off

Instructor: _____ Date:_____

Procedure 33-2
Chemically Preparing, Placing, Curing, and Finishing Composite Resins

Objective: Demonstrate how to prepare, place, cure, and finish a composite restoration.

Equipment and Supplies Needed: composite resin carpules and delivery gun or syringes; mixing wells with lightproof shield; brushes; acid-etch syringe with tips; bonding system; curing light; pluggers/condensers; plastic instruments; carving instruments; rotary instruments with carbide burs and finishing points, discs, and/or cups; sanding strips; matrix system; occlusal paper; and floss.

Notes to the Student:

Skills Assessment Requirements

Read and familiarize yourself with the procedure; complete the minimum practice requirements. Document information when appropriate to demonstrate proper charting techniques. Complete each procedure within a reasonable amount of time, with a minimum of 85% accuracy.

POINT VALUE ♦ = 5 points ＊ = 10 points		PRACTICE TRIAL	GRADED TRIAL # 1	GRADED TRIAL # 2	NOTES:
1. ＊	Select the shade of the tooth to be restored. Use natural light. Fluorescent light will alter the shade selection.				
2. ＊	Confirm moisture control that is necessary for the bonding procedure to occur.				
3. ＊	Place carpule of proper shade into the delivery gun, or syringe the proper shade into a mixing well. Dispense adhesive into well and cover with the lightproof shield.				
4. ＊	Pass the syringe of phosphoric acid to the dentist.				
5. ＊	Rinse and suction etch from the preparation. Dry with air.				

(continued)

POINT VALUE ♦ = 5 points ✳ = 10 points		PRACTICE TRIAL	GRADED TRIAL # 1	GRADED TRIAL # 2	NOTES:
6. ✳	Pass brush with bonding agent to dentist. Thin the adhesive with air from the air/water syringe.				
7. ♦	Light cure adhesive as necessary.				
8. ♦	Pass composite resin material to dentist.				
9. ✳	Pass necessary instruments for material manipulation to dentist.				
10. ✳	Light cure material as necessary during material placement.				
11. ✳	Have carbide burs and polishing items ready and available.				

Document:

Enter the appropriate information in the chart below.

Grading

Points earned	_____		
Points possible	_____	100	100
Percent grade (Points earned/Points possible)	_____		
Pass:	_____	❏ YES ❏ NO ❏ N/A	❏ YES ❏ NO ❏ N/A

Instructor Sign-Off

Instructor:_____ Date:_____

Procedure 33-3
Preparing and Delivering Intermediate Restorative Material

Objective: Demonstrate how to prepare and deliver intermediate restorative material.

Equipment and Supplies Needed: liquid and powder container of IRM with measuring scoop, mixing pad, and spatula.

Notes to the Student:

Skills Assessment Requirements

Read and familiarize yourself with the procedure; complete the minimum practice requirements. Document information when appropriate to demonstrate proper charting techniques. Complete each procedure within a reasonable amount of time, with a minimum of 85% accuracy.

POINT VALUE ♦ = 5 points * = 10 points		PRACTICE TRIAL	GRADED TRIAL # 1	GRADED TRIAL # 2	NOTES:
1. *	Shake the powder prior to dispensing.				
2. *	Dispense powder using the provided measuring scoop onto the mixing pad.				
3. **	Dispense liquid onto the mixing pad. (IRM is made in a 1:1 ratio, meaning one scoop of power to one drop of liquid.)				
4. **	Mix powder into liquid in increments to form a stiff paste. Mixing time should be less than one minute.				
5. **	Roll the IRM into a ball for easy delivery into tooth.				
6. *	Wipe the spatula clean before material sets.				
7. *	Set IRM in the restored tooth.				

(continued)

Document:

Enter the appropriate information in the chart below.

Grading

Points earned	_____		
Points possible	_____	100	100
Percent grade (Points earned/Points possible)	_____		
Pass:	_____	❏ YES ❏ NO ❏ N/A	❏ YES ❏ NO ❏ N/A

Instructor Sign-Off

Instructor: _____ Date:_____

Procedure 33-4
Preparing and Delivering Provisional Restorative Material

Objective: Demonstrate how to prepare and deliver provisional restorative material.

Equipment and Supplies Needed: stint, spatula, delivery gun with material cartridge and tip, mixing pad, and tubes of temporary cement.

Notes to the Student:

Skills Assessment Requirements

Read and familiarize yourself with the procedure; complete the minimum practice requirements. Document information when appropriate to demonstrate proper charting techniques. Complete each procedure within a reasonable amount of time, with a minimum of 85% accuracy.

POINT VALUE ♦ = 5 points ∗ = 10 points		PRACTICE TRIAL	GRADED TRIAL # 1	GRADED TRIAL # 2	NOTES:
1. ∗	Fill stint with provisional material.				
2. ∗∗	Place stint over prepared tooth or teeth. Allow material to cure per manufacturer recommendations.				
3. ∗	Remove stint from the mouth and then remove the provisional material from the stint.				
4. ∗	Trim, finish, and polish the stint so no rough edges are felt.				
5. ∗∗	Mix temporary cement and fill the provisional.				
6. ∗	Seat provisional onto prepared tooth. Allow cement to cure.				
7. ∗	Remove excess cured cement from around the tooth or teeth.				
8. ∗	Check and adjust the occlusion.				

(continued)

Document:

Enter the appropriate information in the chart below.

Grading

Points earned	_____		
Points possible	_____	100	100
Percent grade (Points earned/Points possible)	_____		
Pass:	_____	❏ YES ❏ NO ❏ N/A	❏ YES ❏ NO ❏ N/A

Instructor Sign-Off

Instructor: _____ Date: _____

PROCEDURE 34-1
Applying a Calcium Hydroxide Liner

Objective: Demonstrate the proper application process for a calcium hydroxide liner.

Equipment and Supplies Needed: tubes of calcium hydroxide "catalyst" and "base" (from same manufacturer), small mixing pad (provided by the manufacturer), small spatula, calcium hydroxide applicator instrument, and 2 × 2 gauze pads.

Notes to the Student:

Skills Assessment Requirements

Read and familiarize yourself with the procedure; complete the minimum practice requirements. Document information when appropriate to demonstrate proper charting techniques. Complete each procedure within a reasonable amount of time, with a minimum of 85% accuracy.

POINT VALUE ♦ = 5 points ✳ = 10 points		PRACTICE TRIAL	GRADED TRIAL # 1	GRADED TRIAL # 2	NOTES:
1. ✳	Dispense small equal portions of the catalyst and base onto the special mixing pad.				
2. ✳	Quickly mix the two pastes in a circular motion over a small area with the spatula.				
3. ✳	After a homogenous mixture has been achieved, use a 2 × 2 gauze pad to wipe clean the spatula.				
4. ✳	Using the ball tip of the applicator, pick up a small amount of material and apply in a thin layer directly over the pulp.				
5. ♦	Use the explorer to remove any material that may have gotten onto the enamel.				
6. ♦	Clean and disinfect all equipment.				

(continued)

Document:

Document information for proper charting of this procedure.

Grading

Points earned	_____		
Points possible	_____	50	50
Percent grade (Points earned/Points possible)	_____		
Pass:	_____	❑ YES ❑ NO ❑ N/A	❑ YES ❑ NO ❑ N/A

Instructor Sign-Off

Instructor: _____ Date: _____

PROCEDURE 34-2

Applying a Glass Ionomer Liner

Objective: Demonstrate the proper application of a glass ionomer as a liner.

Equipment and Supplies Needed: glass ionomer cement powder/liquid with manufacturer's scoop, paper mixing pad, small spatula, ball burnisher applicator instrument, and moistened 2 × 2 gauze pads.

Notes to the Student:

Skills Assessment Requirements

Read and familiarize yourself with the procedure; complete the minimum practice requirements. Document information when appropriate to demonstrate proper charting techniques. Complete each procedure within a reasonable amount of time, with a minimum of 85% accuracy.

POINT VALUE ♦ = 5 points ∗ = 10 points		PRACTICE TRIAL	GRADED TRIAL # 1	GRADED TRIAL # 2	NOTES:
1. ∗ ∗	Dispense material per manufacturer's directions.				
2. ∗	Dispense the powder on the other half of the pad.				
3. ∗ ∗	Incorporate the powder and liquid according to the manufacturer's directions.				
4. ∗	Use a 2 × 2 gauze pad to wipe clean the spatula.				
5. ∗ ∗	Apply liner (see Procedure 34-1, step 4).				
6. ∗ ∗	Clean and disinfect all equipment.				

(continued)

Document:

Document information for proper charting of this procedure.

Grading

Points earned	_____		
Points possible	_____	100	100
Percent grade (Points earned/Points possible)	_____		
Pass:	_____	❏ YES ❏ NO ❏ N/A	❏ YES ❏ NO ❏ N/A

Instructor Sign-Off

Instructor:_____ Date: _____

PROCEDURE 34-3

Applying Zinc Oxide Eugenol Cement Liner Using The Two-Paste System

Objective: Demonstrate the proper application of the zinc oxide eugenol cement liner using the two-paste system.

Equipment and Supplies Needed: two-paste zinc oxide eugenol cement liner "accelerator" and "base" (from same manufacturer), small mixing pad (provided by the manufacturer), small cement spatula, small ball burnisher applicator instrument or plastic instrument, and moist 2 × 2 gauze pads.

Notes to the Student:

Skills Assessment Requirements

Read and familiarize yourself with the procedure; complete the minimum practice requirements. Document information when appropriate to demonstrate proper charting techniques. Complete each procedure within a reasonable amount of time, with a minimum of 85% accuracy.

POINT VALUE ♦ = 5 points ∗ = 10 points		PRACTICE TRIAL	GRADED TRIAL # 1	GRADED TRIAL # 2	NOTES:
1. ∗ ∗	Dispense material per manufacturer's directions.				
2. ∗ ∗	Quickly gather the materials and mix the two pastes.				
3. ∗ ∗	Use a moistened 2 × 2 gauze pad to wipe clean the spatula.				
4. ∗ ∗	Apply liner (see Procedure 34-1, step 4).				
5. ∗ ∗	Clean and disinfect all equipment.				

(continued)

Document:

Document information for proper charting of this procedure.

Grading

Points earned	_____		
Points possible	_____	100	100
Percent grade (Points earned/Points possible)	_____		
Pass:	_____	❏ YES ❏ NO ❏ N/A	❏ YES ❏ NO ❏ N/A

Instructor Sign-Off

Instructor: _____ Date: _____

PROCEDURE 34-4
Applying Dental Varnishes

Objective: Demonstrate the proper application of dental varnishes.

Equipment and Supplies Needed: dental varnish, and cotton pliers, cotton pellets or microbrush applicators.

Notes to the Student:

Skills Assessment Requirements

Read and familiarize yourself with the procedure; complete the minimum practice requirements. Document information when appropriate to demonstrate proper charting techniques. Complete each procedure within a reasonable amount of time, with a minimum of 85% accuracy.

POINT VALUE ♦ = 5 points ✳ = 10 points		PRACTICE TRIAL	GRADED TRIAL # 1	GRADED TRIAL # 2	NOTES:
1. ✳ ✳	Open bottle of varnish and saturate the cotton pellet or applicator.				
2. ✳ ✳	Apply to walls and margins of cavity preparation.				
3. ✳	Allow the varnish to air dry.				
4. ✳ ✳	Prepare a second varnish. Saturate the cotton pellet with second varnish if the second varnish is needed.				
5. ✳	Apply second varnish if needed.				
6. ✳ ✳	Clean and disinfect all equipment.				

(continued)

Document:

Document information for proper charting of this procedure.

Grading

Points earned	_____		
Points possible	_____	100	100
Percent grade (Points earned/Points possible)	_____		
Pass:	_____	❑ YES ❑ NO ❑ N/A	❑ YES ❑ NO ❑ N/A

Instructor Sign-Off

Instructor: _____ Date: _____

PROCEDURE 34-5
Applying Dentin Sealers

Objective: Demonstrate the proper application of dentin sealers.

Equipment and Supplies Needed: dental sealer material and microbrush applicators.

Notes to the Student:

Skills Assessment Requirements

Read and familiarize yourself with the procedure; complete the minimum practice requirements. Document information when appropriate to demonstrate proper charting techniques. Complete each procedure within a reasonable amount of time, with a minimum of 85% accuracy.

POINT VALUE ♦ = 5 points ✳ = 10 points		PRACTICE TRIAL	GRADED TRIAL # 1	GRADED TRIAL # 2	NOTES:
1. ✳ ✳	Perform moisture control. Tooth should be dry and clean.				
2. ✳ ✳	Apply saturated applicator to the cavity preparation.				
3. ✳ ✳	Wait 30 seconds. Air dry.				
4. ✳ ✳	Repeat a second application if patient has had sensitivity history.				
5. ✳ ✳	Clean and disinfect all equipment.				

(continued)

Document:

Document information for proper charting of this procedure.

Grading

Points earned	_____		
Points possible	_____	100	100
Percent grade (Points earned/Points possible)	_____		
Pass:	_____	❑ YES ❑ NO ❑ N/A	❑ YES ❑ NO ❑ N/A

Instructor Sign-Off

Instructor: _____ Date: _____

PROCEDURE 34-6
Applying Zinc Oxide Eugenol Cement Base

Objective: Demonstrate the proper application of zinc oxide eugenol cement base.

Equipment and Supplies Needed: zinc oxide powder and scoop dispenser, eugenol liquid and dropper, small mixing pad (provided by the manufacturer), small cement spatula, plastic instrument, amalgam condenser, and 2 × 2 gauze pads.

Notes to the Student:

Skills Assessment Requirements

Read and familiarize yourself with the procedure; complete the minimum practice requirements. Document information when appropriate to demonstrate proper charting techniques. Complete each procedure within a reasonable amount of time, with a minimum of 85% accuracy.

POINT VALUE ♦ = 5 points ✳ = 10 points		PRACTICE TRIAL	GRADED TRIAL # 1	GRADED TRIAL # 2	NOTES:
1. ✳	Dispense the powder and liquid per manufacturer's instruction onto a special mixing pad.				
2. ✳ ✳	Using the spatula, combine half the powder into the liquid and mix thoroughly for about 20 to 30 seconds.				
3. ✳ ✳	Then pull the remaining powder into the mixture, mixing for another 20 to 30 seconds until the material becomes putty-like.				
4. ✳ ✳	Place portion needed in the cavity preparation.				
5. ✳ ✳	Use a moistened 2 × 2 gauze to wipe clean the spatula and condenser.				
6. ✳	Clean and disinfect all equipment.				

(continued)

Document:

Document information for proper charting of this procedure.

Grading

Points earned	_____		
Points possible	_____	100	100
Percent grade (Points earned/Points possible)	_____		
Pass:	_____	❑ YES ❑ NO ❑ N/A	❑ YES ❑ NO ❑ N/A

Instructor Sign-Off

Instructor: _____ Date: _____

PROCEDURE 34-7
Applying Zinc Phosphate

Objective: Demonstrate the proper application of zinc phosphate.

Equipment and Supplies Needed: zinc phosphate powder and liquid with scoop dispenser, chilled glass slab, small cement spatula, amalgam condenser, plastic instrument, and 2 × 2 gauze pads.

Notes to the Student:

Skills Assessment Requirements

Read and familiarize yourself with the procedure; complete the minimum practice requirements. Document information when appropriate to demonstrate proper charting techniques. Complete each procedure within a reasonable amount of time, with a minimum of 85% accuracy.

POINT VALUE ♦ = 5 points ✳ = 10 points		PRACTICE TRIAL	GRADED TRIAL # 1	GRADED TRIAL # 2	NOTES:
1. ✳	Dispense the powder and liquid per manufacturer's directions onto a chilled glass slab.				
2. ✳	Using the spatula, mix small increments of powder into the liquid until the material is a thick or putty consistency. Allow for dissipation of heat.				
3. ♦	Use a moistened 2 × 2 gauze to wipe clean the spatula and condenser.				
4. ✳	Using the condenser, place putty on the end and carry to the dentist for placement.				
5. ♦	Use a moistened 2 × 2 gauze to wipe the condenser tip if necessary.				
6. ✳	Clean and disinfect all equipment.				

(continued)

Document:

Document information for proper charting of this procedure.

Grading

Points earned	_____		
Points possible	_____	50	50
Percent grade (Points earned/Points possible)	_____		
Pass:	_____	❏ YES ❏ NO ❏ N/A	❏ YES ❏ NO ❏ N/A

Instructor Sign-Off

Instructor: _____ Date: _____

PROCEDURE 34-8
Applying a Polycarboxylate Cement Base

Objective: Demonstrate the proper application of polycarboxylate cement base.

Equipment and Supplies Needed: polycarboxylate powder and scoop dispenser, polycarboxylate liquid and dropper, mixing pad (provided by the manufacturer), small cement spatula, plastic instrument, amalgam condenser, and 2 × 2 inch gauze pads.

Notes to the Student:

Skills Assessment Requirements

Read and familiarize yourself with the procedure; complete the minimum practice requirements. Document information when appropriate to demonstrate proper charting techniques. Complete each procedure within a reasonable amount of time, with a minimum of 85% accuracy.

POINT VALUE ♦ = 5 points ∗ = 10 points		PRACTICE TRIAL	GRADED TRIAL # 1	GRADED TRIAL # 2	NOTES:
1. ∗∗	Dispense powder and liquid per manufacturer's directions. Keep in mind that when mixing polycarboxylate the mixture is thicker for a base than when used as a liner or cement.				
2. ∗∗	Using the spatula, combine all the powder into the liquid and mix thoroughly and all at once within 30 seconds.				
3. ∗∗	Roll material into a ball.				
4. ∗∗	Using the condenser, place the putty onto the end and place into the preparation.				
5. ∗∗	Clean and disinfect all equipment.				

(continued)

Document:

Document information for proper charting of this procedure.

Grading

Points earned	_____		
Points possible	_____	100	100
Percent grade (Points earned/Points possible)	_____		
Pass:	_____	❏ YES ❏ NO ❏ N/A	❏ YES ❏ NO ❏ N/A

Instructor Sign-Off

Instructor: _____ Date: _____

PROCEDURE 34-9
Applying a Dental Acid Etchant

Objective: Demonstrate the proper application of acid etchant.

Equipment and Supplies Needed: rubber dam or cotton rolls, dental acid etchant, applicators—syringe, cotton pellets, small applicator tips or microbrush applicators, dappen dish, and timer.

Notes to the Student:

Skills Assessment Requirements

Read and familiarize yourself with the procedure; complete the minimum practice requirements. Document information when appropriate to demonstrate proper charting techniques. Complete each procedure within a reasonable amount of time, with a minimum of 85% accuracy.

POINT VALUE ◆ = 5 points ✳ = 10 points		PRACTICE TRIAL	GRADED TRIAL # 1	GRADED TRIAL # 2	NOTES:
1. ✳✳	Use rubber dam or cotton rolls to isolate the area if necessary.				
2. ✳✳	Clean the surface thoroughly.				
3. ✳✳	Etch the surface following manufacturer's directions.				
4. ✳✳	Go to next procedure in bonding restoration process.				
5. ✳✳	Clean and disinfect all equipment.				

(continued)

Document:

Document information for proper charting of this procedure.

Grading

Points earned	_____		
Points possible	_____	100	100
Percent grade (Points earned/Points possible)	_____		
Pass:	_____	❏ YES ❏ NO ❏ N/A	❏ YES ❏ NO ❏ N/A

Instructor Sign-Off

Instructor: _____ Date: _____

PROCEDURE 34-10
Applying Dental Bonding

Objective: Demonstrate the proper application process for dental bonding.

Equipment and Supplies Needed: rubber dam or cotton rolls (for isolation), bonding system with primer or conditioner/adhesive material, applicators—syringe, cotton pellets, small applicator tips or microbrush applicators, dappen dish, air/water syringe, curing light and shield, and timer.

Notes to the Student:

Skills Assessment Requirements

Read and familiarize yourself with the procedure; complete the minimum practice requirements. Document information when appropriate to demonstrate proper charting techniques. Complete each procedure within a reasonable amount of time, with a minimum of 85% accuracy.

POINT VALUE ♦ = 5 points ✳ = 10 points		PRACTICE TRIAL	GRADED TRIAL # 1	GRADED TRIAL # 2	NOTES:
1.✳✳	Etching has been completed. Move quickly to prevent bacterial contamination of the dentin.				
2. ✳✳	Apply primer if indicated.				
3. ✳✳	Apply bonding resin or composite restoration material. Set with curing light.				
4. ✳✳	Place small increments of bonding resin into the cavity preparation and set in layers until preparation is completely filled.				
5. ✳✳	Clean and disinfect all equipment.				

(continued)

Document:

Document information for proper charting of this procedure.

Grading

Points earned	_____		
Points possible	_____	100	100
Percent grade (Points earned/Points possible)	_____		
Pass:	_____	❏ YES ❏ NO ❏ N/A	❏ YES ❏ NO ❏ N/A

Instructor Sign-Off

Instructor: _____ Date: _____

Procedure 35-1
Mixing ZOE Type I Temporary Cement

Objective: Demonstrate how to properly disinfect a treatment room.

Equipment and Supplies Needed: cotton rolls (for isolation), ZOE two-paste system (temporary bond), treated paper mixing pad, and spatula.

Notes to the Student:

Skills Assessment Requirements

Read and familiarize yourself with the procedure; complete the minimum practice requirements. Document information when appropriate to demonstrate proper charting techniques. Complete each procedure within a reasonable amount of time, with a minimum of 85% accuracy.

POINT VALUE ♦ = 5 points ✳ = 10 points		PRACTICE TRIAL	GRADED TRIAL # 1	GRADED TRIAL # 2	NOTES:
1. ✳ ✳ ♦	Dispense equal lengths of accelerator and base on treated pad.				
2. ✳ ✳ ♦	Spatulate until homogenous.				
3. ✳ ✳ ♦	Place in temporary crown and seat.				
4. ✳ ✳ ♦	Clean and disinfect all equipment.				

(continued)

Document:

Enter the appropriate information in the chart below.

Grading

Points earned	_____		
Points possible	_____	100	100
Percent grade (Points earned/Points possible)	_____		
Pass:	_____	❏ YES ❏ NO ❏ N/A	❏ YES ❏ NO ❏ N/A

Instructor Sign-Off

Instructor: _____ Date: _____

Procedure 35-2
Mixing ZOE Type II Cement for Permanent Cementation

Objective: Demonstrate how to mix ZOE Type II Cement for permanent cementation.

Equipment and Supplies Needed: ZOE powder/liquid, treated paper pad or glass slab, small spatula, and 2 × 2 gauze pads.

Notes to the Student:

Skills Assessment Requirements

Read and familiarize yourself with the procedure; complete the minimum practice requirements. Document information when appropriate to demonstrate proper charting techniques. Complete each procedure within a reasonable amount of time, with a minimum of 85% accuracy.

POINT VALUE ◆ = 5 points ∗ = 10 points		PRACTICE TRIAL	GRADED TRIAL # 1	GRADED TRIAL # 2	NOTES:
1. ∗	Dispense powder and liquid according to manufacturer's directions.				
2. ∗	Divide the powder into increments.				
3. ∗	Dispense the liquid near the powder on the mixing pad.				
4. ∗	Blend the powder and liquid all at once.				
5. ∗ ∗	Check to ensure that the mix has a homogenous color.				
6. ∗	Be sure cavity preparation is dry and clean.				
7. ∗ ∗	The inside of the indirect restoration should be loaded and handed to the dentist.				
8. ∗	Clean and disinfect all equipment.				

(continued)

Document:

Enter the appropriate information in the chart below.

Grading

Points earned	_____		
Points possible	_____	100	100
Percent grade (Points earned/Points possible)	_____		
Pass:	_____	❏ YES ❏ NO ❏ N/A	❏ YES ❏ NO ❏ N/A

Instructor Sign-Off

Instructor: _____ Date: _____

Procedure 35-3
Mixing Zinc Phosphate for Permanent Cementation

Objective: Demonstrate how to mix zinc phosphate for permanent cementation.

Equipment and Supplies Needed: zinc phosphate powder and liquid with dispenser, glass slab, small spatula, and 2 × 2 gauze pads.

Notes to the Student:

Skills Assessment Requirements

Read and familiarize yourself with the procedure; complete the minimum practice requirements. Document information when appropriate to demonstrate proper charting techniques. Complete each procedure within a reasonable amount of time, with a minimum of 85% accuracy.

POINT VALUE ◆ = 5 points ∗ = 10 points		PRACTICE TRIAL	GRADED TRIAL # 1	GRADED TRIAL # 2	NOTES:
1. ∗	Measure powder according to manufacturer's directions and dispense the powder at one end of the slab and the liquid at the other end.				
2. ∗	Divide the powder into increments.				
3. ∗	Incorporate each powder increment into the liquid.				
4. ∗	Using the spatula, mix thoroughly, using large figure 8 type strokes over entire glass slab ensuring that each increment of powder is mixed thoroughly before adding another increment of powder.				
5. ∗	Test mix for correct cementation consistency. The cement should string up and break about one inch from the slab.				

(continued)

POINT VALUE ♦ = 5 points ✳ = 10 points		PRACTICE TRIAL	GRADED TRIAL # 1	GRADED TRIAL # 2	NOTES:
6. ✳	Fill the casting by gathering cement mix onto the spatula.				
7. ✳	Slide the edge of the spatula along the margin, allowing the cement to flow from the spatula into the casting, or use a Woodson for lining smaller castings.				
8. ✳	Place the tip of the spatula or Woodson into the restoration and move the mixture so that it completely covers all the inside walls.				
9. ✳	Turn the casting over in your palm and transfer to the dentist.				
10. ✳	Clean and disinfect all equipment.				

Document:

Enter the appropriate information in the chart below.

Grading

Points earned	_____		
Points possible	_____	100	100
Percent grade (Points earned/Points possible)	_____		
Pass:	_____	❑ YES ❑ NO ❑ N/A	❑ YES ❑ NO ❑ N/A

Instructor Sign-Off

Instructor: _____ Date: _____

Procedure 35-4
Mixing Polycarboxylate Cement

Objective: Demonstrate how to mix polycarboxylate cement.

Equipment and Supplies Needed: polycarboxylate powder/liquid and dispenser, oil-resistant treated paper pad or glass slab, small spatula, two 2 × 2 gauze pads.

Notes to the Student:

Skills Assessment Requirements

Read and familiarize yourself with the procedure; complete the minimum practice requirements. Document information when appropriate to demonstrate proper charting techniques. Complete each procedure within a reasonable amount of time, with a minimum of 85% accuracy.

POINT VALUE ♦ = 5 points ✳ = 10 points		PRACTICE TRIAL	GRADED TRIAL # 1	GRADED TRIAL # 2	NOTES:
1. ✳	Dispense powder and liquid according to the manufacturer's directions.				
2. ✳ ✳	Mix the powder into the liquid quickly with the flat side of the spatula, all at one time, to a homogenous consistency.				
3. ✳ ✳	Check to ensure that the consistency of the cement is correct. It should be somewhat thick and have a shiny, glossy surface.				
4. ✳	With the casting inner opening facing upward, gather cement mix onto the spatula and slide the edge of the spatula along the margin, allowing the cement to flow into the casting.				

(continued)

POINT VALUE ♦ = 5 points ✳ = 10 points		PRACTICE TRIAL	GRADED TRIAL # 1	GRADED TRIAL # 2	NOTES:
5. ✳	Place the tip of the spatula or a Woodson to move the mixture so that it completely covers all inside walls of the casting with a thin lining of cement.				
6. ✳	Turn the casting over in your palm and transfer it to the dentist.				
7. ✳	Transfer a cotton roll to the dentist for the patient to bite down on to help seat the casting and disburse the excess cement.				
8. ✳	Clean and disinfect all equipment.				

Document:

Enter the appropriate information in the chart below.

Grading

Points earned	_____		
Points possible	_____	100	100
Percent grade (Points earned/Points possible)	_____		
Pass:	_____	❏ YES ❏ NO ❏ N/A	❏ YES ❏ NO ❏ N/A

Instructor Sign-Off

Instructor: _____ Date: _____

Procedure 35-5

Mixing Glass Ionomer Cement

Objective: Demonstrate how to mix glass ionomer cement.

Equipment and Supplies Needed: glass ionomer cement powder and dispenser, glass ionomer cement liquid and dropper, treated oil-resistant paper pad or glass slab, small spatula, and 2 × 2 gauze pads.

Notes to the Student:

Skills Assessment Requirements

Read and familiarize yourself with the procedure; complete the minimum practice requirements. Document information when appropriate to demonstrate proper charting techniques. Complete each procedure within a reasonable amount of time, with a minimum of 85% accuracy.

POINT VALUE ♦ = 5 points ✳ = 10 points		PRACTICE TRIAL	GRADED TRIAL # 1	GRADED TRIAL # 2	NOTES:
1. ✳ ✳	Dispense the powder and liquid according to manufacturer's directions.				
2. ✳ ✳	Mix the powder into the liquid one increment at a time until all is mixed.				
3. ✳ ✳	Check to ensure that the consistency of the cement is correct. It should be somewhat thick and have a shiny, glossy surface.				
4. ✳ ✳	Place cement into the restoration.				
5. ✳ ✳	Clean and disinfect equipment.				

(continued)

Document:

Enter the appropriate information in the chart below.

Grading

Points earned	_____		
Points possible	_____	100	100
Percent grade (Points earned/Points possible)	_____		
Pass:	_____	❏ YES ❏ NO ❏ N/A	❏ YES ❏ NO ❏ N/A

Instructor Sign-Off

Instructor: _____ Date: _____

Procedure 35-6
Mixing Commercial Resin Cements

Objective: Demonstrate how to mix commercial resin cements.

Equipment and Supplies Needed: resin cement powder/liquid or syringe type, etching system and bonding system, applicators—syringe, cotton pellets, small applicator tips or microbrush applicators, plastic instrument, small spatula, treated oil-resistant paper pad, and 2 × 2 gauze pads.

Notes to the Student:

Skills Assessment Requirements

Read and familiarize yourself with the procedure; complete the minimum practice requirements. Document information when appropriate to demonstrate proper charting techniques. Complete each procedure within a reasonable amount of time, with a minimum of 85% accuracy.

POINT VALUE ♦ = 5 points * = 10 points		PRACTICE TRIAL	GRADED TRIAL # 1	GRADED TRIAL # 2	NOTES:
1. *	Apply etchant to enamel and dentin, rinse, air dry.				
2. * *	Apply a bonding adhesive to enamel and dentin, and dry gently.				
3. *	Light cure each surface for 10 seconds.				
4. * *	Apply primer to etched porcelain.				
5. * *	Dispense ratio of powder-to-liquid onto a mixing pad and mix. Apply a thin layer of mixture into the prepared surface of the restoration.				
6. *	Seat crown, light cure margins for 40 seconds.				
7. *	Clean and disinfect all equipment.				

(continued)

Document:

Enter the appropriate information in the chart below.

Grading

Points earned	_____		
Points possible	_____	100	100
Percent grade (Points earned/Points possible)	_____		
Pass:	_____	❏ YES ❏ NO ❏ N/A	❏ YES ❏ NO ❏ N/A

Instructor Sign-Off

Instructor: _____ Date: _____

Procedure 35-7
Removing Excess Cement

Objective: Demonstrate how to properly remove excess cement.

Equipment and Supplies Needed: mirror, explorer, and dental floss.

Notes to the Student:

Skills Assessment Requirements

Read and familiarize yourself with the procedure; complete the minimum practice requirements. Document information when appropriate to demonstrate proper charting techniques. Complete each procedure within a reasonable amount of time, with a minimum of 85% accuracy.

POINT VALUE ♦ = 5 points ✳ = 10 points		PRACTICE TRIAL	GRADED TRIAL # 1	GRADED TRIAL # 2	NOTES:
1. ✳ ✳ ♦	Use the explorer to examine remaining cement to ensure it has properly set.				
2. ✳ ✳ ♦	Carefully run the edge of the explorer in a horizontal direction just under the cement's edge, pulling the excessive material away from the tooth and casting.				
3. ✳ ✳ ♦	Tie a knot in the middle of the dental floss, and floss the contacts by passing the knot through both the mesial and distal contacts. This helps remove excess cement from the interproximal area.				
4. ✳ ✳ ♦	Clean and disinfect all equipment.				

(continued)

Document:

Enter the appropriate information in the chart below.

Grading

Points earned	_____		
Points possible	_____	100	100
Percent grade (Points earned/Points possible)	_____		
Pass:	_____	❏ YES ❏ NO ❏ N/A	❏ YES ❏ NO ❏ N/A

Instructor Sign-Off

Instructor: _____ Date: _____

Procedure 36-1
Obtaining an Alginate Impression

Objective: Demonstrate how to properly obtain an alginate impression.

Equipment and Supplies Needed: alginate canister, plastic measuring cup for powder, plastic measuring cup for water, flexible rubber bowl, flexible broad blade lab spatula, paper towels, proper size sterile trays, water, small plastic bag, and utility wax (if necessary).

Notes to the Student:

Skills Assessment Requirements

Read and familiarize yourself with the procedure; complete the minimum practice requirements. Document information when appropriate to demonstrate proper charting techniques. Complete each procedure within a reasonable amount of time, with a minimum of 85% accuracy.

POINT VALUE ◆ = 5 points ✳ = 10 points		PRACTICE TRIAL	GRADED TRIAL # 1	GRADED TRIAL # 2	NOTES:
1. ◆	Tumble the container to gently fluff powder. Explain the procedure to the patient.				
2. ✳	Select and/or prepare suitable impression tray. Rigid rim-lock or perforated trays are recommended. Try the mandibular and maxillary trays in the patient's mouth to ensure proper fit and comfort.				
3. ◆	Dip supplied scoop lightly into powder until scoop is full. Do not pack scoop. Tap scoop against rim to ensure that a full measure without voids has been scooped out. Scrape excess off with spatula to achieve level scoop.				

(continued)

	POINT VALUE ♦ = 5 points ✳ = 10 points	PRACTICE TRIAL	GRADED TRIAL # 1	GRADED TRIAL # 2	NOTES:
4. ♦	Empty two scoops of powder into a clean dry mixing bowl for the mandibular impression, and three scoops of powder for a maxillary impression. For a single-use pouch, tear open and empty its contents into the bowl.				
5. ♦	For two scoops, add two-thirds measurement of the alginate powder measuring cup of room temperature water. For each three scoops of powder, add one full measure of water so that all three increments on the water measuring cup are used.				
6. ✳	Mix water and powder carefully until all powder is wet. Once all powder is incorporated, continue to spatulate in a vigorous fashion. Do not whip or stir the alginate material. The spatula should be flattened using pressure against the bowl to reduce incorporating air. Spatulate regular set material for one minute and fast set material for 45 seconds.				
7. ♦	Once the alginate appears homogenous and creamy (i.e., without lumps), put it into the tray. To minimize the trapping of air, wipe the loaded spatula against the tray rim, allowing material to flow from the spatula into the tray. Load the mandibular tray from the lingual sides and use the flat side of the blade to condense the material firmly in the tray. Place the majority of the alginate in the anterior portion of the tray.				

POINT VALUE ♦ = 5 points ∗ = 10 points		PRACTICE TRIAL	GRADED TRIAL # 1	GRADED TRIAL # 2	NOTES:
8. ♦	Use a wet finger to smooth the alginate surface, to eliminate any air pockets trapped near the surface, and to remove excess material from posterior areas. Ask the patient to relax and take a deep breath through the nose and to keep breathing through the nose during the entire procedure. An optional method is to use a finger to place some alginate material on the occlusal surfaces of the teeth first.				
9. ∗	Insert filled tray into the mouth. Use the side of the tray to push one side of the cheek out of the way and a finger on the other side to do the same thing, and then slide the tray into the mouth. For an impression of the mandibular arch, ask the patient to lift the tongue as the tray is inserted. Press the tray gently into position centered over the arch, placing the posterior portion first to form a seal so the material flows forward and not down the throat.				
10. ∗	Push firmly up when seating the maxillary tray and firmly down when seating the mandibular tray. Do not overseat or press the tray to touch the teeth. Immediately lift the patient's lips loosely over the tray so impressions of the oral vestibule and frenula will be captured. Hold the seated tray immovable for one minute or until alginate is no longer sticky.				
11. ∗	Once the material has set, gently break the seal by moving the tray up and down or using the side of a finger at the periphery. Snap the tray loose from the arch and remove the impression tray from the patient's mouth, protecting the opposite arch with a finger.				

(continued)

Procedure 36-1 **643**

POINT VALUE ◆ = 5 points ✳ = 10 points		PRACTICE TRIAL	GRADED TRIAL # 1	GRADED TRIAL # 2	NOTES:
12. ✳	Check for and remove any residual material from the mouth, between the teeth, or from around the patient's face. Give the patient a damp tissue and have her or him rinse with warm water.				
13. ✳	Rinse impression thoroughly under running water. Spray with disinfectant solution, wrap in a wet paper towel, and place in a labeled plastic bag before pouring. Do not store impression submerged in water.				

Document:

Enter the appropriate information in the chart below.

Grading

Points earned	_____		
Points possible	_____	100	100
Percent grade (Points earned/Points possible)	_____		
Pass:	_____	❑ YES ❑ NO ❑ N/A	❑ YES ❑ NO ❑ N/A

Instructor Sign-Off

Instructor: _____ Date: _____

Procedure 36-2
Obtaining a Vinyl Polysiloxane Cartridge Single-Phase Impression

Objective: Demonstrate how to properly obtain a vinyl polysiloxane impression.

Equipment and Supplies Needed: metal tray, firm disposable tray or custom tray, adhesive, low-viscosity cartridge material, high-viscosity cartridge material, two cartridge dispensing guns, two cartridge syringe tips, one intraoral tip, and 2 × 2 gauze squares.

Notes to the Student:

Skills Assessment Requirements

Read and familiarize yourself with the procedure; complete the minimum practice requirements. Document information when appropriate to demonstrate proper charting techniques. Complete each procedure within a reasonable amount of time, with a minimum of 85% accuracy.

POINT VALUE ♦ = 5 points ✴ = 10 points		PRACTICE TRIAL	GRADED TRIAL # 1	GRADED TRIAL # 2	NOTES:
1. ♦	Select and prepare suitable tray. Use rigid trays of sufficient size to provide at least a 2- to 3-mm thickness of impression material. Dual-arch trays may be used to record the opposing dentition and bite registration of the two arches.				
2. ✴	Brush a thin layer of tray adhesive onto the rigid tray following manufacturer's instructions.				
3. ♦	Raise the release lever vertically upward on the cartridge dispensing gun, while simultaneously pulling the plunger all the way back in the dispenser handle.				

(continued)

POINT VALUE ♦ = 5 points ∗ = 10 points		PRACTICE TRIAL	GRADED TRIAL # 1	GRADED TRIAL # 2	NOTES:
4. ♦	Load the cartridge by opening the cartridge lock using the top clasp. Orient and insert the cartridge with notches aligned as necessary. Close the top clasp to lock the cartridge into the dispenser gun.				
5. ∗	Remove the cartridge cap by turning it 90 degrees in the counterclockwise direction. The cap can be replaced on the cartridge when storing after initial use, or the used mixing tip can be left in place until the next use after disinfection to serve as a self-sealing cap.				
6. ∗	Dispense a small amount of base and catalyst material onto a 2 × 2 gauze square before installing the mixing tip to ensure an even flow from the cartridge. Use gentle pressure. Be sure a mixed material plug does not exist. If a plug exists, clear it away with an instrument. Wipe away excess material from the cartridge carefully so the base and catalyst do not cross-contaminate each other and cause obstruction of the nozzle.				
7. ♦	Install a mixing tip in both the light-body and heavy-body cartridge by lining up the notch on the outside rim of the mixing tip with the notch on the cartridge flange. Ensure the holes are aligned properly. Turn the tip to align it in the cap.				
8. ♦	When notches are aligned, turn the mixing cap 90 degrees in the clockwise direction to lock it in place. Attach the intraoral tip to the end of the light-body mixing tip for direct intraoral syringing around the gingival sulcus.				

POINT VALUE ♦ = 5 points ✳ = 10 points		PRACTICE TRIAL	GRADED TRIAL # 1	GRADED TRIAL # 2	NOTES:
9. ✳	Clean the tooth with an air/water spray. Remove excess water with suction. Do not desiccate or overdry the tooth.				
10. ♦	The assistant should pass the dispensing gun with the wash material and intraoral tip to the dentist and receive the cotton rolls that were used to keep the working area dry.				
11. ✳	The assistant dispenses tray material into the tray, ensuring that the least amount of air has been incorporated into the material. For best results the dispensing tip should be submerged in the impression material during extrusion to prevent introducing air bubbles into the mix. The tray must be loaded within 35 seconds from the time of first syringing the wash material.				
12. ♦	At the same time as the assistant is loading the tray, the dentist injects syringe material into any existing anatomy and continues syringing around the preparation until it is completely covered with syringe material.				
13. ♦	The assistant passes the loaded tray to the dentist and receives the cartridge gun. The dentist or assistant holds the tray in position in the patient's mouth until the material is firmly set. The minimum removal time for fast set is three minutes from the start of the mix. Higher temperatures reduce work times, and lower temperatures increase the time.				

(continued)

POINT VALUE ♦ = 5 points ✳ = 10 points		PRACTICE TRIAL	GRADED TRIAL # 1	GRADED TRIAL # 2	NOTES:
14. ✳	The impression should be removed from the mouth by pulling slowly to break the seal, and then snapped out along the long axis of the tooth. The patient's mouth should be rinsed and the impression should be rinsed under cold water and disinfected according to manufacturer's instructions.				

Document:

Enter the appropriate information in the chart below.

Grading

Points earned	_____		
Points possible	_____	100	100
Percent grade (Points earned/Points possible)	_____		
Pass:	_____	❑ YES ❑ NO ❑ N/A	❑ YES ❑ NO ❑ N/A

Instructor Sign-Off

Instructor: _____ Date: _____

Procedure 36-3
Obtaining a Vinyl Polysiloxane Bite Registration

Objective: Demonstrate how to properly obtain a vinyl polysiloxane bite registration.

Equipment and Supplies Needed: bite registration cartridge material, cartridge dispensing gun, one cartridge syringe tip, vinyl gloves, and one intraoral tip.

Notes to the Student:

Skills Assessment Requirements

Read and familiarize yourself with the procedure; complete the minimum practice requirements. Document information when appropriate to demonstrate proper charting techniques. Complete each procedure within a reasonable amount of time, with a minimum of 85% accuracy.

POINT VALUE ♦ = 5 points ✳ = 10 points		PRACTICE TRIAL	GRADED TRIAL # 1	GRADED TRIAL # 2	NOTES:
1. ✳	Ensure the patient is sitting in an upright position. Ask the patient to close her back teeth together. Tell the patient that this is how you need her to close with the bite registration material in place. Observe how both sides of the arches occlude.				
2. ✳✳	Place the bite registration material cartridge into the dispensing gun.				
3. ✳✳	Dispense material onto the occlusal surface of the patient's arch starting in the posterior molars on one side and continuing to syringe the material onto the anterior teeth and around to the molars on the opposite side. A full-arch bite registration will ensure an accurate occlusal record.				

(continued)

POINT VALUE ♦ = 5 points ✳ = 10 points		PRACTICE TRIAL	GRADED TRIAL #1	GRADED TRIAL #2	NOTES:
4. ✳	Have the patient close her mouth, or guide the patient's jaw into the proper position.				
5. ✳	Most vinyl polysiloxane bite registration materials will set in 20 to 30 seconds.				
6. ✳ ✳	Remove the bite registration from the mouth. Rinse the material, dry, and disinfect according to manufacturer's instructions.				
7. ✳	Be sure to avoid contact with any chemicals known to inhibit setting of vinyl polysiloxane such as latex gloves and acrylic residues. Wear vinyl gloves during this procedure.				

Document:

Enter the appropriate information in the chart below.

Grading

Points earned	_____		
Points possible	_____	100	100
Percent grade (Points earned/Points possible)	_____		
Pass:	_____	❑ YES ❑ NO ❑ N/A	❑ YES ❑ NO ❑ N/A

Instructor Sign-Off

Instructor: _____ Date: _____

Procedure 37-1
Pouring Dental Models Using the Inverted Pour Method

Objective: Demonstrate how to pour dental models using the inverted pour method.

Equipment and Supplies Needed: maxillary or mandibular alginate impression, flexible rubber mixing bowl, lab spatula, tile or glass slab, plaster, water, and vibrator.

Notes to the Student:

Skills Assessment Requirements

Read and familiarize yourself with the procedure; complete the minimum practice requirements. Document information when appropriate to demonstrate proper charting techniques. Complete each procedure within a reasonable amount of time, with a minimum of 85% accuracy.

POINT VALUE ♦ = 5 points ✳ = 10 points		PRACTICE TRIAL	GRADED TRIAL # 1	GRADED GRADED # 2	NOTES:
1. ♦	Measure room temperature water and weigh the powder. Add water to a clean, dry, rubber bowl. Add powder to the water and use a clean wide lab spatula to gently but quickly incorporate all the powder evenly into the mix until it is uniform and creamy. Avoid whipping the mix because whipping could incorporate air bubbles into the model, which is undesirable.				
2. ✳	Turn the vibrator on. Vibrate the mixing bowl for 30 seconds to one minute to bring any air pockets to the surface.				

(continued)

POINT VALUE ♦ = 5 points ✳ = 10 points		PRACTICE TRIAL	GRADED TRIAL # 1	GRADED TRIAL # 2	NOTES:
3. ♦	Hold the impression tray by the handle so that it rests on the vibrator. Place a small amount of plaster onto the impression at one end of the arch and let it quickly flow to the other side of the arch. Place another small amount of mixed plaster into the impression, ensuring that each tooth depression is filled in as gravity is used to cause the material to move around the impression. Touch the impression to the vibrator each time additional plaster is added.				
4. ✳	After filling all teeth and covering critical surfaces of the impression, progressively larger amounts of the mix should be added. The intensity of the vibrator should be enough to cause the material to flow across the surface of the impression but not so intense that it creates bubbles.				
5. ✳	Continue filling the impression to a level slightly above the height of the impression walls. Do not overfill. The plaster should not flow over the outside of the tray because it will interfere with separating the model from the tray.				
6. ♦	Set the impression down and turn off the vibrator. Using the spatula, place all of the remaining plaster from the bowl onto the tile or glass slab. If the plaster is thin, a small amount of powder may be mixed into the base material to make it stronger. Shape the base portion, utilizing the spatula to flatten it into an even patty with flat sides and just a larger width than the impression.				

POINT VALUE ♦ = 5 points ✳ = 10 points		PRACTICE TRIAL	GRADED TRIAL # 1	GRADED TRIAL # 2	NOTES:
7. ♦	Invert the impression with the anatomic portion of plaster and place it onto the plaster patty. Bring up the posterior portion of the base material to meet the anatomic portion and smooth out the side and front of the base. Do not bring the sides of the base up to the tray because that could cause the tray to become embedded and locked into the base. For a mandibular cast use a narrow spatula to smooth and contour the tongue area of the base to ensure that it is flat while the plaster is still soft.				

Document:

Enter the appropriate information in the chart below.

Grading

Points earned	_____		
Points possible	_____	50	50
Percent grade (Points earned/Points possible)	_____		
Pass:	_____	❏ YES ❏ NO ❏ N/A	❏ YES ❏ NO ❏ N/A

Instructor Sign-Off

Instructor:_____ Date: _____

Procedure 37-2
Trimming Diagnostic Cast Models

Objective: Demonstrate how to trim diagnostic cast models.

Equipment and Supplies Needed: cast stone or plaster models, pencil, laboratory knife, bowl of water, eye protection, and model trimmer.

Notes to the Student:

Skills Assessment Requirements

Read and familiarize yourself with the procedure; complete the minimum practice requirements. Document information when appropriate to demonstrate proper charting techniques. Complete each procedure within a reasonable amount of time, with a minimum of 85% accuracy.

POINT VALUE ◆ = 5 points ✳ = 10 points		PRACTICE TRIAL	GRADED TRIAL # 1	GRADED TRIAL # 2	NOTES:
1. ◆	After the heat from the setting process dissipates completely (approximately 45 minutes), trim any excess gypsum material from the outside of the tray with a lab knife and carefully separate the cast from the impression. Do not force the tray, or teeth may be broken during the process. The knife should be placed between the gypsum material and the tray to gently pry it loose all the way around the tray before separating the tray from the model.				
2. ✳	Soak stone casts in room temperature water for at least 30 minutes before trimming.				

(continued)

POINT VALUE ♦ = 5 points ✳ = 10 points		PRACTICE TRIAL	GRADED TRIAL # 1	GRADED TRIAL # 2	NOTES:
3. ✳	Mark the maxillary cast with trimming marks between the central incisors, at the center of the cuspids, and posterior of the tuberosities. The mandibular cast will be trimmed to the shape of the maxillary cast.				
4. ✳	Put on eye protection and turn on the water to the model trimmer. Adjust water as needed to keep the wheel wet and turn on the model trimmer motor. Begin trimming the maxillary cast by placing the model onto the trimmer table and cut just enough on the posterior to create a flat surface. Cut to approximately ¼ inch behind the maxillary tuberosities.				
5. ✳	Set the maxillary model on the counter to determine how even the base is and then place the model on the trimmer with the base of the model against the blade and put pressure where needed to even the base on the maxillary model. Make sure that when the anatomic portion of the model is placed on the table or counter the art portion is parallel with the countertop. (See top left image from page 590.)				
6. ✳	Cut the sides of the maxillary model using the cuspid as a guide so that the cut is parallel to the alveolar ridge, flared at the molar areas, and approximately ¼ inch wide.				
7. ♦	Turn the model using the lateral incisors and the line between the central incisors as a guide and trim until there is a point at the canine eminence. Do the same on the next front cut, watching as you create a point between the central incisors and a point at the cuspid.				

POINT VALUE ♦ = 5 points ✳ = 10 points		PRACTICE TRIAL	GRADED TRIAL # 1	GRADED TRIAL # 2	NOTES:
8. ✳	Trim the posterior of the mandibular model to at least ¼ inch beyond the retromolar pads, then trim to even the base. Whichever model has the longest arch, the maxillary or mandibular, will be the guide for making the posterior cut even. Do not cut too close or the maxillary and mandibular landmarks will be ruined.				
9. ✳	Put the maxillary and mandibular models together in proper occlusion. A bite registration may be necessary to provide an accurate occlusal relationship.				
10. ♦	Place both models together and, using the maxillary cuts as a guide, trim the two sides and two front cuts of the mandibular model.				
11. ♦	Separate the models and round the anterior portion of the mandibular model, keeping the canine eminence points created by the maxillary model guide.				
12. ♦	Put the two models together again in proper occlusion and trim the heel on each side of the model to approximately ½ inch at an angle, ensuring that the maxillary tuberosities and mandibular retromolar areas are unharmed. (*Hint:* If the first side cuts are kept wide enough, these cuts will not damage the posterior arch landmarks.)				
13. ♦	With the models together ensure that the posterior cuts are still even. Rinse both models well making sure that any debris from trimming is removed from the models or it will dry and create an inaccurate surface. Use a soft toothbrush and a moderate stream of water to gently remove any filing debris, but do not scrub the model because it may destroy the model and create holes—especially on plaster models.				

(continued)

POINT VALUE ♦ = 5 points ✳ = 10 points		PRACTICE TRIAL	GRADED TRIAL # 1	GRADED TRIAL # 2	NOTES:
14.	Deposits from saliva bubbles should be broken off the surface of the models with a small instrument. Be extremely careful not to cause damage to the models. Rinse the models well again, dry, and label each model with the patient's name and date. Run water through the model trimmer to clean the pipe, and wipe down the outside of the trimmer.				

Document:

Enter the appropriate information in the chart below.

Grading

Points earned	_____		
Points possible	_____	100	100
Percent grade (Points earned/Points possible)	_____		
Pass:	_____	❏ YES ❏ NO ❏ N/A	❏ YES ❏ NO ❏ N/A

Instructor Sign-Off

Instructor:_____ Date: _____

Procedure 37-3
Curing a VLC Impression Tray

Objective: Demonstrate how to cure a VLC impression tray.

Equipment and Supplies Needed: cast stone model, pencil, baseplate wax, laboratory knife, petroleum jelly, opaque container of visible light cure resin, paper cup, plastic measuring vial, bowl of water, and crown and bridge scissors.

Notes to the Student:

Skills Assessment Requirements

Read and familiarize yourself with the procedure; complete the minimum practice requirements. Document information when appropriate to demonstrate proper charting techniques. Complete each procedure within a reasonable amount of time, with a minimum of 85% accuracy.

POINT VALUE ♦ = 5 points ✳ = 10 points		PRACTICE TRIAL	GRADED TRIAL # 1	GRADED TRIAL # 2	NOTES:
1. ♦	Outline the casts for the custom edentulous tray. Warm a piece of pink baseplate wax and apply it over the tissue-bearing areas of the cast. Trim wax layer to the tray outline. Place additional wax in any area that appears to have an undercut, which could get filled in with custom tray material and not allow it to release.				
2. ✳	For stops, remove a small amount of wax from the residual ridge area at the midline and on each molar area with a blunt instrument. These will become tissue stops.				
3. ♦	Coat the wax with a layer of model release agent or petroleum jelly.				

(continued)

POINT VALUE ♦ = 5 points ✻ = 10 points		PRACTICE TRIAL	GRADED TRIAL #1	GRADED TRIAL #2	NOTES:
4. ✻	Remove a sheet of visible light cure (VLC) material from its protective pouch. Pull off a small piece and press into each of the holes in the wax spacers to serve as tissue stops. Lay the rest of the VLC material over the tissue surface of the cast. Form into a two-inch wafer for a maxillary tray and mold into a U-shape for a mandibular tray.				
5. ✻	Give the material a moment to slump, or droop, onto the impression surface of the cast.				
6. ✻	With wet or petroleum jellycoated fingers, gently press material into place with no voids, onto the palate, the periphery rolls, and/or the lingual areas. Be sure the retromolar areas distal of the mandibular ridge and the maxillary tuberosity are completely covered.				
7. ♦	Using a sharp instrument and/or scissors, trim excess material up to the custom tray outline. The material may be cut lightly beyond the outline and trimmed back after curing. Never trim the custom tray short of the outline on the cast.				
8. ♦	Fabricate handles. Be careful because they may slump. Avoid placing tray handle material where it might cause distortion of the frenum and lip.				
9. ✻	Put the cast with tray material into the visible light cure unit and process for two minutes.				
10. ✻	Remove the cast and tray from the unit. Separate the cast and custom tray. Carefully remove the wax from inside the custom tray.				

POINT VALUE ♦ = 5 points ∗ = 10 points		PRACTICE TRIAL	GRADED TRIAL # 1	GRADED TRIAL # 2	NOTES:
11. ∗	Return the tray to the curing unit and process for an additional six minutes.				
12. ∗	Adjust and finish the borders of the tray to the outline drawn on the cast. Scrub tray with soap and water.				

Document:

Enter the appropriate information in the chart below.

Grading

Points earned	_____		
Points possible	_____	100	100
Percent grade (Points earned/Points possible)	_____		
Pass:	_____	❏ YES ❏ NO ❏ N/A	❏ YES ❏ NO ❏ N/A

Instructor Sign-Off

Instructor: _____ Date: _____

Procedure 37-4
Constructing an Acrylic Custom Tray

Objective: Demonstrate how to construct an acrylic custom tray.

Equipment and Supplies Needed: cast stone model, pencil, baseplate wax, laboratory knife, petroleum jelly, bowl of water, auto-polymerization acrylic tray and baseplate material powder and liquid, paper cup, plastic measuring vial, and slow speed handpiece with acrylic bur.

Notes to the Student:

Skills Assessment Requirements

Read and familiarize yourself with the procedure; complete the minimum practice requirements. Document information when appropriate to demonstrate proper charting techniques. Complete each procedure within a reasonable amount of time, with a minimum of 85% accuracy.

POINT VALUE ♦ = 5 points ∗ = 10 points		PRACTICE TRIAL	GRADED TRIAL # 1	GRADED TRIAL # 2	NOTES:
1. ∗	For spacer, adapt one thickness of baseplate wax to the model. For stops remove small amount of wax from ridge area with a blunt instrument.				
2. ∗	Soak model in room temperature water.				
3. ∗	Fluff powder. Add one full measurement of powder to one vial of liquid in paper mixing cup. Mix with wood tongue depressor for one minute.				
4. ∗	When mixture becomes stringy, remove and incorporate cold water. This will reduce exothermic heat when curing and prevent sticking.				

(continued)

POINT VALUE ♦ = 5 points ✳ = 10 points		PRACTICE TRIAL	GRADED TRIAL # 1	GRADED TRIAL # 2	NOTES:
5. ✳	With wet or petroleum jelly-coated fingers, knead for 30 seconds and then form into a 2-inch disc for a maxillary tray. For a mandibular tray, form into a U-shape. Save a small piece of the mix for a handle.				
6. ✳	Place wafer on palatal area, overlapping the ridge, and gently push over the ridge to the periphery. Push excess toward posterior until proper and even thickness is formed. Trim excess with a knife.				
7. ✳	Use the saved piece of material to form a handle and press into position with a drop of acrylic liquid. The handle, if used, should be positioned in the midline of the tray at an angle to avoid interfering with the upper lip or frenula.				
8. ✳	If retention holes are desired, use a blunt instrument to perforate before the material sets.				
9.	Allow to cure for three minutes. To accelerate cure, place in hot water. To prevent wax spacer from melting, place in cool water.				
10. ✳	An optional technique is to place a piece of foil on the model between the wax and the acrylic material. This prevents the wax from melting. If making stops, the dental assistant must remember to match cuts in the foil to the cuts in the wax spacer.				
11. ✳	Trim with acrylic bur. Polish or flame to smooth edges if desired. Use acrylic bur to remove material at frenum landmarks.				

Document:

Enter the appropriate information in the chart below.

Grading

Points earned	_____		
Points possible	_____		
Percent grade (Points earned/Points possible)	_____	100	100
Pass:	_____	❏ YES ❏ NO ❏ N/A	❏ YES ❏ NO ❏ N/A

Instructor Sign-Off

Instructor: _____ Date: _____

Procedure 38-1

Assisting with a Class I Composite Restoration

Objective: Demonstrate how to assist during a Class I composite restoration.

Equipment and Supplies Needed: restorative tray for appropriate dental material to be used including basic setup, hand-cutting instruments, amalgam carrier, condensers, burnishers, carvers, plastic instrument, articulating paper holder; local anesthetic setup (some patients do not require anesthetic), dental dam setup (some doctors do not use the dental dam), high volume evacuator (HVE) and saliva ejector, high-speed and low-speed rotary handpieces, burs—often in a block (each dentist has preferences), cotton products (pellets, rolls, 2 × 2 gauze squares, and dry angles), dental liner, base, bonding agent and caries indicator dye, permanent restorative material of choice, articulating paper, polishing items, and dental floss.

Notes to the Student:

Skills Assessment Requirements

Read and familiarize yourself with the procedure; complete the minimum practice requirements. Document information when appropriate to demonstrate proper charting techniques. Complete each procedure within a reasonable amount of time, with a minimum of 85% accuracy.

POINT VALUE ♦ = 5 points ✳ = 10 points		PRACTICE TRIAL	GRADED TRIAL # 1	GRADED TRIAL # 2	NOTES:
1. ♦	Deliver mouth mirror and explorer to dentist. (Dentist must examine tooth to be restored.)				
2. ♦	Assist dentist in the delivery of anesthetic, topical and local.				
3. ♦	Place isolation items, cotton rolls, or dental dam (state permitting).				
4. ♦	Deliver mouth mirror to dentist and inform dentist of the type of bur on the handpiece.				
5. ♦	Adjust the light, retract the patient's cheek or tongue, and use the HVE and air/water syringe to keep the working area clear for the dentist.				

(continued)

POINT VALUE ♦ = 5 points * = 10 points		PRACTICE TRIAL	GRADED TRIAL # 1	GRADED TRIAL # 2	NOTES:
6. ♦	Transfer the necessary instruments to the dentist during the preparation as needed.				
7. ♦	Rinse and dry prepared tooth for the dentist to evaluate.				
8. ♦	Deliver caries indicator dye to the preparation, wait, rinse, and dry. (Repeat until tooth is clear of caries.)				
9. ♦	If the preparation requires a base or liner, mix and deliver to the dentist.				
10. ♦	Deliver etch and rinse. Then deliver bond and light cure.				
11. ♦	Place an appropriate amount of composite resin on a paper pad and protect from light.				
12. ♦	Deliver the composite to the dentist with the composite placement instrument of the dentist's choice. The dentist will add material in increments, each followed by use of the curing light.				
13. ♦	The dentist will use a high-speed handpiece with finishing burs to carve the restoration.				
14. ♦	The dental assistant will continue to use the HVE to remove particles and for retraction during the continued occlusal adjustments and finishing of the composite.				
15. ♦	The assistant must still use the HVE to remove any pieces of composite as well as continue to retract the cheek, lip, or tongue.				
16. ♦	Remove all cotton and the dental dam. Rinse and dry the area.				

POINT VALUE ♦ = 5 points ✳ = 10 points		PRACTICE TRIAL	GRADED TRIAL # 1	GRADED TRIAL # 2	NOTES:
17. ♦	Place articulating paper between the maxillary and mandibular teeth to check the occlusion. The dentist will continue to adjust the occlusion until the bite is correct. Heavy colored marks will appear on the restoration in areas needing adjustment.				
18. ♦	Inform the patient the composite material is cured and chewing is possible immediately.				
19. ♦	If the patient received anesthetic, inform her to avoid chewing until the anesthetic is gone so as to avoid biting her cheeks or tongue.				
20. ♦	Inform the patient to call the office if she finds her occlusion is incorrect. She will need to return to the office for an occlusal adjustment.				

Document:

Enter the appropriate information in the chart below.

Grading

Points earned	_____		
Points possible	_____	100	100
Percent grade (Points earned/Points possible)	_____		
Pass:	_____	❏ YES ❏ NO ❏ N/A	❏ YES ❏ NO ❏ N/A

Instructor Sign-Off

Instructor: _____ Date: _____

Procedure 38-1
Assisting with a Class I Amalgam Restoration

Objective: Demonstrate how to assist during a Class I amalgam restoration.

Equipment and Supplies Needed: restorative tray for appropriate dental material to be used including basic setup, hand-cutting instruments, amalgam carrier, condensers, burnishers, carvers, plastic instrument, articulating paper holder; local anesthetic setup (some patients do not require anesthetic), dental dam setup (some doctors do not use the dental dam), high volume evacuator (HVE), saliva ejector, high-speed and low-speed rotary handpieces, burs—often in a block (each dentist has preferences), cotton products (pellets, rolls, 2 × 2 gauze squares, dry angles), dental liner, base, bonding agent, caries indicator dye, permanent restorative material of choice, articulating paper, polishing items, and dental floss.

Notes to the Student:

Skills Assessment Requirements

Read and familiarize yourself with the procedure; complete the minimum practice requirements. Document information when appropriate to demonstrate proper charting techniques. Complete each procedure within a reasonable amount of time, with a minimum of 85% accuracy.

POINT VALUE ♦ = 5 points ✳ = 10 points		PRACTICE TRIAL	GRADED TRIAL # 1	GRADED TRIAL # 2	NOTES:
1. ♦	Deliver mouth mirror and explorer to dentist. (Dentist must examine tooth to be restored.)				
2. ♦	Assist dentist in the delivery of anesthetic, topical and local.				
3. ♦	Place isolation items, cotton rolls, or dental dam (state permitting).				
4. ♦	Deliver mouth mirror to dentist and inform dentist of the type of bur on the handpiece.				
5. ♦	Adjust the light, retract the patient's cheek or tongue, and use the HVE and air/water syringe to keep the working area clear for the dentist.				

(continued)

	POINT VALUE ♦ = 5 points ∗ = 10 points	PRACTICE TRIAL	GRADED TRIAL # 1	GRADED TRIAL # 2	NOTES:
6. ♦	Transfer the necessary instruments to the dentist during the preparation as needed.				
7. ♦	Rinse and dry prepared tooth for the dentist to evaluate.				
8. ♦	Deliver caries indicator dye to the preparation, wait, rinse, and dry. (Repeat until tooth is clear of caries.)				
9. ♦	If the preparation requires a base or liner, mix and deliver to the dentist.				
10. ♦	Activate amalgam capsule and triturate.				
11. ♦	Fill the smaller end of the amalgam carrier and transfer to the dentist. The dentist may want both ends of the carrier filled. Alternate the condenser with the carrier. Continue to supply the dentist with more amalgam until the preparation is slightly overfilled.				
12. ♦	Exchange the condenser for the burnisher so the dentist can burnish the excess mercury to the tooth surface.				
13. ♦	Deliver the carving instruments of dentist's choice until the restoration is complete.				
14. ♦	The dental assistant will continue to use the HVE to remove particles and for retraction during the continued carving and burnishing.				
15. ♦	The assistant must still use the HVE to remove any pieces of amalgam as well as continue to retract the cheek, lip, or tongue.				
16. ♦	Remove all cotton and the dental dam. Rinse and dry the area.				

POINT VALUE ♦ = 5 points ✳ = 10 points		PRACTICE TRIAL	GRADED TRIAL # 1	GRADED TRIAL # 2	NOTES:
17. ♦	Place articulating paper between the maxillary and mandibular teeth to check the occlusion. The patient should bite down carefully and gently so as to not fracture the new restoration. The dentist will continue to adjust the occlusion until the bite is correct. Heavy colored marks will appear on the restoration in areas needing adjustment.				
18. ♦	Inform the patient not to chew on that side of his mouth. The amalgam will continue to harden for several hours after placement.				
19. ♦	If the patient received anesthetic, inform him to avoid chewing until the anesthetic is gone so as to avoid biting his cheeks or tongue.				
20. ♦	Inform the patient to call the office if he finds his occlusion is incorrect. He will need to return to the office for an occlusal adjustment.				

Document:

Enter the appropriate information in the chart below.

(continued)

Grading

Points earned	_____		
Points possible	_____	100	100
Percent grade (Points earned/Points possible)	_____		
Pass:	_____	❑ YES ❑ NO ❑ N/A	❑ YES ❑ NO ❑ N/A

Instructor Sign-Off

Instructor: _____ Date: _____

Procedure 38-2
Assisting with a Class II Composite Restoration

Objective: Demonstrate how to assist with a Class II composite restoration.

Equipment and Supplies Needed: restorative tray for appropriate dental material to be used including basic setup; hand-cutting instruments, amalgam carrier, condensers, burnishers, carvers; plastic instrument, articulating paper holder; local anesthetic setup (some patients do not require anesthetic), dental dam setup (some doctors do not use the dental dam), high volume evacuator (HVE), saliva ejector, high-speed and low-speed rotary handpieces, burs—often in a block (each dentist has preferences), cotton products (pellets, rolls, 2 × 2 gauze squares, dry angles), matrix system setup, dental liner, base, bonding agent, caries indicator dye, permanent restorative material of choice, articulating paper, polishing items, and dental floss.

Notes to the Student:

Skills Assessment Requirements

Read and familiarize yourself with the procedure; complete the minimum practice requirements. Document information when appropriate to demonstrate proper charting techniques. Complete each procedure within a reasonable amount of time, with a minimum of 85% accuracy.

POINT VALUE ♦ = 5 points ✳ = 10 points		PRACTICE TRIAL	GRADED TRIAL # 1	GRADED TRIAL # 2	NOTES:
1. ♦	Deliver mouth mirror and explorer to dentist. (Dentist must examine tooth to be restored.)				
2. ♦	Assist dentist in the delivery of anesthetic, topical and local.				
3. ♦	Place isolation items, cotton rolls, dry angle, or dental dam (state permitting).				
4. ♦	Deliver mouth mirror to dentist and inform dentist of the type of bur on the handpiece.				
5. ♦	Adjust the light, retract the patient's cheek or tongue, and use the HVE and air/water syringe to keep the working area clear for the dentist.				

(continued)

POINT VALUE ♦ = 5 points ✳ = 10 points		PRACTICE TRIAL	GRADED TRIAL # 1	GRADED TRIAL # 2	NOTES:
6. ♦	Transfer the necessary instruments to the dentist during the preparation as needed.				
7. ♦	Rinse and dry prepared tooth for the dentist to evaluate.				
8. ♦	Deliver caries indicator dye to the preparation, wait, rinse, and dry. (Repeat until tooth is clear of caries.)				
9. ♦	Deliver to the dentist the matrix system of the dentist's choice. If state regulations permit, the dental assistant may place the matrix system.				
10. ♦	If the preparation requires a base or liner, mix and deliver to the dentist.				
11. ♦	Deliver etch and rinse. Then deliver bond and light cure.				
12. ♦	Place an appropriate amount of composite resin on a paper pad and protect from light.				
13. ♦	Deliver the composite to the dentist with the composite placement instrument of the dentist's choice. The dentist will add material in increments, each followed by use of the curing light.				
14. ♦	The dentist will use a high-speed handpiece with finishing burs to carve the restoration.				
15. ♦	The assistant must still use the HVE to remove any pieces of composite as well as continue to retract the cheek, lip, or tongue.				
16. ♦	Remove all cotton and the dental dam. Rinse and dry the area.				

POINT VALUE ♦ = 5 points ✳ = 10 points		PRACTICE TRIAL	GRADED TRIAL #1	GRADED TRIAL #2	NOTES:
17. ♦	Place articulating paper between the maxillary and mandibular teeth to check the occlusion. The patient should bite down carefully and gently so as to not fracture the new restoration, especially when the marginal ridge is too high. The dentist will continue to adjust the occlusion until the bite is correct. Heavy colored marks will appear on the restoration in areas needing adjustment.				
18. ♦	The dental assistant will continue to use the HVE to remove particles and for retraction during the continued carving.				
19. ♦	Inform the patient the composite material is cured and chewing is possible immediately.				
20. ♦	If the patient received anesthetic, inform her to avoid chewing until the anesthetic is gone so as to avoid biting her cheeks or tongue. Inform her to call the office if she finds her occlusion is incorrect. She will need to return to the office for an occlusal adjustment.				

Document:

Enter the appropriate information in the chart below.

(continued)

Grading

Points earned	_____		
Points possible	_____	100	100
Percent grade (Points earned/Points possible)	_____		
Pass:	_____	❑ YES ❑ NO ❑ N/A	❑ YES ❑ NO ❑ N/A

Instructor Sign-Off

Instructor: _____ Date: _____

Procedure 38-2
Assisting with a Class II Amalgam Restoration

Objective: Demonstrate how assist with a Class II amalgam restoration.

Equipment and Supplies Needed: restorative tray for appropriate dental material to be used including basic setup; hand-cutting instruments, amalgam carrier, condensers, burnishers, carvers; plastic instrument, articulating paper holder; local anesthetic setup (some patients do not require anesthetic), dental dam setup (some doctors do not use the dental dam), high volume evacuator (HVE), saliva ejector, high-speed and low-speed rotary handpieces, burs—often in a block (each dentist has preferences), cotton products (pellets, rolls, 2×2 gauze squares, dry angles), matrix system setup, dental liner, base, bonding agent, caries indicator dye, permanent restorative material of choice, articulating paper, polishing items, and dental floss.

Notes to the Student:

Skills Assessment Requirements

Read and familiarize yourself with the procedure; complete the minimum practice requirements. Document information when appropriate to demonstrate proper charting techniques. Complete each procedure within a reasonable amount of time, with a minimum of 85% accuracy.

POINT VALUE ♦ = 5 points ✳ = 10 points		PRACTICE TRIAL	GRADED TRIAL #1	GRADED TRIAL #2	NOTES:
1. ♦	Deliver mouth mirror and explorer to dentist. (Dentist must examine tooth to be restored.)				
2. ♦	Assist dentist in the delivery of anesthetic, topical and local.				
3. ♦	Place isolation items, cotton rolls, dry angle, or dental dam (state permitting).				
4. ♦	Deliver mouth mirror to dentist and inform dentist of the type of bur on the handpiece.				
5. ♦	Adjust the light, retract the patient's cheek or tongue, and use the HVE and air/water syringe to keep the working area clear for the dentist.				

(continued)

	POINT VALUE ♦ = 5 points ✳ = 10 points	PRACTICE TRIAL	GRADED TRIAL # 1	GRADED TRIAL # 2	NOTES:
6. ♦	Transfer the necessary instruments to the dentist during the preparation as needed.				
7. ♦	Rinse and dry prepared tooth for the dentist to evaluate.				
8. ♦	Deliver caries indicator dye to the preparation, wait, rinse, and dry. (Repeat until tooth is clear of caries.)				
9. ♦	Deliver to the dentist the matrix system of the dentist's choice. If state regulations permit, the dental assistant may place the matrix system.				
10. ♦	If the preparation requires a base or liner, mix and deliver to the dentist.				
11. ♦	Activate amalgam capsule and triturate.				
12. ♦	Fill the smaller end of the amalgam carrier and transfer to the dentist. The dentist may want both ends of the carrier filled. Alternate the condenser with the carrier. Continue to supply the dentist with more amalgam until the preparation is slightly overfilled.				
13. ♦	Exchange the condenser for the burnisher so the dentist can burnish the excess mercury to the tooth surface.				
14. ♦	Deliver the carving instruments of dentist's choice until the restoration is complete.				
15. ♦	The assistant must still use the HVE to remove any pieces of amalgam as well as continue to retract the cheek, lip, or tongue.				
16. ♦	Remove all cotton and the dental dam. Rinse and dry the area.				

POINT VALUE ♦ = 5 points ∗ = 10 points		PRACTICE TRIAL	GRADED TRIAL # 1	GRADED TRIAL # 2	NOTES:
17. ♦	Place articulating paper between the maxillary and mandibular teeth to check the occlusion. The patient should bite down carefully and gently so as to not fracture the new restoration. The dentist will continue to adjust the occlusion until the bite is correct. Heavy colored marks will appear on the restoration in areas needing adjustment.				
18. ♦	The dental assistant will continue to use the HVE to remove particles and for retraction during the continued carving.				
19. ♦	Inform the patient not to chew on that side of his mouth. The amalgam will continue to harden for several hours after placement.				
20. ♦	If the patient received anesthetic, inform him to avoid chewing until the anesthetic is gone so as to avoid biting his cheeks or tongue. Inform the patient to call the office if he/she finds his occlusion is incorrect. He will need to return to the office for an occlusal adjustment.				

Document:

Enter the appropriate information in the chart below.

(continued)

Grading

Points earned	_____		
Points possible	_____	100	100
Percent grade (Points earned/Points possible)	_____		
Pass:	_____	❑ YES ❑ NO ❑ N/A	❑ YES ❑ NO ❑ N/A

Instructor Sign-Off

Instructor: _____ Date: _____

Procedure 38-3
Assisting with a Chair-Side Veneer

Objective: Demonstrate how to assist with a chair-side veneer.

Equipment and Supplies Needed: restorative tray for appropriate dental material to be used including basic setup; hand-cutting instruments; condensers; carvers; plastic instrument; articulating paper holder; patient safety glasses; local anesthetic setup (some patients do not require anesthetic), dental dam setup (some doctors do not use the dental dam), high volume evacuator (HVE) and saliva ejector, high-speed and low-speed rotary handpieces, curing light and protective shield, burs—often in a block (each dentist has preferences), cotton products (pellets, rolls, 2 × 2 gauze squares), delivery brushes and mixing wells, mylar matrix system, composite resin shade guide, dental liner, base, etch, bonding agent, caries indicator dye, permanent restorative (composite resin and delivery gun), dental floss, articulating paper, finishing carbide burs, and polishing items including abrasive strips, discs, cups, and polishing paste.

Notes to the Student:

Skills Assessment Requirements

Read and familiarize yourself with the procedure; complete the minimum practice requirements. Document information when appropriate to demonstrate proper charting techniques. Complete each procedure within a reasonable amount of time, with a minimum of 85% accuracy.

POINT VALUE ◆ = 5 points ✳ = 10 points		PRACTICE TRIAL	GRADED TRIAL # 1	GRADED TRIAL # 2	NOTES:
1. ◆	Shade selection. The dentist may choose several shades to emulate the various areas of natural teeth.				
2. ◆	Assist in the delivery of topical and local anesthetic if necessary.				
3. ◆	Place moisture control items such as cotton rolls and dental dam (state permitting).				
4. ◆	Deliver mouth mirror to dentist and inform dentist of the type of bur on the handpiece.				

(continued)

	POINT VALUE ♦ = 5 points ✳ = 10 points	PRACTICE TRIAL	GRADED TRIAL # 1	GRADED TRIAL # 2	NOTES:
5. ♦	Adjust the light, retract the patient's lip, and use the HVE and air/water syringe to keep the working area clear for the dentist.				
6. ♦	Transfer the necessary instruments to the dentist during the preparation as needed.				
7. ♦	Rinse and dry prepared tooth for the dentist to evaluate.				
8. ♦	Place mylar matrix system.				
9. ♦	When placing composite resin, deliver etch and rinse. Then deliver bond and light cure.				
10. ♦	Place an appropriate amount of composite resin on a paper pad and protect from light. Numerous shades may be used. Manage the materials carefully so as to give the dentist the correct shade at the correct moment.				
11. ♦	Pass the dentist the instrument of choice for composite material. The plastic instrument is the most often utilized.				
12. ♦	Have bonding agent available. The dentist may use a bonding agent to help manipulate the material.				
13. ♦	Due to the thin layer, the composite may or may not be cured in layers. The dentist will give direction as to when to light cure.				
14. ♦	The dentist will use a high-speed handpiece with finishing burs to carve the restoration.				
15.	The low-speed handpiece is used with a mandrel or attachment to place the final polish.				

POINT VALUE ♦ = 5 points * = 10 points		PRACTICE TRIAL	GRADED TRIAL # 1	GRADED TRIAL # 2	NOTES:
16. ♦	The assistant must still use the HVE to remove any pieces of composite as well as continue to retract the lip.				
17. ♦	Remove all cotton and the dental dam. Rinse and dry the area.				
18. ♦	Provide a large mirror for the patient to approve the restoration.				
19. ♦	If the patient received anesthetic, inform her to avoid chewing until the anesthetic is gone so as to avoid biting her lips.				
20. ♦	Provide the patient with oral hygiene instructions and advise her of the need to keep regular dental visits to help maintain the new veneers.				
21. ♦	Inform the patient that composite resin will stain over time with the foods and liquids she eats and drinks. Chair-side veneers have limited longevity. They may chip and wear over time. Inform the patient to never bite into hard items such as ice or hard candy; such actions can fracture the bonding.				

Document:

Enter the appropriate information in the chart below.

(continued)

Grading

Points earned	_____		
Points possible	_____	100	100
Percent grade (Points earned/Points possible)	_____		
Pass:	_____	❑ YES ❑ NO ❑ N/A	❑ YES ❑ NO ❑ N/A

Instructor Sign-Off

Instructor: _____ Date: _____

Procedure 39-1
Preparing the Tofflemire Matrix System

Objective: Demonstrate how to prepare the Tofflemire matrix system.

Equipment and Supplies Needed: basic setup (mouth mirror, explorer, cotton pliers), hemostat, Tofflemire retainer, Tofflemire matrix band, burnisher, paper pad, and assortment of wedges

Notes to the Student:

Skills Assessment Requirements

Read and familiarize yourself with the procedure; complete the minimum practice requirements. Document information when appropriate to demonstrate proper charting techniques. Complete each procedure within a reasonable amount of time, with a minimum of 85% accuracy.

POINT VALUE ♦ = 5 points ✳ = 10 points		PRACTICE TRIAL	GRADED TRIAL # 1	GRADED TRIAL # 2	NOTES:
1. ✳	Examine the preparation with a mirror and note the location in the mouth and the depth of the proximal box.				
2. ✳✳	Choose the type of matrix band to be used, for example, universal or extension. Consider the size of the tooth.				
3. ✳	Burnish the middle of the band on a paper pad until the ends begin to curl to create a thinner area for proper contact. The spindle is released from the locking vise by turning the short knob toward yourself.				
4. ✳	Hold the retainer so the diagonal slot and the U-guides are up. Turn the short knob away from you so the spindle is not visible in the diagonal slot.				
5. ✳	Turn the long knob so the U-guides are close to the locking vise.				

(continued)

POINT VALUE ♦ = 5 points ✳ = 10 points		PRACTICE TRIAL	GRADED TRIAL # 1	GRADED TRIAL # 2	NOTES:
6. ✳	Make a loop with the band to form the occlusal and gingival edges. The occlusal edge is the larger of the two edges.				
7. ✳	With the diagonal slot of the retainer facing up, place the joined ends of the band into the diagonal slot of the locking vise, occlusal edge first.				
8. ✳	Place the band into the proper guide slots. The location of the tooth to be restored determines which way to place the band into the guide slots, for example, maxillary, mandibular, right, or left.				
9. ✳	Tighten the short knob to screw the spindle into the locking vise in order to hold the band in the retainer.				

Document:

Enter the appropriate information in the chart below.

Grading

Points earned	_____		
Points possible	_____	100	100
Percent grade (Points earned/Points possible)	_____		
Pass:	_____	❑ YES ❑ NO ❑ N/A	❑ YES ❑ NO ❑ N/A

Instructor Sign-Off

Instructor: _____ Date: _____

Procedure 39-2

Placing and Removing a Retainer, Matrix Band, and Wedge for a Class II Restoration by an Expanded Duties Dental Assistant

Objective: Demonstrate how to place and remove a retainer, matrix band, and wedge for a Class II restoration.

Equipment and Supplies Needed: basic setup (mouth mirror, explorer, cotton pliers, hemostat), Tofflemire retainer with matrix in place, burnisher, wedge, cotton rolls, and floss.

Notes to the Student:

Skills Assessment Requirements

Read and familiarize yourself with the procedure; complete the minimum practice requirements. Document information when appropriate to demonstrate proper charting techniques. Complete each procedure within a reasonable amount of time, with a minimum of 85% accuracy.

POINT VALUE ♦ = 5 points ✳ = 10 points		PRACTICE TRIAL	GRADED TRIAL # 1	GRADED TRIAL # 2	NOTES:
A.	**Procedure Steps for Preparation of the Matrix Band**				
1. ♦	The band often gets folded upon placement into the retainer. If this should occur, use the handle of a mouth mirror to open the loop.				
2. ♦	Survey the size of the tooth and adjust the band accordingly by turning the long knob.				

(continued)

	POINT VALUE ♦ = 5 points ✳ = 10 points	PRACTICE TRIAL	GRADED TRIAL # 1	GRADED TRIAL # 2	NOTES:
B.	**Procedure Steps for Placement of the Retainer and Matrix Band**				
1. ♦	Place the retainer along the buccal side of the tooth to be restored and lightly slide the band around the tooth with a rocking motion to get past the other proximal contact (if only one contact was removed in preparation). Leave a 1.0- to 1.5-mm lip along the occlusal surface.				
2. ♦	Hold the band in place with one finger on the occlusal surface and tighten the band around the tooth by turning the long knob.				
3. ✳	Check the contour of the band to the tooth with the explorer. The band can catch on the proximal box, creating a poor margin in the box.				
4. ✳	Use the ball burnisher to adapt the band to the proximal tooth for a tight contact.				
C.	**Procedure Steps for Placement of the Wedge**				
1. ✳	Select the proper wedge. The size of the embrasure will determine the size of the wedge.				
2. ♦	Use the cotton pliers to hold the wedge with the flat edge toward the gingival. With moderate pressure, place the wedge from the lingual into the embrasure space. If both mesial and distal contacts need to be restored, then two wedges are needed.				
3. ♦	Check the gingival floor in the proximal box to ensure that the band is tight against the tooth to seal the band to the wall of the tooth.				

POINT VALUE ♦ = 5 points ∗ = 10 points		PRACTICE TRIAL	GRADED TRIAL # 1	GRADED TRIAL # 2	NOTES:
D.	**Procedure Steps for Removal of the Retainer, Matrix Band, and Wedge**				
1. ∗	Once the tooth has been filled and initially carved, loosen the retainer from the band by turning the short knob.				
2. ♦	Place a finger over the occlusal surface and matrix band. Remove the retainer from the mouth by gently lifting it toward the occlusal surface, leaving the matrix band around the tooth.				
3. ♦	With the cotton pliers, remove the wedge.				
4. ∗	Remember that the amalgam is still soft. Very carefully remove the band by using a light seesaw motion to prevent the restoration from fracturing.				
5. ♦	Final carving of the restoration is performed.				
6. ♦	After the initial set of the restorative material, use floss to check the contact with the proximal tooth.				

Document:

Enter the appropriate information in the chart below.

(continued)

Grading

Points earned	_____		
Points possible	_____	100	100
Percent grade (Points earned/Points possible)	_____		
Pass:	_____	❏ YES ❏ NO ❏ N/A	❏ YES ❏ NO ❏ N/A

Instructor Sign-Off

Instructor: _____ Date: _____

Procedure 39-3

Placing a Clear Polyester Matrix for Class III and IV Restorations

Objective: Demonstrate how to place a clear polyester matrix for Class III and IV restorations.

Equipment and Supplies Needed: basic setup (mouth mirror, explorer, cotton pliers), clear matrix strip, wedges, cotton rolls, and floss.

Notes to the Student:

Skills Assessment Requirements

Read and familiarize yourself with the procedure; complete the minimum practice requirements. Document information when appropriate to demonstrate proper charting techniques. Complete each procedure within a reasonable amount of time, with a minimum of 85% accuracy.

POINT VALUE ♦ = 5 points ✳ = 10 points		PRACTICE TRIAL	GRADED TRIAL # 1	GRADED TRIAL # 2	NOTES:
1. ✳	Examine the tooth and preparation to be restored.				
2. ✳ ✳	Contour the matrix band as necessary for the curvature of the tooth.				
3. ✳ ✳	Place the matrix band interproximally, ensuring that the band extends beyond the gingival wall of the preparation.				
4. ✳	Place the wedge into the embrasure using the cotton pliers.				
5. ✳	After curing the composite, the wedge and matrix are removed and discarded.				
6. ✳ ✳	Use floss to check for appropriate contact with the adjacent tooth.				
7. ✳	The composite is then finished and polished.				

(continued)

Document:

Enter the appropriate information in the chart below.

Grading

Points earned	_____		
Points possible	_____	100	100
Percent grade (Points earned/Points possible)	_____		
Pass:	_____	❏ YES ❏ NO ❏ N/A	❏ YES ❏ NO ❏ N/A

Instructor Sign-Off

Instructor: _____ Date: _____

Procedure 40-1

Placing and Removing a Gingival Retraction Cord

Objective: Demonstrate how to place and remove a gingival retraction cord.

Equipment and Supplies Needed: Mouth mirror, explorer, cotton pliers, cord-packing instrument, gingival cords of dentist's preference, scissors, hemostatic agent, dappen dish, and cotton rolls.

Notes to the Student:

Skills Assessment Requirements

Read and familiarize yourself with the procedure; complete the minimum practice requirements. Document information when appropriate to demonstrate proper charting techniques. Complete each procedure within a reasonable amount of time, with a minimum of 85% accuracy.

POINT VALUE ♦ = 5 points ✳ = 10 points		PRACTICE TRIAL	GRADED TRIAL # 1	GRADED TRIAL # 2	NOTES:
1. ✳	Gently rinse and dry the preparation; this allows for better visibility of the margins.				
2. ✳	Isolate the quadrant with cotton rolls.				
3. ✳	Cut an appropriate length of cord—longer for molars and shorter for anterior teeth. (*Hint:* Use the circumference of your little finger to gauge the length of cord for a molar.)				
4. ♦	Place the cord or cotton pellets into the hemostatic solution if there is hemorrhaging of the tissue.				
5. ✳	If using a hemostatic agent, inform the patient that the chemicals will taste bad.				

(continued)

POINT VALUE ♦ = 5 points ✳ = 10 points		PRACTICE TRIAL	GRADED TRIAL # 1	GRADED TRIAL # 2	NOTES:
6. ♦	Using the cotton pliers, make a loop with the cord and gently lay it around the prepared tooth at the margin or opening of the sulcus with the ends of the loop on the buccal side of the preparation. This placement allows for easy removal of the cords.				
7. ✳	With the cord-packing instrument, gently pack the cord with light pressure into the sulcus. (*Hint:* Try to lightly push back toward the portion of the cord last inserted into the sulcus. Pushing forward stretches and drags the cord around the tooth.)				
8. ♦	Once the cord is fully placed, the ends of the loop should be end to end. If the cord is too long, it can be cut with scissors. If it is too short, a new cord should be placed. Placing a small piece is not appropriate because it often gets left in the sulcus, creating a periodontal problem.				
9. ✳	Depending on the dentist's preference, two cords of differing sizes may be used. Place the smaller of the cords first followed by the larger cord.				
10. ♦	The cords should be left in the sulcus for approximately five minutes but not longer than seven minutes. (*Hint:* Set a timer.) Instruct the patient to remain still so as to keep the area dry and the hemostatic agent off the tongue. (*Hint:* Time is dependent on the type of hemostatic agent. Read the manufacturer's information on the agent.)				

POINT VALUE ♦ = 5 points ✳ = 10 points		PRACTICE TRIAL	GRADED TRIAL # 1	GRADED TRIAL # 2	NOTES:
11. ✳	When time is up, the operator removes the cotton and the second cord while the assistant fills the impression tray. The operator removes the cord with the cotton pliers by grasping the end of the cord on the buccal side of the preparation. The cord is not removed until the impression is ready to be taken. The operator must keep the sulcus and preparation dry before the placement of the impression.				
12. ✳	After the impression, the first cord must be removed. Do not forget about the cord—a severe periodontal problem can develop in a short amount of time if a cord is not removed.				

Document:

Enter the appropriate information in the chart below.

Grading

Points earned	_____		
Points possible			
	_____		
Percent grade (Points earned/Points possible)	_____	100	100
Pass:	_____	❑ YES ❑ NO ❑ N/A	❑ YES ❑ NO ❑ N/A

Instructor Sign-Off

Instructor: _____ Date: _____

PROCEDURE 40-2
Assisting with a Crown or Bridge Restoration

Objective: Demonstrate how to assist with a crown or bridge restoration procedure.

Equipment and Supplies Needed: restorative kit (mouth mirror, explorer, cotton pliers, air/water syringe, spoon excavator, scissors, hemostat, spatula, other instruments required by the dentist), local anesthetic setup, gingival retraction setup, provisional coverage setup, impression and bite registration setup including the impression trays, high-speed and contra-angle handpieces and burs, shade guide, high volume evacuator (HVE) and saliva ejector, cotton products (pellets, rolls, 2 × 2 sterile gauze squares, dry angles), articulating paper and holder, and dental floss.

Notes to the Student:

Skills Assessment Requirements

Read and familiarize yourself with the procedure; complete the minimum practice requirements. Document information when appropriate to demonstrate proper charting techniques. Complete each procedure within a reasonable amount of time, with a minimum of 85% accuracy.

POINT VALUE ♦ = 5 points ✳ = 10 points		PRACTICE TRIAL	GRADED TRIAL # 1	GRADED TRIAL # 2	NOTES:
A.	**Procedure Steps Prior to Preparation of the Tooth**				
1.	Assist in administration of local anesthetic.				
2.	If an alginate impression is needed for use in making the provisional or for the opposer (the opposite arch from which the restorative work is to be completed), take it at this time.				
3. ♦	If a stint for making of the provisional is needed, take it at this time. A stint is a small impression of the tooth prior to preparation that is usually made with an alginate impression, bite registration, or a small thermoplastic disc. It is used to make the temporary crown after preparation.				

(continued)

POINT VALUE ♦ = 5 points ✳ = 10 points		PRACTICE TRIAL	GRADED TRIAL # 1	GRADED TRIAL # 2	NOTES:
4. ♦	If the final impression requires a two-stage silicone impression, take the first stage impression at this time.				
5. ♦	If the final restoration is tooth colored, take the shade at this time.				
B.	**Procedure Steps for Preparation of the Tooth**				
1. ♦	Maintain a clear operating field with use of the HVE to retract the lips and tongue and to remove water and debris.				
2.	The dentist uses diamond burs to quickly cut away decayed or fractured portions of the tooth. Other shaped burs define the appropriate shape of the preparation.				
3. ♦	The dentist or dental assistant places the gingival retraction cords.				
4. ♦	Ready the final impression materials.				
5. ♦	Rinse and dry the preparation.				
6. ♦	Transfer the cotton pliers to the dentist for cord removal.				
7. ♦	Assist the dentist or other assistant in placement of the light-body impression materials.				
8. ♦	Fill the impression tray with heavy-body impression material.				
9. ♦	Receive the light-body delivery system (usually a syringe or impression gun) from the dentist while delivering to the dentist the impression tray in correct alignment for the dentist to grasp and insert directly onto the prepared area in the patient's mouth.				

POINT VALUE ♦ = 5 points ✳ = 10 points		PRACTICE TRIAL	GRADED TRIAL #1	GRADED TRIAL #2	NOTES:
10. ♦	Watch the clock for the appropriate setting time according to the recommendations of the impression material's manufacturer.				
11. ♦	The dentist or the dental assistant can remove the impression tray. Check the state regulations.				
12. ♦	Rinse the patient's mouth. Many impression materials have a poor taste.				
13. ♦	Take the bite registration.				
14. ♦	Remove any remaining gingival retraction cords.				
15. ♦	Fabricate the provisional restoration and cement with temporary cement.				
16. ♦	Give the patient provisional restoration care instructions.				
17. ♦	Schedule the patient for the permanent cementation appointment.				
18. ♦	After the dentist writes the laboratory prescription, prepare the case for delivery to the laboratory technician.				

Document:

Enter the appropriate information in the chart below.

(continued)

Grading

Points earned	_____		
Points possible	_____	100	100
Percent grade (Points earned/Points possible)	_____		
Pass:	_____	❏ YES ❏ NO ❏ N/A	❏ YES ❏ NO ❏ N/A

Instructor Sign-Off

Instructor:_____ Date:_____

PROCEDURE 40-3
Assisting in the Cementation of a Fixed Prosthesis

Objective: Demonstrate how to assist in the cementation of a fixed prosthesis.

Equipment and Supplies Needed: restorative kit (including mouth mirror, explorer, cotton pliers, air/water syringe, spoon excavator, scissors, hemostat, spatula, and other instruments required by the dentist), cast or milled restoration delivered from the laboratory, bonding setup and/or cementation setup (per dentist's preference), high-speed and low-speed rotary handpieces, high volume evacuator (HVE) and saliva ejector, articulating paper and holder, cotton products (pellets, rolls, 2 × 2 sterile gauze squares, dry angles), scaler to remove excess cement, burs, porcelain or gold polishers, and dental floss.

Notes to the Student:

Skills Assessment Requirements

Read and familiarize yourself with the procedure; complete the minimum practice requirements. Document information when appropriate to demonstrate proper charting techniques. Complete each procedure within a reasonable amount of time, with a minimum of 85% accuracy.

POINT VALUE ♦ = 5 points ∗ = 10 points		PRACTICE TRIAL	GRADED TRIAL # 1	GRADED TRIAL # 2	NOTES:
1. ♦	Place restoration onto the model returned from the dental laboratory for inspection by the dentist. If the crown is not returned from the lab as "disinfected," the dental assistant must disinfect it prior to the dentist placing it in the patient's mouth.				
2. ∗	Transfer the restoration to the dentist for placement onto the prepared tooth.				
3. ♦	Transfer the mouth mirror and explorer to the dentist.				
4. ∗	Hold the restoration in place with cotton pliers for the dentist to check the contacts of the restoration with the adjacent tooth.				

(continued)

POINT VALUE ♦ = 5 points ✳ = 10 points		PRACTICE TRIAL	GRADED TRIAL # 1	GRADED TRIAL # 2	NOTES:
5. ♦	Place cotton rolls to help keep the preparation dry.				
6. ✳	When the dentist signals, mix the cement and quickly apply the cement in a thin layer to the internal surface of the restoration.				
7. ♦	Transfer the restoration to the dentist for placement.				
8. ✳	The dentist places the restoration with firm finger pressure. The patient then bites on a cotton roll or wooden stick to seat the restoration completely.				
9. ✳	Once the cement reaches its initial set after three to five minutes, the excess may be removed. Use a controlled fulcrum to maintain stability when removing the excess cement.				
10. ✳	Use the tip of the explorer or scaler to slightly extend into the sulcus to lift up on the excess cement. Use lateral pressure against the restoration. This procedure often requires the removal of cement subgingivally. Many states do not allow the dental assistant to use any instrument subgingivally. Check state regulations for allowed dental assistant duties.				
11. ✳	To remove the excess cement in the embrasure space, tie a knot in a piece of dental floss and carefully pull the knot through the embrasure space to dislodge the cement.				
12. ✳	After the cement is removed, the dentist checks the occlusion, adjusts if necessary, and polishes the restoration with the contra-angle and slow-speed polishers.				

Document:

Enter the appropriate information in the chart below.

Grading

Points earned	_____		
Points possible	_____	100	100
Percent grade (Points earned/Points possible)	_____		
Pass:	_____	❏ YES ❏ NO ❏ N/A	❏ YES ❏ NO ❏ N/A

Instructor Sign-Off

Instructor:_____ Date:_____

PROCEDURE 41-1

Fabricating and Placing a Custom Provisional Bridge

Objective: Demonstrate how to assist with custom provisional bridge placement.

Equipment and Supplies Needed: basic setup (mirror, explorer, cotton pliers), cement spatula, mixing pad, temporary cement, saliva ejector, high volume evacuator (HVE) tip, air/water syringe tip, crown and bridge scissors, Bis-Acryl auto mix cartridge and delivery system, slow-speed motor, assortment of acrylic burs, discs, and mandrels, high-speed handpiece with diamond burs, articulating paper, and dental floss.

Notes to the Student:

Skills Assessment Requirements

Read and familiarize yourself with the procedure; complete the minimum practice requirements. Document information when appropriate to demonstrate proper charting techniques. Complete each procedure within a reasonable amount of time, with a minimum of 85% accuracy.

POINT VALUE ♦ = 5 points ✳ = 10 points		PRACTICE TRIAL	GRADED TRIAL # 1	GRADED TRIAL # 2	NOTES:
1. ✳	Prior to preparation for the bridge, while the anesthetic is taking effect, take a quadrant impression with alginate impression material. Cut out the pontic area with a scalpel blade. Remove any interdental gingival areas to provide bulk for the temporary restoration and so the impression will seat correctly later. Wrap the impression in a wet paper towel to keep moist so it does not distort when drying out.				
2. ♦	Inform the patient that you are going to make a temporary bridge, which will allow the teeth to function normally while the permanent bridge is being fabricated by the dental laboratory. Select a tooth shade if appropriate.				

(continued)

POINT VALUE ♦ = 5 points ✳ = 10 points		PRACTICE TRIAL	GRADED TRIAL # 1	GRADED TRIAL # 2	NOTES:
3. ✳	Clean and dry the teeth. Fill the impression with the Bis-Acryl provisional material, placing extra material into the pontic area. To prevent air bubbles, dispense provisional material onto the occlusal (or incisal) surfaces and then bring the tip of the material gingivally, slightly overbuilding it.				
4. ✳	Insert the impression back into the mouth over the prepared teeth. Hold firmly in place for approximately two to three minutes. Check that the material is still in its rubbery stage with an instrument. If left to set too rigid, removal may be difficult.				
5. ✳	Remove the provisional bridge together with the impression from the prepared teeth. While still rubbery, excess material may be cut with crown and bridge scissors. Allow five additional minutes for the material to set. Evaluate the provisional bridge for fit, voids, and thin areas.				
6. ✳	Mark the margins and proximal contact with a pencil to ensure these areas do not get trimmed away. Trim the margin areas to shape with slow-speed acrylic burs. Trim the embrasure areas with discs on a mandrel while using a fulcrum and eye protection.				
7. ♦	Place the bridge onto the prepared teeth and ask the patient to carefully close the teeth together while you hold articulating paper between the maxilla and mandible. Note high spots and adjust the occlusion with slow-speed round burs. Polish with a wet rag-wheel and pumice. Rinse and dry the abutment teeth well.				

POINT VALUE ♦ = 5 points ✳ = 10 points		PRACTICE TRIAL	GRADED TRIAL # 1	GRADED TRIAL # 2	NOTES:
8. ♦	Rinse the patient's tooth to clean it and dry it well. Place cotton rolls on the buccal and lingual areas and instruct the patient to hold her mouth open while you mix the cement.				
9. ✳	Mix the temporary cement or place automix temporary cement into the abutment teeth. Line the provisional abutments and place the temporary bridge on the prepared teeth. Tell the patient to bite down firmly on a cotton roll.				
10. ♦	Allow the temporary cement to set. Remove excess cement from around the margin.				
11. ✳	Floss the gingival sulcus to remove cement from under the gingiva. Pull the floss out through the side so the temporary bridge will not be loosened. Use a bridge threader to floss under the pontic. Rinse the area well.				
12. ✳	Give the patient a mirror and show her how to clean under the pontic and abutment areas. Provide postoperative instructions.				

Document:

Enter the appropriate information in the chart below.

(continued)

Grading

Points earned	_____		
Points possible	_____	100	100
Percent grade (Points earned/Points possible)	_____		
Pass:	_____	❏ YES ❏ NO ❏ N/A	❏ YES ❏ NO ❏ N/A

Instructor Sign-Off

Instructor:_____ Date:_____

PROCEDURE 41-2

Fabricating and Placing an Aluminum Shell Provisional Restoration

Objective: Demonstrate how to assist with aluminum shell provisional placement.

Equipment and Supplies Needed: basic setup (mirror, explorer, cotton pliers), cement spatula, mixing pad, temporary cement, saliva ejector, high volume evacuator (HVE) tip, air/water syringe tip, assortment of aluminum shells, crown, and bridge scissors, contouring pliers, hemostats, dappen dish, methy-methacrylate acrylic powder and liquid, slow-speed handpiece, assortment of acrylic burs, green stones, and discs, articulating paper, and dental floss.

Notes to the Student:

Skills Assessment Requirements

Read and familiarize yourself with the procedure; complete the minimum practice requirements. Document information when appropriate to demonstrate proper charting techniques. Complete each procedure within a reasonable amount of time, with a minimum of 85% accuracy.

POINT VALUE ♦ = 5 points * = 10 points		PRACTICE TRIAL	GRADED TRIAL # 1	GRADED TRIAL # 2	NOTES:
1. ♦	Inform the patient that you are going to make a temporary crown that will allow the tooth to function normally while the permanent crown is being fabricated by the dental laboratory.				
2. ♦	Use the measurement device included in the aluminum shell kit to measure the mesiodistal distance of the tooth needing the temporary. If a shell is selected that is slightly larger or smaller than necessary, it is soft enough to be shaped to the proper proportions with the contouring pliers.				

(continued)

POINT VALUE ♦ = 5 points ✳ = 10 points		PRACTICE TRIAL	GRADED TRIAL # 1	GRADED TRIAL # 2	NOTES:
3. ✳	Use cotton pliers to remove aluminum crowns from the box so as not to cross-contaminate the container. Try the shell on the prepared tooth. If the shell is too large, the proximal contact areas can be adjusted with the green stone. If the shell is too small, place the aluminum crown on the stretching block provided with the temporary crown kit, and stretch the margins slightly. Contouring pliers may also be used to stretch the aluminum crown to size. Disinfect any crown that has been tried on.				
4. ♦	Aluminum shells must be trimmed from the marginal areas on the mesial and distal sides in order to seat completely on the tooth preparation. Using crown and bridge scissors, cut small, slivered shapes from these areas. Trim the mesial and distal margins of the shell until the occlusal height of the crown is correct. Be sure to follow the contour of the gingival tissue.				
5. ♦	Try the shell back on the prepared tooth. It should extend to or slightly past the finish line of the preparation. Trim away any areas on the aluminum crown that impede upon the gingival tissues enough to cause them to blanch.				
6. ✳	Using the contouring pliers, smooth the aluminum crown and contour it so that it is wider at the proximal contact and narrower at the gingiva. Pulling the pliers side to side will also smooth rough edges.				
7. ♦	Use a green stone and/or discs to ensure all jagged edges are smooth.				

POINT VALUE ♦ = 5 points ∗ = 10 points		PRACTICE TRIAL	GRADED TRIAL # 1	GRADED TRIAL # 2	NOTES:
8. ♦	Place powder and liquid acrylic into the large end of the dappen dish and mix to the consistency of honey. Place the acrylic resin into the aluminum crown form.				
9. ∗	Place the crown form with acrylic onto the tooth and press firmly into place. When the excess resin feels rubbery, remove the crown matrix carefully. For the next 2–3 minutes, continue placing the aluminum crown on and off the tooth. If it remains on the tooth, the acrylic resin will become too hot for the tooth pulp to tolerate. If left off the tooth for too long, the acrylic will shrink and will no longer fit on the tooth.				
10. ♦	When the acrylic is hardened, remove the aluminum shell by cutting with crown and bridge scissors and bending with the hemostats until it is completely removed. Try it on the tooth and have the patient close his/her teeth together on the articulating paper. Adjust the occlusion with the acrylic bur or green stone.				
11. ∗	Using a lathe, a wet rag wheel, and pumice, polish the temporary crown until it is smooth. Rinse it well.				
12. ∗	Rinse the patient's tooth to clean it and dry it well. Place cotton rolls on the buccal and lingual areas, and instruct the patient to stay open while you mix the cement. Mix the temporary cement.				
13. ♦	Fill the provisional crown and place it on the prepared tooth. Tell the patient to bite down firmly on a cotton roll.				

(continued)

POINT VALUE ◆ = 5 points ✳ = 10 points		PRACTICE TRIAL	GRADED TRIAL # 1	GRADED TRIAL # 2	NOTES:
14. ◆	Allow the temporary cement to set. Remove excess cement from around the margin. Floss the gingival sulcus to remove cement from under the gingiva. Pull the floss out through the side. Rinse the area well.				
15. ◆	Give the patient a mirror and show him/her how to clean the provisional with floss by pulling it out the sides of the crown. Also give postoperative instructions.				

Document:

Enter the appropriate information in the chart below.

Grading

Points earned	_____		
Points possible	_____	100	100
Percent grade (Points earned/Points possible)	_____		
Pass:	_____	❏ YES ❏ NO ❏ N/A	❏ YES ❏ NO ❏ N/A

Instructor Sign-Off

Instructor: _____ Date:_____

PROCEDURE 42-1
Making a Final Impression for a Partial Denture

Objective: Demonstrate how to properly take a final impression for a partial denture.

Equipment and Supplies Needed: basic setup, mouthwash, custom tray or stock tray, tray adhesive, periphery wax for border molding, tooth shade guide, bite registration material, dispensing gun, mixing tips, mixing pad, spatula, and lab prescription form.

Notes to the Student:

Skills Assessment Requirements

Read and familiarize yourself with the procedure; complete the minimum practice requirements. Document information when appropriate to demonstrate proper charting techniques. Complete each procedure within a reasonable amount of time, with a minimum of 85% accuracy.

POINT VALUE ♦ = 5 points ✳ = 10 points		PRACTICE TRIAL	GRADED TRIAL # 1	GRADED TRIAL # 2	NOTES:
1.	The dentist places the custom or stock tray in the patient's mouth to determine fit.				
2.	The dentist places periphery wax on the rim of the impression tray for contouring.				
3. ✳ ✳	The dental assistant applies tray adhesive to the inside and borders of the impression tray and lets it completely dry.				
4. ✳ ✳	The dental assistant mixes the impression material using either a two-part or cartridge method and loads the impression tray. (The dentist places the impression tray.)				
5. ✳ ✳	The dentist removes the impression tray from the patient's mouth when the impression material has completely set.				

(continued)

POINT VALUE ♦ = 5 points ✳ = 10 points		PRACTICE TRIAL	GRADED TRIAL # 1	GRADED TRIAL # 2	NOTES:
6. ✳✳	The dentist takes the occlusal bite registration and selects the tooth shade.				
7. ✳✳	The dental assistant disinfects the impression and occlusal bite registration by spraying it with a disinfecting solution and placing it in a sealed container for the dental lab to pick up and process.				
8.	The dentist completes the lab prescription form informing the dental lab technician what is needed for the denture case. The prescription form must be signed by the dentist in order for the dental lab technician to process the denture case.				

Document:

Document information for proper charting of this procedure.

Grading

Points earned	_____		
Points possible	_____	100	100
Percent grade (Points earned/Points possible)	_____		
Pass:	_____	❑ YES ❑ NO ❑ N/A	❑ YES ❑ NO ❑ N/A

Instructor Sign-Off

Instructor: _____ Date: _____

PROCEDURE 44-1
Assisting with an Endodontic Procedures

Objective: Demonstrate how to assist during endodontic procedures.

Equipment and Supplies Needed: basic setup (mirror, explorer, locking cotton pliers), anesthetic setup, rubber dam setup, saliva ejector, high volume evacuator (HVE) tip, air/water syringe tip, slow-speed handpiece and a #4 or #6 round bur, assortment of acrylic burs, discs, and mandrels, high-speed handpiece with #556 or #557 bur or burs (as preferred by the dentist), broaches, files, reamers, endodontic spoon excavator, spreader, condenser, woodson, articulating paper, floss, irrigating syringe, irrigating solution, bead sterilizer, butane torch or other heat source, paper points, small cotton pellets, medication, temporary filling material, endodontic ruler and stops, x-ray film, lead apron, and thyroid collar.

Notes to the Student:

Skills Assessment Requirements

Read and familiarize yourself with the procedure; complete the minimum practice requirements. Document information when appropriate to demonstrate proper charting techniques. Complete each procedure within a reasonable amount of time, with a minimum of 85% accuracy.

POINT VALUE ♦ = 5 points ✳ = 10 points		PRACTICE TRIAL	GRADED TRIAL # 1	GRADED TRIAL # 2	NOTES:
1. ♦	The dental assistant passes the mirror and explorer to the dentist and then passes a 2 × 2 gauze to dry the muccobuccal fold and the topical anesthetic. The dental assistant passes the anesthetic syringe. When the dentist completes the anesthetic, the dental assistant rinses the area with the air/water syringe and aspirates excess water with the HVE tip.				

(continued)

	POINT VALUE ♦ = 5 points ✳ = 10 points	PRACTICE TRIAL	GRADED TRIAL # 1	GRADED TRIAL # 2	NOTES:
2. ♦	The dental assistant or dentist places the rubber dam on the affected tooth. The dental assistant should inform the patient of the purpose of the dental dam and if there are any concerns to let the dental team know.				
3. ♦	The dentist creates an opening in the tooth with the high-speed handpiece and bur. The dental assistant should keep the rubber dam free of debris but be sure to stay out of the dentist's line of vision.				
4. ♦	The dentist uses the slow-speed handpiece and round bur to remove caries and to access the pulp chamber. The dental assistant may quickly rinse the area to improve the dentist's field of view.				
5. ♦	The dentist may want to use the endodontic spoon excavator to remove caries and the endodontic explorer to locate the pulp chamber and canal openings.				
6. ♦	The dental assistant passes a barbed broach for the dentist to remove pulpal tissues from within the root canal. The dentist may want several broaches, especially if the tooth has more than one root.				
7. ♦	The dental assistant passes a #10 or #15 reamer with stoppers to measure the length of each canal. The dental assistant exposes a radiograph so the dentist can measure the length of each canal with the file(s) or reamer(s) in place. The radiograph and working length of each canal are recorded in the patient's chart.				

		PRACTICE TRIAL	GRADED TRIAL # 1	GRADED TRIAL # 2	NOTES:
POINT VALUE ♦ = 5 points ∗ = 10 points					
8. ♦	The dental assistant passes additional files in progression until the proper width and length of the canal are achieved. The size and length of the final file used are recorded in the patient's chart.				
9. ♦	The dental assistant passes the irrigating syringe with irrigating solution to the dentist. The dentist then irrigates the canal(s). The dental assistant must keep the tip of the HVE very close to the tooth so the irrigating solution is efficiently aspirated and not allowed to splash the patient or the dental team.				
10. ♦	The dental assistant passes paper points with locking cotton pliers to the dentist and continues to pass paper points until the canal(s) are completely dry.				
11. ♦	The dental assistant passes a small cotton pellet containing medication to the dentist who places it in the tooth. (At this point the dentist places a temporary filling material into the tooth or continues to obturate the canal(s) and completes the root canal treatment. If a tooth is severely infected, the dentist may elect to have the patient return at a later date to complete the endodontic therapy.)				
12. ♦	A master gutta percha point is selected that matches the width size of the last file used in each canal. The dental assistant exposes a radiograph to verify the proper length and seal.				

(continued)

POINT VALUE ♦ = 5 points ✳ = 10 points		PRACTICE TRIAL	GRADED TRIAL # 1	GRADED TRIAL # 2	NOTES:
13. ♦	The dental assistant mixes the endodontic sealer to a creamy consistency and passes it to the dentist, so he or she can coat the tip of the master gutta percha point. The dentist places the gutta percha with cement into the canal. (Some dentists will use a lentulo spiral to place the endodontic sealer deep into the canal(s) before placing the gutta percha point.)				
14. ♦	The dental assistant passes the endodontic spreader and additional accessory gutta percha points to the dentist and continues to pass the spreader and an additional point until each canal is full.				
15. ♦	The dental assistant passes the endodontic condenser and prepares the torch. The dental assistant holds some 2 × 2 gauze squares and holds the HVE tip close to the tooth.				
16. ♦	The dentist heats the tip of the endodontic condenser and melts off the excess gutta percha material. It is important to adequately heat the instrument to avoid removal of the gutta percha filling from the canal. The dental assistant ensures that the HVE tip aspirates any smoke and receives the melted gutta percha from the dentist with a 2 × 2 gauze.				
17. ♦	The dental assistant prepares the temporary filling material and passes the Woodson to the dentist. The dentist places the filling. The dental assistant passes a lightly dampened cotton applicator to the dentist, who uses it to smooth the temporary restoration.				

POINT VALUE ♦ = 5 points ✳ = 10 points		PRACTICE TRIAL	GRADED TRIAL # 1	GRADED TRIAL # 2	NOTES:
18. ♦	The dental assistant uses the HVE and air/water syringe to ensure that the rubber dam is rinsed free of debris. The rubber dam is removed and the dental assistant freshens the patient's mouth by rinsing and aspirating.				
19. ♦	The dental assistant dries the tooth and passes the articulating paper to the dentist who will ask the patient to lightly tap the teeth together. If necessary, the dentist will adjust the occlusion with the Woodson, cotton applicator, or a round bur and slow-speed handpiece.				
20. ♦	The dental assistant exposes a final radiograph and provides postoperative instructions to the patient.				

Document:

Enter the appropriate information in the chart below.

(continued)

Grading

Points earned	_____		
Points possible	_____	100	100
Percent grade (Points earned/Points possible)	_____		
Pass:	_____	❑ YES ❑ NO ❑ N/A	❑ YES ❑ NO ❑ N/A

Instructor Sign-Off

Instructor:_____ Date: _____

PROCEDURE 44-2
Assisting with an Apicoectomy and Retrograde Filling

Objective: Demonstrate how to assist during an apicoectomy and retrograde filling.

Equipment and Supplies Needed: surgical setup (mirror, scalpel and blade handle, periosteal elevator, curette), retrograde filling instruments and material, surgical high volume evacuator (HVE) tip, air/water syringe tip, slow-speed handpiece, and high-speed handpiece with surgical burs.

Notes to the Student:

Skills Assessment Requirements

Read and familiarize yourself with the procedure; complete the minimum practice requirements. Document information when appropriate to demonstrate proper charting techniques. Complete each procedure within a reasonable amount of time, with a minimum of 85% accuracy.

POINT VALUE ♦ = 5 points ✻ = 10 points		PRACTICE TRIAL	GRADED TRIAL # 1	GRADED TRIAL # 2	NOTES:
1. ✻✻	The dentist makes a flap in the gingival tissue. The assistant may be asked to retract while the dentist creates a window in the bone at the apex of the root.				
2. ✻✻	When the root tip is exposed, the dentist uses the high-speed handpiece and surgical bur to cut and section the apex of the tooth and uses the surgical curette to remove all diseased alveolar bone tissue. The assistant should have several squares of 2 × 2 gauze available and continue to rinse the area and aspirate debris as necessary.				

.(*continued*)

POINT VALUE ♦ = 5 points ✳ = 10 points		PRACTICE TRIAL	GRADED TRIAL # 1	GRADED TRIAL # 2	NOTES:
3. ✳ ✳	The dentist prepares the apex of the tooth with the high-speed bur or with other technology such as ultrasonics.				
4. ✳ ✳	The assistant mixes and passes the retrograde filling material to the dentist, who places it into the opening in the apex of the tooth.				
5. ✳ ✳	The area is cleaned and sutures placed.				

Document:

Enter the appropriate information in the chart below.

Grading

Points earned	_____		
Points possible	_____	100	100
Percent grade (Points earned/Points possible)	_____		
Pass:	_____	❑ YES ❑ NO ❑ N/A	❑ YES ❑ NO ❑ N/A

Instructor Sign-Off

Instructor:_____ Date: _____

Procedure 46-1
Completing a Surgical Scrub

Objective: Demonstrate how to properly perform a surgical scrub.

Equipment and Supplies Needed: antimicrobial soap, sterile surgical scrub brush, and sterile disposable towels.

Notes to the Student:

Skills Assessment Requirements

Read and familiarize yourself with the procedure; complete the minimum practice requirements. Document information when appropriate to demonstrate proper charting techniques. Complete each procedure within a reasonable amount of time, with a minimum of 85% accuracy.

POINT VALUE ♦ = 5 points ✳ = 10 points		PRACTICE TRIAL	GRADED TRIAL # 1	GRADED TRIAL # 2	NOTES:
1.	Remove all jewelry from hands and arms.				
2. ♦	Wet hands and forearms up to the elbow with warm water for 30 seconds.				
3. ♦	Dispense about 5mL of an antimicrobial soap into cupped hands and rub all over the wet area to make lather for 30 seconds.				
4. ♦	Clean under fingernails with a nail stick or sterile scrub brush. (*Note:* Fingernails must be clipped.)				
5. ♦	Rinse thoroughly for 30 seconds under tap water.				
6. ♦	Repeat the procedure with soap but now without the scrub brush for another 30 seconds. (*Note:* Do not use a scrub brush on the skin because it is too stiff and may cause microscopic abrasions.)				

(continued)

POINT VALUE ♦ = 5 points ✳ = 10 points		PRACTICE TRIAL	GRADED TRIAL # 1	GRADED TRIAL # 2	NOTES:
7. ♦	Finally rinse with warm water, beginning at the finger tips and moving the hands and forearms through the water and up so that the water drains off the forearms last. This is done to prevent hands from recontamination.				
8. ♦	Close the tap either by pedal control or by the end of the elbow. Motion-sensitive taps are a good option. Do not touch anything with bare, cleaned hands. (*Note:* Once the hands have been washed, they must be kept above the navel level, because the area below the navel is considered unclean in a hospital surgical setting.)				
9. ♦	Dry hands and forearms thoroughly with disposable sterile towels.				
10. ♦	Apply antimicrobial lotion. This is recommended before gloving because it protects the skin from drying and cracking.				
11. ♦	Don sterile gloves (see Procedure 46-2).				

Document:

Document information for proper charting of this procedure.

Grading

Points earned	_____		
Points possible	_____	50	50
Percent grade (Points earned/Points possible)	_____		
Pass:	_____	❑ YES ❑ NO ❑ N/A	❑ YES ❑ NO ❑ N/A

Instructor Sign-Off

Instructor: _____ Date: _____

Procedure 46-2
Donning Surgical Gloves

Objective: Demonstrate how to properly don surgical gloves.

Equipment and Supplies Needed: pair of double-wrapped, sterile, appropriately sized surgical gloves; and hand cream (if needed, prior to gloving).

Notes to the Student:

Skills Assessment Requirements

Read and familiarize yourself with the procedure; complete the minimum practice requirements. Document information when appropriate to demonstrate proper charting techniques. Complete each procedure within a reasonable amount of time, with a minimum of 85% accuracy.

POINT VALUE ◆ = 5 points ✳ = 10 points		PRACTICE TRIAL	GRADED TRIAL # 1	GRADED TRIAL # 2	NOTES:
1. ✳	Perform surgical scrub (see Procedure 46-1).				
2. ◆	Select the appropriate glove size and inspect the package to make sure it is intact, dry, and sealed.				
3. ◆	Check the expiration date on the package.				
4. ✳	Place the sterile package on a clean, dry surface above waist height with the cuffed end of the gloves toward you. (*Note:* Consider anything held below the waist level contaminated.) Do not place a sterile glove package on a wet surface.				
5. ✳	Open the sterile glove wrapper by touching the outside of the pack only. Do not touch the outside of the glove with your bare hands or the inside of the glove with a gloved hand.				

(continued)

POINT VALUE ♦ = 5 points ✱ = 10 points		PRACTICE TRIAL	GRADED TRIAL # 1	GRADED TRIAL # 2	NOTES:
6. ✱	Keep hands inside gown sleeves while grasping the cuff of the glove for the dominant hand.				
7. ✱	Lay glove on forearm of the dominant (right) hand, with the palm of the glove facing down, glove fingers pointed toward elbow, and glove thumb positioned on thumb side of dominant hand (right) hand.				
8. ♦	Grasp the inside glove cuff with the right hand.				
9. ♦	With the nondominant (left) hand, pull the dominant (right) hand glove cuff over the cuff of the gown by grasping the folded inside edge of the cuff, because the folded inside edge will be placed against the skin and thus will be contaminated. The outside portion of the glove must not be touched by an ungloved hand because it must remain sterile.				
10. ♦	Pull the cuff onto the dominant hand using the thumb and fingers of the nondominant hand to avoid touching the rest of the glove.				
11. ♦	Place second glove on the forearm of the nondominant (left) hand with the palm of the gloved dominant (right) hand with fingers pointed toward the elbow, and gloved thumb on thumb side of the nondominant (left) hand.				
12. ✱	Grasp the inside glove cuff with the nondominant hand through the gown, being careful to keep fingers inside the gown.				

POINT VALUE ♦ = 5 points ✳ = 10 points		PRACTICE TRIAL	GRADED TRIAL # 1	GRADED TRIAL # 2	NOTES:
13. ✳	Grasp the sleeve of the gown and the cuff of the glove and pull the glove onto the nondominant (left) hand, making sure that the thumb of the right gloved hand is not touching the cuff. Do not try to adjust the fit until you have donned both gloves.				
14.	Adjust the fingers in both gloves.				

Document:

Document information for proper charting of this procedure.

Grading

Points earned	_____		
Points possible	_____	100	100
Percent grade (Points earned/Points possible)	_____		
Pass:	_____	❏ YES ❏ NO ❏ N/A	❏ YES ❏ NO ❏ N/A

Instructor Sign-Off

Instructor: _____ Date: _____

Procedure 47-1
Applying Fluoride for the Pediatric Patient

Objective: Demonstrate how to properly administer topical fluoride for the pediatric patient.

Equipment and Supplies Needed: mirror, explorer, cotton pliers, HVE, saliva ejector, air/water syringe, 2 × 2 gauze sponges, fluoride solution (gel, foam, or rinse), fluoride trays (correct size), and clock or watch.

Notes to the Student:

Skills Assessment Requirements

Read and familiarize yourself with the procedure; complete the minimum practice requirements. Document information when appropriate to demonstrate proper charting techniques. Complete each procedure within a reasonable amount of time, with a minimum of 85% accuracy.

POINT VALUE ♦ = 5 points ✳ = 10 points		PRACTICE TRIAL	GRADED TRIAL # 1	GRADED TRIAL # 2	NOTES:
1. ♦	Fluoride should be applied after a coronal polish for best results.				
2. ♦	Ensure the patient has no allergic reaction to fluoride (review health history).				
3. ✳	Instruct patient not to swallow fluoride.				
4. ♦	Place napkin and shield glasses on the patient.				
5. ✳	Select correct tray size making sure all teeth are covered.				
6. ✳	Place fluoride into tray about one-third full.				
7. ✳	Dry patient's teeth with air or gauze sponge and instruct patient to hold the mouth open while the tray is inserted.				

(continued)

POINT VALUE ♦ = 5 points ✳ = 10 points		PRACTICE TRIAL	GRADED TRIAL # 1	GRADED TRIAL # 2	NOTES:
8. ♦	Place tray onto teeth and place salvia ejector between the maxillary and mandibular trays to remove excess fluoride.				
9. ♦	Have patient close the mouth gently around the trays and saliva ejector.				
10. ✳	Check the clock or watch for desired time according to the manufacturer's instructions.				
11. ♦	When time has elapsed, remove the saliva ejector and trays from the patient's mouth.				
12. ✳	Quickly remove excess fluoride from the mouth with the saliva ejector.				
13. ♦	Instruct the patient not to eat, drink, or rinse for 30 minutes.				
14. ♦	Document in the chart the type of fluoride used.				

Document:

Document information for proper charting of this procedure.

Grading

Points earned	_____	100	100
Points possible	_____		
Percent grade (Points earned/Points possible)	_____		
Pass:	_____	❑ YES ❑ NO ❑ N/A	❑ YES ❑ NO ❑ N/A

Instructor Sign-Off

Instructor: _____ Date: _____

Procedure 47-2
Assisting with a Pulpotomy on a Pediatric Patient

Objective: Demonstrate how to assist with performing a pulpotomy on a pediatric patient.

Equipment and Supplies Needed: dental dam setup; cotton pellets; medication (formocresol); anesthetic; cement (IRM or ZOE); composite, amalgam, or stainless steel crown setup; and burs (dentist's preference).

Notes to the Student:

Skills Assessment Requirements

Read and familiarize yourself with the procedure; complete the minimum practice requirements. Document information when appropriate to demonstrate proper charting techniques. Complete each procedure within a reasonable amount of time, with a minimum of 85% accuracy.

POINT VALUE ♦ = 5 points ✳ = 10 points	PRACTICE TRIAL	GRADED TRIAL # 1	GRADED TRIAL # 2	NOTES:
1. ♦ Place topical and dispense anesthetic.				
2. ♦ Put on dental dam.				
3. ♦ With a high-speed handpiece, access the pulp chamber through the occlusal surface of the tooth.				
4. ♦ Remove the coronal portion of the pulp with the spoon excavator.				
5. ♦ Dip cotton pellet into formocresol bottle, blot off excess with 2 × 2 gauze, and place inside pulp cavity for 5 minutes.				
6. ♦ Remove cotton. Rinse and dry pulp cavity.				
7. ♦ Prepare cement to a thick base consistency and put a layer over remaining pulp.				

(continued)

POINT VALUE ♦ = 5 points ✳ = 10 points		PRACTICE TRIAL	GRADED TRIAL # 1	GRADED TRIAL # 2	NOTES:
8. ♦	Place the restorative material (temporary or permanent) or stainless steel crown.				
9. ✳	Remove the dental dam and check occlusion with articulating paper. Tip the patient's chin toward the floor to alleviate swallowing of the fluoride.				
10.	Freshen patient's mouth (rinse and dry).				
11.	Provide postoperative instructions to the patient and his/her parent or guardian.				

Document:

Document information for proper charting of this procedure.

Grading

Points earned	_____		
Points possible	_____	50	50
Percent grade (Points earned/Points possible)	_____		
Pass:	_____	❑ YES ❑ NO ❑ N/A	❑ YES ❑ NO ❑ N/A

Instructor Sign-Off

Instructor: _____ Date: _____

Procedure 47-3

Assisting with Placement of Stainless Steel Crowns on a Pediatric Patient

Objective: Demonstrate how to place stainless steel crowns.

Equipment and Supplies Needed: explorer, mirror, cotton pliers, spoon excavator, crown and bridge scissors, spatula, contouring pliers, articulating paper holder, high- and slow-speed handpieces, diamond burs, green stones, polishing wheels, various sizes of stainless steel crowns, 2 × 2 gauze sponges, cotton rolls, paper pad and cement, floss, HVE, salvia ejector, and articulating paper.

Notes to the Student:

Skills Assessment Requirements

Read and familiarize yourself with the procedure; complete the minimum practice requirements. Document information when appropriate to demonstrate proper charting techniques. Complete each procedure within a reasonable amount of time, with a minimum of 85% accuracy.

POINT VALUE ♦ = 5 points ✳ = 10 points		PRACTICE TRIAL	GRADED TRIAL # 1	GRADED TRIAL # 2	NOTES:
1. ✳	Place topical in the *muccobuccal* fold. The dentist will dispense anesthetic near tooth to be restored.				
2.	Remove decay and reduce elevation and perimeter structure of the tooth with diamond burs (DENTIST).				
3. ✳	Select correct size stainless steel crown for prepared tooth and place on tooth to ensure fit.				
4. ✳	Use the crown and bridge scissors to adjust the height of crown, making contact with the mesial and distal surfaces. Try adjusted crown on tooth to ensure fit.				

(continued)

POINT VALUE ♦ = 5 points ✳ = 10 points		PRACTICE TRIAL	GRADED TRIAL # 1	GRADED TRIAL # 2	NOTES:
5. ✳	Smooth jagged edges made by the scissors with a green stone and adjust shape with contouring pliers.				
6. ✳	Polish smooth with polishing wheels.				
7. ✳	Seat crown on the tooth. Check bite with the articulating paper.				
8. ✳	Mix permanent cement and place it inside the crown. Pass the crown to the dentist, who seats it in position. Ask the patient to bite down on a cotton roll.				
9. ✳	Once cement is dry, remove excess around the gingival margin with an explorer. Remove interproximal cement with floss by snapping between contacts, gliding the floss back and fourth in the embrasure area to dislodge cement, and pulling the floss out toward the buccal side instead of back out through the contact.				
10. ✳	Provide a final rinse to remove any small pieces of cement and refresh he patient's mouth.				
11. ✳	Provide postoperative instructions to the patient and his/her parent or guardian.				

Document:

Document information for proper charting of this procedure.

Grading

Points earned	_____		
Points possible	_____	100	100
Percent grade (Points earned/Points possible)	_____		
Pass:	_____	❏ YES ❏ NO ❏ N/A	❏ YES ❏ NO ❏ N/A

Instructor Sign-Off

Instructor: _____ Date: _____

PROCEDURE 48-1
Coronal Polishing

Objective: Demonstrate how to perform a coronal polishing.

Equipment and Supplies Needed: basic setup (mirror, explorer, cotton pliers), saliva ejector, air/water tip, disclosing agent (liquid or tablet), polishing paste (fine or extra fine), dental floss, bridge threader, 2 × 2 sterile gauze squares, cotton tip applicator, prophy angle (disposable or sterile), prophy brush (disposable or sterile), slow-speed handpiece, patient hand mirror, patient toothbrush, red or blue pencil, and dental tooth chart.

Notes to the Student:

Skills Assessment Requirements

Read and familiarize yourself with the procedure; complete the minimum practice requirements. Document information when appropriate to demonstrate proper charting techniques. Complete each procedure within a reasonable amount of time, with a minimum of 85% accuracy.

POINT VALUE ♦ = 5 points ＊ = 10 points		PRACTICE TRIAL	GRADED TRIAL # 1	GRADED TRIAL # 2	NOTES:
1. ♦	Review the patient's medical and dental history.				
2. ♦	Greet and seat the patient. Place a napkin and eyewear on the patient and explain the procedure to the patient.				
3. ♦	Check the patient's oral cavity for appliances and abnormal lumps or lesions (remove appliances).				
4. ＊	Use a cotton tip applicator to place disclosing agent on the facial, buccal, lingual, and occlusal surfaces.				
5. ♦	Once all tooth structures have been covered with the disclosing agent, rinse the patient's mouth.				

(continued)

	POINT VALUE ♦ = 5 points ✳ = 10 points	PRACTICE TRIAL	GRADED TRIAL # 1	GRADED TRIAL # 2	NOTES:
6. ✳	Use a hand mirror to show the patient where plaque is present.				
7. ✳	Identify on the dental tooth chart with red pencil the surfaces the patient has been missing when brushing. Provide the tooth chart to the patient when polishing is finished to review and correct any missed areas.				
8. ♦	Take the toothbrush and have the patient hold the hand mirror while you show the patient how to correctly clean all tooth surfaces.				
9. ✳	Pick up the prophy angle and fill the prophy cup with polishing paste; spread the paste across up to three teeth to polish.				
10. ♦	The operator can begin in the right maxillary quadrant on the posterior teeth or where the operator chooses as long as no areas are missed. Establish a fulcrum on the incisors or close to the area on which the operator is working. Use a mouth mirror for retraction.				
11. ♦	Moving from the right maxillary posterior toward the anterior facial surface, retract the lip with a finger and establish a fulcrum on the teeth next to the tooth being polished.				
12. ♦	When the midline is reached, switch over onto the lingual surface of the maxillary right central moving toward the posterior area, using the mirror for indirect vision and making the fulcrum on the buccal surfaces of the maxillary.				

POINT VALUE ♦ = 5 points ✳ = 10 points		PRACTICE TRIAL	GRADED TRIAL #1	GRADED TRIAL #2	NOTES:
13. ♦	After polishing the last lingual surface of the most posterior tooth present, move onto the occlusal surface polishing the pits and fissures of the teeth moving from posterior to anterior. (A prophy brush can be used to clean this surface.)				
14. ♦	When the midline is reached, rinse the patient's mouth two or three times and repeat steps until all quadrants have been polished.				
15. ♦	When the teeth have been polished and rinsed, floss the interproxmial surfaces of all teeth.				
16. ♦	After completing the polishing procedure, dismiss the patient with a new toothbrush, floss, completed tooth chart, and any remaining instructions. (Fluoride treatment may be provided but only to children or patients with sensitive teeth).				

Document:

Enter the appropriate information in the chart below.

(continued)

Grading

Points earned	_____		
Points possible	_____	100	100
Percent grade (Points earned/Points possible)	_____		
Pass:	_____	❏ YES ❏ NO ❏ N/A	❏ YES ❏ NO ❏ N/A

Instructor Sign-Off

Instructor: _____ Date: _____

PROCEDURE 49-1
Applying Dental Sealants

Objective: Demonstrate how to place dental sealants.

Equipment and Supplies Needed: mirror, explorer, cotton pliers, saliva ejector, HVE tip, air/water tip, slow-speed handpiece, light-curing unit, white Arkansas stone (finishing bur), pumice, dappen dish, prophy angle (disposable or sterile), cotton rolls and/or dry angles, etchant, sealant material, articulating paper, and fluoride gel or foam.

Notes to the Student:

Skills Assessment Requirements

Read and familiarize yourself with the procedure; complete the minimum practice requirements. Document information when appropriate to demonstrate proper charting techniques. Complete each procedure within a reasonable amount of time, with a minimum of 85% accuracy.

POINT VALUE ♦ = 5 points ✳ = 10 points		PRACTICE TRIAL	GRADED TRIAL # 1	GRADED TRIAL # 2	NOTES:
1. ♦	Review the patient's medical and dental history.				
2. ♦	Greet and seat the patient. Place a napkin and eyewear on the patient and tell her about the procedure. Instruct the patient on the importance of keeping the mouth open during the procedure to maintain a dry field (or place a dental dam).				
3.	The dentist checks the tooth to ensure no decay is present.				
4. ✳	Moisten pumice with water to create a slurry consistency. Always make sure that the cleaning agent does not have any fluoride in it, because that would not allow the sealant to bond completely to the enamel rods.				

(continued)

	POINT VALUE ♦ = 5 points ✳ = 10 points	PRACTICE TRIAL	GRADED TRIAL #1	GRADED TRIAL #2	NOTES:
5. ✳	Clean the occlusal surface with pumice and rinse thoroughly.				
6. ✳	Place a cotton roll on the lingual and buccal surfaces. Dry the tooth completely with the air tip. Prior to using the air tip, be sure to clean out the air line by testing it on the patient's napkin or glove.				
7. ✳	Place acid etchant into the pits and grooves of the occlusal surface. Leave on for 30 to 45 seconds or according to the manufacturer's instructions.				
8. ♦	Completely rinse the tooth for a full 60 seconds.				
9. ♦	Carefully replace cotton rolls as needed to ensure that no moisture gets on the etched surface.				
10. ♦	Ensure teeth are completely dry, then dab the sealant on the occlusal surface covering all pits and fissures. Make sure the sealant is evenly placed across the surface. Light cure for 60 seconds.				
11. ♦	Check the sealant surface with the explorer for hardness.				
12. ♦	Remove cotton rolls.				
13. ✳	Check the occlusion with the articulating paper.				
14.	The dentist will make adjustments if necessary.				
15. ♦	Fluoride may be applied to help remineralize the enamel.				
16. ♦	Freshen the patient's mouth.				
17. ♦	Give the patient postoperative instructions.				

Document:

Enter the appropriate information in the chart below.

Grading

Points earned	_____		
Points possible	_____		
Percent grade (Points earned/Points possible)	_____	100	100
Pass:	_____	❏ YES ❏ NO ❏ N/A	❏ YES ❏ NO ❏ N/A

Instructor Sign-Off

Instructor: _____ Date: _____

PROCEDURE 50-1
Placing and Removing Brass Wire Separators

Objective: Demonstrate how to place and remove brass wire separators.

Equipment and Supplies Needed: basic setup (mouth mirror, explorer, cotton pliers), soft 20-mm brass wire, hemostat, ligature wire cutter, and orthodontic scaler or condenser.

Notes to the Student:

Skills Assessment Requirements

Read and familiarize yourself with the procedure; complete the minimum practice requirements. Document information when appropriate to demonstrate proper charting techniques. Complete each procedure within a reasonable amount of time, with a minimum of 85% accuracy.

POINT VALUE ♦ = 5 points ✳ = 10 points		PRACTICE TRIAL	GRADED TRIAL # 1	GRADED TRIAL # 2	NOTES:
A.	**Procedure Steps for Placing Brass Wire Separators**				
1. ✳	Bend brass wire into a C-shape or hook shape leaving a tail.				
2. ✳	Use a hemostat to hold the brass wire. Insert the hook into the lingual interproximal space (usually between the second premolar and first and second molars).				
3. ✳ ✳	Grab the tail of the brass wire and fold it over the contact by bringing it over to the facial.				
4. ✳ ✳	Bring the ends of the wire together and twist using the hemostat. Make sure that the wire is not too tight or too loose.				

(continued)

POINT VALUE ♦ = 5 points ✳ = 10 points		PRACTICE TRIAL	GRADED TRIAL # 1	GRADED TRIAL # 2	NOTES:
5. ✳✳	Cut the wire using a ligature cutter. Fold the wire and tuck into the embrasure area using the orthodontic scaler or condenser.				
B.	**Procedure Steps for Removing Brass Wire Separators**				
1. ✳	Using the ligature wire cutter, carefully lift the brass wire to the occlusal surface and cut the wire.				
2. ✳	Use the hemostat to carefully remove both sections of the wire on the facial side.				

Document:

Document information for proper charting of this procedure.

Grading

Points earned	_____		
Points possible	_____	100	100
Percent grade (Points earned/Points possible)	_____		
Pass:	_____	❏ YES ❏ NO ❏ N/A	❏ YES ❏ NO ❏ N/A

Instructor Sign-Off

Instructor: _____ Date: _____

PROCEDURE 50-2
Placing and Removing Steel Separating Springs

Objective: Demonstrate how to properly place and remove steel separating springs.

Equipment and Supplies Needed: basic setup (mouth mirror, explorer, cotton pliers), steel separating springs, bird-beak (No. 139) pliers, and an orthodontic scaler.

Notes to the Student:

Skills Assessment Requirements

Read and familiarize yourself with the procedure; complete the minimum practice requirements. Document information when appropriate to demonstrate proper charting techniques. Complete each procedure within a reasonable amount of time, with a minimum of 85% accuracy.

POINT VALUE ♦ = 5 points ∗ = 10 points		PRACTICE TRIAL	GRADED TRIAL # 1	GRADED TRIAL # 2	NOTES:
A.	**Procedure Steps for Placing Steel Separating Springs**				
1. ∗∗	Grasp the spring at the base of the shorter leg using the bird-beak pliers.				
2. ∗∗	Place the bent end or curve hook end into the lingual embrasure. Pull the spring open to allow the shorter leg of the spring to slip beneath the contact from the lingual side to the facial side.				
3. ∗∗	Carefully slip the spring into place with the helix or coiled side on the facial.				
B.	**Procedure Steps for Removing Steel Separating Springs**				
1. ∗	Operator should place one finger of one hand over the spring to prevent it from coming off and injuring the patient.				

(continued)

POINT VALUE ♦ = 5 points ✳ = 10 points		PRACTICE TRIAL	GRADED TRIAL # 1	GRADED TRIAL # 2	NOTES:
2. ✳ ✳	Place the orthodontic scaler into the coil or helix and lift upward until there is space between the upper arm and the occlusal aspect of the marginal ridge.				
3. ✳	While supporting the separator on the helix with the index finger, remove the upper arm of the spring and pull it toward the facial surface of the embrasure.				

Document:

Document information for proper charting of this procedure.

Grading

Points earned	_____		
Points possible	_____	100	100
Percent grade (Points earned/Points possible)	_____		
Pass:	_____	❑ YES ❑ NO ❑ N/A	❑ YES ❑ NO ❑ N/A

Instructor Sign-Off

Instructor: _____ Date: _____

PROCEDURE 50-3
Placing and Removing Elastomeric Ring Separators

Objective: Demonstrate how to properly place and remove elastomeric ring separators.

Equipment and Supplies Needed: basic setup (mouth mirror, explorer, cotton pliers), elastomeric separators, dental floss, separating pliers, orthodontic scaler, and patient protective eyewear.

Notes to the Student:

Skills Assessment Requirements

Read and familiarize yourself with the procedure; complete the minimum practice requirements. Document information when appropriate to demonstrate proper charting techniques. Complete each procedure within a reasonable amount of time, with a minimum of 85% accuracy.

POINT VALUE ♦ = 5 points ✳ = 10 points		PRACTICE TRIAL	GRADED TRIAL # 1	GRADED TRIAL # 2	NOTES:
A.	**Procedure Steps for Placing Elastomeric Ring Separators**				
1. ✳ ✳	Place the elastic separator over the beaks of the separating pliers, making sure to squeeze the pliers to ensure the separator is secure.				
2. ✳	Stretch and squeeze the ring separator, allowing one side of the separator to be inserted between the contact areas. This can be done by using a back-and-forth motion, similar to flossing.				
3. ✳ ✳	Release the tension of the pliers and disengage from the separator. Repeat this process on all teeth that will be receiving metal bands.				

(continued)

POINT VALUE ♦ = 5 points ✳ = 10 points		PRACTICE TRIAL	GRADED TRIAL # 1	GRADED TRIAL # 2	NOTES:
B.	**Procedure Steps for Removing Elastomeric Ring Separators**				
1. ✳ ✳	Using an orthodontic scaler, slip one end into the ring of the elastic separator.				
2. ✳ ✳	Hold one finger of the hand over the separator so that it does not snap and hurt the patient.				
3. ✳	Carefully pull the elastic separator using slight pressure to release it from the contact area.				

Document:

Document information for proper charting of this procedure.

Grading

Points earned	_____		
Points possible	_____	100	100
Percent grade (Points earned/Points possible)	_____		
Pass:	_____	❑ YES ❑ NO ❑ N/A	❑ YES ❑ NO ❑ N/A

Instructor Sign-Off

Instructor: _____ Date: _____

PROCEDURE 50-4

Assisting in the Fitting and Cementation of Orthodontic Bands

Objective: Demonstrate how to assist in the fitting and cementation of orthodontic bands.

Equipment and Supplies Needed: basic setup (mouth mirror, explorer, cotton pliers), cotton rolls or gauze squares, preselected orthodontic bands, chilled glass slab or paper pad, cement spatula (stainless steel), band pusher, band seater, bite stick, scaler, band remover, and ChapStick, toothpaste, or utility wax.

Notes to the Student:

Skills Assessment Requirements

Read and familiarize yourself with the procedure; complete the minimum practice requirements. Document information when appropriate to demonstrate proper charting techniques. Complete each procedure within a reasonable amount of time, with a minimum of 85% accuracy.

POINT VALUE ♦ = 5 points ✳ = 10 points		PRACTICE TRIAL	GRADED TRIAL # 1	GRADED TRIAL # 2	NOTES:
A.	**Preparation**				
1. ♦	Once the separators have been removed, polish the teeth with a rubber cup.				
2. ♦	Rinse the patient's mouth and air dry teeth. Cotton rolls are placed lingual and buccal to isolate the molars and keep the area dry.				
3. ✳	Preselected bands are placed on a small square of masking tape with the occlusal surface down on tape and with the gingival margin upright.				
4. ✳	Buccal tubes and any attachments are wiped with ChapStick, toothpaste, or utility wax to prevent cement from getting into them.				

(continued)

POINT VALUE ♦ = 5 points ✳ = 10 points		PRACTICE TRIAL	GRADED TRIAL # 1	GRADED TRIAL # 2	NOTES:
B.	**Procedure Steps for Mixing and Placing Cement**				
1. ♦	Once the orthodontist is ready to put the bands on, the assistant will mix the cement on the glass slab or mixing pad, carefully following the manufacturer's directions. The mixture should be thoroughly homogenous.				
2. ✳	Load the first band by holding it by the margin of the masking tape, making sure that the gingival surface is upright.				
3. ✳	While placing the spatula with cement over the margin, allow the cement to flow into the circumference of the band.				
4. ✳	Transfer the band to the orthodontist, who will invert the band over the tooth. (*Note:* There are various ways that the orthodontist may want to transfer the bands; however, the transfer should be as smooth as possible. The bands must always be positioned so that they are handed to the orthodontist in the correct sequential order).				
5. ✳	Transfer the band seater, bite stick, or any other instrument that the orthodontist might request until the band is properly seated. The patient is instructed to bite down gently, forcing the band down onto the middle third of the crown.				
6. ✳	At this point, excess cement is forced out from under the gingival and occlusal margins of the bands and allowed to dry.				

POINT VALUE ♦ = 5 points ✳ = 10 points		PRACTICE TRIAL	GRADED TRIAL #1	GRADED TRIAL #2	NOTES:
C.	**Procedure Steps for Removing Excess Cement**				
1. ✳	After the cement has reached the final stage of setting, remove the excess with an orthodontic scaler or explorer.				
2. ♦	Thoroughly rinse any cement from the patient's mouth.				

Document:

Document information for proper charting of this procedure.

Grading

Points earned	_____		
Points possible	_____	100	100
Percent grade (Points earned/Points possible)	_____		
Pass:	_____	❏ YES ❏ NO ❏ N/A	❏ YES ❏ NO ❏ N/A

Instructor Sign-Off

Instructor: _____ Date: _____

PROCEDURE 50-5

Assisting in the Direct Bonding of Orthodontic Brackets

Objective: Demonstrate how to assist in the direct bonding of orthodontic brackets.

Equipment and Supplies Needed: basic setup (mouth mirror, explorer, cotton pliers), brackets, cotton rolls or lip retractors, pumice, slow-speed handpiece with prophy angle and rubber cup, bonding setup (acid etching and bonding agent), and orthodontic scaler.

Notes to the Student:

Skills Assessment Requirements

Read and familiarize yourself with the procedure; complete the minimum practice requirements. Document information when appropriate to demonstrate proper charting techniques. Complete each procedure within a reasonable amount of time, with a minimum of 85% accuracy.

POINT VALUE ◆ = 5 points ✷ = 10 points		PRACTICE TRIAL	GRADED TRIAL # 1	GRADED TRIAL # 2	NOTES:
A.	**Preparation**				
1. ✷	First clean the teeth by using a prophy cup with pumice. (*Note:* A prophy paste without fluoride is acceptable. The use of fluoride will interfere with the bonding process.)				
2. ✷	Rinse and dry the teeth. Place cotton rolls for isolation, and position lip retractors.				
3. ✷ ✷	Dab the acid etchant solution onto the facial surface of the tooth that is to receive bonding. This solution remains on the tooth for a specific time according to the manufacturer's direction.				
4. ✷	Dry the tooth, noticing the chalky appearance caused by the etching material.				

(continued)

POINT VALUE ♦ = 5 points ✳ = 10 points		PRACTICE TRIAL	GRADED TRIAL # 1	GRADED TRIAL # 2	NOTES:
B.	**Procedure Steps for Bonding the Brackets**				
1.	The orthodontist applies a liquid sealant (usually the monomer of the bonding agent) to the prepared tooth surface.				
2. ✳	The assistant places a small quantity of bonding material on the back of the specified bracket.				
3. ✳	The assistant uses bracket placement forceps to transfer the bracket to the orthodontist.				
4.	The orthodontist places the bracket on approximately the middle third of the tooth.				
5. ✳	Remove excess bonding agent with the scaler.				
6. ✳	Bond the brackets to the teeth with a curing light.				
7. ✳	Remove the cotton rolls and lip retractors from the mouth.				

Document:

Document information for proper charting of this procedure.

Grading

Points earned	_____		
Points possible	_____	100	100
Percent grade (Points earned/Points possible)	_____		
Pass:	_____	❑ YES ❑ NO ❑ N/A	❑ YES ❑ NO ❑ N/A

Instructor Sign-Off

Instructor: _____ Date: _____

PROCEDURE 50-6
Placing the Arch Wire and Ligature Ties

Objective: Demonstrate how to place the arch wire and ligature ties.

Equipment and Supplies Needed: basic setup (mouth mirror, explorer, cotton pliers), gauze and cotton rolls, high volume evacuator and/or saliva ejector, arch wire selected to fit, Weingart pliers, bird-beak pliers, ligature wire and/or elastics, ligature-cutting pliers, ligature-tying pliers, and distal-end cutting pliers.

Notes to the Student:

Skills Assessment Requirements

Read and familiarize yourself with the procedure; complete the minimum practice requirements. Document information when appropriate to demonstrate proper charting techniques. Complete each procedure within a reasonable amount of time, with a minimum of 85% accuracy.

POINT VALUE ♦ = 5 points * = 10 points		PRACTICE TRIAL	GRADED TRIAL # 1	GRADED TRIAL # 2	NOTES:
A.	**Procedure Steps for Placing the Arch Wire**				
1. *	Insert the prefitted arch wire onto the brackets and into the buccal arch wire slot of the molar bands.				
2. *	Securely fit the wire into the horizontal slots in the middle of the brackets. Tie the brackets with elastomeric ties or ligature wire.				
3. *	The elastomeric ties are placed over the brackets using a hemostat or ligature tying pliers. The ring ties are spread and placed on the gingival side of the bracket. They are then pulled down over the arch wire and wrapped around the occlusal side of the bracket.				

(continued)

POINT VALUE ♦ = 5 points ∗ = 10 points		PRACTICE TRIAL	GRADED TRIAL # 1	GRADED TRIAL # 2	NOTES:
B.	**Procedure Steps for Placing Ligature Wire Ties**				
1.∗	While holding the ligature wire between the thumb and index finger, wrap the wire around the occlusal and gingival wings of the bracket, going in a distal to mesial direction. Twist the ends of the wires together, using a hemostat or ligature tying pliers.				
2. ∗	Using the pliers or hemostat, twist the ends of the ties for several rotations. Do not twist the wire too tight causing it to break.				
3.	Repeat the process until the entire arch wire is tied.				
4. ∗	The twisted ends of the ligature ties, or "pigtails" as they are often called, are cut with ligature wire cutting pliers to about 3 to 4 mm.				
5. ∗	The orthodontist places the bracket on approximately the middle third of the tooth.				
6. ∗	The pigtail is bent to allow it to be placed into the embrasure with a condenser.				
7. ∗	After cutting and tucking the wire into the embrasure, run your finger over the area to check for sharps ends.				
8.∗	Check the distal ends of the arch wire, making sure you bend any leftover wire toward the tooth leaving only 1 mm of the wire extending out.				

Document:

Document information for proper charting of this procedure.

Grading

Points earned	_____		
Points possible	_____	100	100
Percent grade (Points earned/Points possible)	_____		
Pass:	_____	❑ YES ❑ NO ❑ N/A	❑ YES ❑ NO ❑ N/A

Instructor Sign-Off

Instructor: _____ Date: _____

PROCEDURE 50-7
Assisting at a Completion Appointment

Objective: Demonstrate how to assist at a completion appointment.

Equipment and Supplies Needed: basic setup (mouth mirror, explorer, cotton pliers), gauze and cotton rolls, scaler, ligature wire-cutting pliers, bracket and bonding material, removal pliers, posterior band remover, ultrasonic scaler (optional), prophy angle, prophy paste with fluoride, and alginate impression material. (preselected tray)

Notes to the Student:

Skills Assessment Requirements

Read and familiarize yourself with the procedure; complete the minimum practice requirements. Document information when appropriate to demonstrate proper charting techniques. Complete each procedure within a reasonable amount of time, with a minimum of 85% accuracy.

POINT VALUE ♦ = 5 points ✳ = 10 points		PRACTICE TRIAL	GRADED TRIAL # 1	GRADED TRIAL # 2	NOTES:
A.	**Procedure Steps for Removing Elastic Bands**				
1. ✳	The elastic ties or bands are lifted and removed with a scaler. The elastic bands are then rolled over the bracket wings.				
B.	**Procedure Steps for Removing Ligature Wire Ties**				
1. ✳	Using a ligature cutter, place the beaks of the cutter where the ligature wire is exposed. Cut the wire, making sure that you have hold of the wire.				
2. ✳	Remove the wire from the wings of the bracket. Repeat this procedure on each bracket until all are removed.				

(continued)

POINT VALUE ♦ = 5 points ✳ = 10 points		PRACTICE TRIAL	GRADED TRIAL #1	GRADED TRIAL #2	NOTES:
3.✳	The entire arch wire can now be removed by using a pair of Weingart pliers. Remove the arch wire by first pulling it out of the buccal tube on one end. Then, holding it securely, remove it from the opposite end.				
C.	**Procedure Steps for Removing Brackets**				
1.✳	Remove the brackets using bracket-removing pliers. The lower beak of the pliers with the sharp edge is placed on the gingival edge of the bracket; the upper beak with the softer nylon tip is placed on the occlusal edge of the bracket. The pliers are then squeezed together, causing the sharp end of the pliers to break the bond and remove some of the cement.				
D.	**Procedure Steps for Removing Bands**				
1.✳	To remove the posterior bands, a pair of band-removing pliers is used. The cushioned end is placed on the buccal cusp of the tooth. The end with the blade is placed against the gingival edge of the band. The pliers are squeezed and the band is gently lifted toward the occlusal surface.				
2.✳	This same process is repeated on the lingual surfaces until the cement bond releases the band.				
3.✳	After all brackets and bands have been removed, the teeth are scaled with a hand or ultrasonic scaler to remove excess cement and bonding material.				
4.✳	Polish with a rubber cup and take completion photographs (intra- and extraoral).				

POINT VALUE ♦ = 5 points ✳ = 10 points		PRACTICE TRIAL	GRADED TRIAL #1	GRADED TRIAL #2	NOTES:
5.✳	After the teeth have been scaled and polished and there are no signs of cement or bonding material present, an alginate impression is taken on both arches for fabrication of retainers.				
6.	The patient is given an appointment for placement of the retainers. This may be later that day or in a week depending on the orthodontist's schedule. At this time, the patient is given instructions for wearing the retainer.				

Document:

Document information for proper charting of this procedure.

Grading

Points earned	_____		
Points possible	_____	100	100
Percent grade (Points earned/Points possible)	_____		
Pass:	_____	❑ YES ❑ NO ❑ N/A	❑ YES ❑ NO ❑ N/A

Instructor Sign-Off

Instructor: _____ Date: _____

Procedure 51-1
Performing the ABCs of CPR

Objective: Demonstrate how to effectively perform CPR.

Equipment and Supplies Needed: approved mannequin, gloves, ventilator mask, mouth guard.

Notes to the Student:

Skills Assessment Requirements

Read and familiarize yourself with the procedure; complete the minimum practice requirements. Document information when appropriate to demonstrate proper charting techniques. Complete each procedure within a reasonable amount of time, with a minimum of 85% accuracy.

POINT VALUE ♦ = 5 points ✳ = 10 points		PRACTICE TRIAL	GRADED TRIAL #1	GRADED TRIAL #2	NOTES:
1. ✳	*Determine unresponsiveness:* Tap the patient's shoulder and shout: "Are you OK, are you OK?" Speak loudly and clearly.				
2. ✳	*Activate EMS/obtain the AED:* Direct someone to call 911 and get the AED. (For an adult victim, phone first; for a child phone after one minute of CPR.) If you witness a child going unconscious, activate EMS, then begin CPR if necessary.				
3. ✳	*Open the airway:* Use the head-tilt/chin-lift maneuver. Place one hand on the forehead, the other under the chin. The mouth should not be completely closed.				

(continued)

	POINT VALUE ♦ = 5 points ✳ = 10 points	PRACTICE TRIAL	GRADED TRIAL # 1	GRADED TRIAL # 2	NOTES:
4. ✳	*Check for breathing:* Look, listen, and feel for breathing. Look for the chest to rise, listen for breathing sounds, and feel for air on your cheek. Continue for 5 seconds, but no more than 10 seconds.				
5. ✳✳	*Provide two full breaths (each breath should take one second):* Put mouth over patient's mouth and pinch the nostrils. Use a pocket mask if available. If the chest does not rise, reposition the airway and try again. If the patient has a loose denture, remove it. If the denture fits, leave it in, because it will help with the mouth-to-mouth seal.				
6. ✳	*Check the pulse:* Place two three fingers on windpipe to (Adam's apple) and slide fingers into the groove on the side of the neck nearest you. Check the carotid artery for 5 to 10 seconds along with signs of circulation/movement.				
7. ✳	*If no pulse, begin chest compressions:* Deliver 30 chest compressions in less than 23 seconds. Using the heel of one hand with the other hand clasped on top, place the hands on the lower half of the sternum. Push hard and fast. Allow the chest to return to normal between compressions.				
8. ✳	Continue the compression-to-ventilation ratio of 30:2 until the emergency crew arrives. After three cycles, check the pulse and reassess.				
9. ✳	Document the emergency information and procedures in patient's dental health record.				

Document:

Document information for proper charting of this procedure.

Grading

Points earned	_____		
Points possible	_____	100	100
Percent grade (Points earned/Points possible)	_____		
Pass:	_____	❑ YES ❑ NO ❑ N/A	❑ YES ❑ NO ❑ N/A

Instructor Sign-Off

Instructor: _____ Date: _____

Procedure 51-2
Operating the Automated External Defibrillator

Objective: Demonstrate how to operate the automated external defibrillator.

Equipment and Supplies Needed: approved mannequin, gloves, automatic external defibrillator, ventilator mask, mouth guard.

Notes to the Student:

Skills Assessment Requirements

Read and familiarize yourself with the procedure; complete the minimum practice requirements. Document information when appropriate to demonstrate proper charting techniques. Complete each procedure within a reasonable amount of time, with a minimum of 85% accuracy.

POINT VALUE ♦ = 5 points ∗ = 10 points		PRACTICE TRIAL	GRADED TRIAL # 1	GRADED TRIAL # 2	NOTES:
1. ∗	If there is no pulse, follow the ABCs of CPR (see Procedure 51-1).				
2. ∗	Place electrodes on the patient's chest. (Follow AED instructions on machine.)				
3. ∗	Press *Analyze* on the AED.				
4. ∗	Announce "Everyone stand clear" while the machine analyzes the patient's heart rhythms.				
5. ∗	If the AED unit indicates a shock is needed, make sure everyone is standing clear.				
6. ∗	Give the shocks indicated by the unit.				
7. ∗	Check the patient's pulse.				

(continued)

POINT VALUE ♦ = 5 points ✳ = 10 points		PRACTICE TRIAL	GRADED TRIAL # 1	GRADED TRIAL # 2	NOTES:
8. ✳	If a pulse is present, assess vital signs and keep patient comfortable until emergency services arrive.				
9. ✳	If no pulse is present, press *Analyze* again and repeat the shock procedure if indicated. *Safety note:* Ensure that no bystanders or rescuers are touching the victim while the shock is being administered.				
10. ✳	Document the emergency procedures in the patient's dental health record.				

Document:

Enter the appropriate information in the chart below.

Grading

Points earned	_____		
Points possible	_____	100	100
Percent grade (Points earned/Points possible)	_____		
Pass:	_____	❑ YES ❑ NO ❑ N/A	❑ YES ❑ NO ❑ N/A

Instructor Sign-Off

Instructor: _____ Date: _____

Procedure 51-3
Administering Oxygen

Objective: Demonstrate how to administer oxygen.

Equipment and Supplies Needed: oxygen cylinder, oxygen mask or nasal cannula, and ambu-bag.

Notes to the Student:

Skills Assessment Requirements

Read and familiarize yourself with the procedure; complete the minimum practice requirements. Document information when appropriate to demonstrate proper charting techniques. Complete each procedure within a reasonable amount of time, with a minimum of 85% accuracy.

POINT VALUE ♦ = 5 points ✳ = 10 points	PRACTICE TRIAL	GRADED TRIAL # 1	GRADED TRIAL # 2	NOTES:
1. ✳ Position the patient in the supine or subsupine position. The supine position is when the patient is lying down with his head, chest, and knees at the same level. The subsupine position is when the patient's head is lower than his heart and feet. This position is often used in emergencies.				
2. ✳ Reassure the patient and explain the treatment being performed.				
3. ♦ Ensure the green oxygen cylinder contains oxygen by opening the main valve at the top until gas starts to come out. Then close the valve immediately.				
4. ✳ Attach the regulator by aligning the pin with the cylinder holes.				

(continued)

POINT VALUE ♦ = 5 points ✳ = 10 points		PRACTICE TRIAL	GRADED TRIAL # 1	GRADED TRIAL # 2	NOTES:
5. ✳	Open the valve two full turns. Check the pressure gauge to ensure that it reads 2,000 pounds per square inch (psi).				
6. ✳	Attach the tubing from the mask or nasal cannula.				
7. ✳	Position the mask over the patient's face. Ensure the mask forms a tight seal.				
8. ✳	Attach the ambu-bag if needed.				
9. ✳	Start the flow of oxygen with the regulator control. The gauge should be set to flow at two to six liters per minute.				
10. ✳	Observe the patient's color and response to the oxygen.				
11. ✳	Document the emergency procedures in the patient's dental health record.				

Document:

Enter the appropriate information in the chart below.

Grading

Points earned	_____		
Points possible	_____	100	100
Percent grade (Points earned/Points possible)	_____		
Pass:	_____	❏ YES ❏ NO ❏ N/A	❏ YES ❏ NO ❏ N/A

Instructor Sign-Off

Instructor: _____ Date: _____

Procedure 51-4
Managing an Obstructed Airway

Objective: Demonstrate how to clean an obstructed airway.

Equipment and Supplies Needed: none.

Notes to the Student:

Skills Assessment Requirements

Read and familiarize yourself with the procedure; complete the minimum practice requirements. Document information when appropriate to demonstrate proper charting techniques. Complete each procedure within a reasonable amount of time, with a minimum of 85% accuracy.

POINT VALUE ♦ = 5 points ✳ = 10 points		PRACTICE TRIAL	GRADED TRIAL # 1	GRADED TRIAL # 2	NOTES:
1. ♦	Determine whether the patient is choking by asking "Are you choking?" "May I help you?" (The patient may have her hands on her throat, which is the universal signal for choking.)				
2. ♦	Position yourself behind the patient, place one of your legs between the patient's (for stability), and wrap your arms around her abdomen (see Figure 51.11). Let the person know that you are there to help so she does not panic.				
3. ♦	Place the thumb side of your hand between the navel and the xiphoid process (the notch at the end of the lower part of the sternum). Grasp hands together. (For pregnant or obese people, wrap your arms around the chest, just under the armpits.)				

(continued)

POINT VALUE ♦ = 5 points ✱ = 10 points		PRACTICE TRIAL	GRADED TRIAL #1	GRADED TRIAL #2	NOTES:
4. ✱	Give quick inward, upward thrusts until the obstruction is expelled or the patient becomes unconscious.				
5. ✱	If the patient becomes unconscious, lower her to the floor, check the airway, straddle her, and provide chest thrusts (similar to CPR chest compressions).				
6. ✱	If the obstruction is relieved, but the victim is not breathing or does not have a pulse, call 911 and begin CPR.				
7. ♦	Document the emergency procedures in the patient's dental health record.				

Document:

Enter the appropriate information in the chart below.

Grading

Points earned	_____		
Points possible	_____	50	50
Percent grade (Points earned/Points possible)	_____		
Pass:	_____	❏ YES ❏ NO ❏ N/A	❏ YES ❏ NO ❏ N/A

Instructor Sign-Off

Instructor: _____ Date: _____

PROCEDURE 54-1

Managing Financial Transactions

Objective: Demonstrate how to properly manage basic financial transactions.

Equipment and Supplies Needed: dental charts for the day, daily appointment schedule, insurance information, day sheet, pen/pencil, and computer if forms are computerized.

Notes to the Student:

Skills Assessment Requirements

Read and familiarize yourself with the procedure; complete the minimum practice requirements. Document information when appropriate to demonstrate proper charting techniques. Complete each procedure within a reasonable amount of time, with a minimum of 85% accuracy.

POINT VALUE ♦ = 5 points ✳ = 10 points		PRACTICE TRIAL	GRADED TRIAL # 1	GRADED TRIAL # 2	NOTES:
1. ✳ ♦	On the day prior to the patient's appointment, the business assistant should: • Pull and review the patient's chart. • Confirm the appointment.				
2. ✳ ♦	On the day of the appointment, the business assistant should: • Check the schedule. • Review dental charts. • When patient arrives, update financial and insurance information. • When treatment is complete, post transactions and schedule next appointment.				

(continued)

POINT VALUE ♦ = 5 points ✳ = 10 points		PRACTICE TRIAL	GRADED TRIAL #1	GRADED TRIAL #2	NOTES:
3. ✳ ✳	At the end of the day, the business assistant should: • Complete posting of daily transactions. • Process any mail payments. • Balance the day sheet and produce reports. • Complete an audit report. • Complete insurance processing.				

Document:

Enter the appropriate information in the chart below.

Grading

Points earned	_____		
Points possible	_____	50	50
Percent grade (Points earned/Points possible)	_____		
Pass:	_____	❏ YES ❏ NO ❏ N/A	❏ YES ❏ NO ❏ N/A

Instructor Sign-Off

Instructor: _____ Date: _____

PROCEDURE 54-2
Writing Checks

Objective: Demonstrate how to properly write a check.

Equipment and Supplies Needed: writing pen, typewriter/computer, checks or printable check paper, and checkbook ledger.

Notes to the Student:

Skills Assessment Requirements

Read and familiarize yourself with the procedure; complete the minimum practice requirements. Document information when appropriate to demonstrate proper charting techniques. Complete each procedure within a reasonable amount of time, with a minimum of 85% accuracy.

POINT VALUE ♦ = 5 points ✳ = 10 points		PRACTICE TRIAL	GRADED TRIAL # 1	GRADED TRIAL # 2	NOTES:
1. ✳	Always use ink because it cannot be altered. The ink can come from a pen, typewriter, or computer. Checks are printed on special paper that helps avoid the possibility of the check being altered or counterfeited.				
2. ✳ ✳ ♦	Write accurately and neatly.				
3. ✳ ✳ ♦	Enter the name of the person or company receiving the check in the **Payee** section. Write the complete company name as it appears on the statement. Titles such as Dr., Mr., and Mrs. are not used when writing a check.				

(continued)

POINT VALUE ♦ = 5 points ✳ = 10 points		PRACTICE TRIAL	GRADED TRIAL # 1	GRADED TRIAL # 2	NOTES:
4. ✳ ✳	Annotate the amount of the check in alpha and numeric form, for instance, "$233.24" and "Two hundred thirty-three and 24/100 dollars."				
5. ✳ ✳	After the check has been written, have it signed by an authorized person (usually the dentist or office manager).				

Document:

Enter the appropriate information in the chart below.

Grading

Points earned	_____		
Points possible	_____	100	100
Percent grade (Points earned/Points possible)	_____		
Pass:	_____	❑ YES ❑ NO ❑ N/A	❑ YES ❑ NO ❑ N/A

Instructor Sign-Off

Instructor: _____ Date: _____

PROCEDURE 56-1

Preparing a Professional Resume and Cover Letter

Objective: Demonstrate how to properly prepare a professional resume and cover letter.

Notes to the Student:

Skills Assessment Requirements

Read and familiarize yourself with the procedure; complete the minimum practice requirements. Document information when appropriate to demonstrate proper charting techniques. Complete each procedure within a reasonable amount of time, with a minimum of 85% accuracy.

POINT VALUE ♦ = 5 points ✳ = 10 points		PRACTICE TRIAL	GRADED TRIAL # 1	GRADED TRIAL # 2	NOTES:
	Procedure Steps				
1. ✳	Gather education and past employment information.				
2. ✳	Type résumé following the sample format provided in Figure 56.2.				
3. ✳	Use a 12-point font and a common, easy-to-read typeface.				
4. ✳	Tailor the résumé to the specific job.				
5. ✳	Avoid embellishing any information.				
6. ✳	Proofread the résumé for any errors.				
7. ✳	Have another individual proofread the résumé.				
8. ✳	Ensure résumé is free of errors prior to printing.				

(continued)

POINT VALUE ♦ = 5 points ✱ = 10 points		PRACTICE TRIAL	GRADED TRIAL # 1	GRADED TRIAL # 2	NOTES:
9. ✱	Print on standard 8½ × 11 inch white or ivory heavy paper.				
10. ✱	Prepare cover letter specifically for the job position following the sample shown in Figure 56.3.				

Document:

Enter the appropriate information in the chart below.

Grading

Points earned	_____		
Points possible	_____	100	100
Percent grade (Points earned/Points possible)	_____		
Pass:	_____	❏ YES ❏ NO ❏ N/A	❏ YES ❏ NO ❏ N/A

Instructor Sign-Off

Instructor: _____ Date: _____